Women with Epilepsy

Women with Epilepsy

A Practical Management Handbook

Edited by

Esther Bui
University of Toronto

P. Emanuela Voinescu
Brigham and Women's Hospital

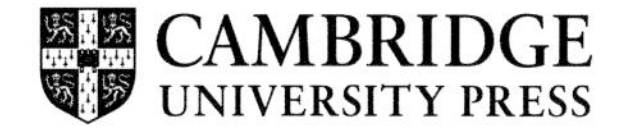

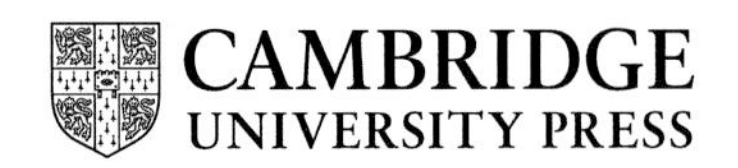

Shaftesbury Road, Cambridge CB2 8EA, United Kingdom

One Liberty Plaza, 20th Floor, New York, NY 10006, USA

477 Williamstown Road, Port Melbourne, VIC 3207, Australia

314–321, 3rd Floor, Plot 3, Splendor Forum, Jasola District Centre,
New Delhi – 110025, India

103 Penang Road, #05–06/07, Visioncrest Commercial, Singapore 238467

Cambridge University Press is part of Cambridge University Press & Assessment,
a department of the University of Cambridge.

We share the University's mission to contribute to society through the pursuit of
education, learning and research at the highest international levels of excellence.

www.cambridge.org
Information on this title: www.cambridge.org/9781009009072

DOI: 10.1017/9781009006903

First published 2014
Second edition 2024

A catalogue record for this publication is available from the British Library

Library of Congress Cataloging-in-Publication Data
Names: Bui, Esther, editor. | Voinescu, P. Emanuela (Paula Emanuela), editor.
Title: Women with epilepsy : a practical management handbook / edited by Esther Bui,
P. Emanuela Voinescu.
Other titles: Women with epilepsy (2014)
Description: Second edition. | Cambridge, United Kingdom ; New York, NY : Cambridge University Press,
2024. | Includes bibliographical references and index.
Identifiers: LCCN 2023052013 | ISBN 9781009009072 (paperback) | ISBN 9781009006903 (ebook)
Subjects: MESH: Epilepsy | Women's Health | Pregnancy Complications
Classification: LCC RC372 | NLM WL 385 | DDC 616.85/30082–dc23/eng/20231214
LC record available at https://lccn.loc.gov/2023052013

ISBN 978-1-009-00907-2 Paperback

This book is dedicated to all the courageous women and their families who have faced the challenges of epilepsy, often quietly and stoically, to come out defined not by their illness, but by their *courage, resilience and grace*. Someone once wrote "just because we carry it well, doesn't mean it isn't heavy". Despite the weight of their diagnosis, women with epilepsy and their families are the true drivers of change in the work we do. I want to thank my husband Carlo, my children M & J who have supported me in the long hours of work to bring this book to fruition, my co-editor Dr. Emma Voinescu who worked in the trenches with me to refine and build a new edition, the authors of each chapter who generously contributed their expertise and time to update this book, Julianne Hazlewood and Brandy McFadden both determined visionaries who long recognized the value of our collective stories, and last but certainly not least, my dear friend Dr. Autumn Klein, who co-edited the first edition of this book and shared the vision that women's health and priorities should be a fundamental and forefront part of epilepsy care.

Esther Bui

Contents

Contributors

Paula Alcaide Leon
Department of Medical Imaging
University of Toronto
Toronto, ON, Canada

Danielle M. Andrade
Adult Genetic Epilepsy Program
University of Toronto
Toronto, ON, Canada

Leah J. Blank
Departments of Neurology and Population Health Science and Policy
Mount Sinai School of Medicine
New York, NY, USA

Naveed Chaudhry
Department of Neurology
Johns Hopkins School of Medicine
Baltimore, MD, USA

Lidia Di Vito
IRCCS Istituto delle Scienze Neurologiche di Bologna, European Reference Network for Rare and Complex Epilepsies (EpiCARE), Bologna, Italy.

Tadeu Fantaneanu
The Ottawa Hospital
University of Ottawa
Ottawa Hospital Research Institute
Ottawa, ON, Canada

Abrar O. al-Faraj
Boston Medical Center
Boston University School of Medicine
Boston, MA, USA

Elizabeth E. Gerard
Department of Neurology
Feinberg School of Medicine
Northwestern University
Chicago, IL, USA

Cecil D. Hahn
Division of Neurology
The Hospital for Sick Children and
Department of Paediatrics
University of Toronto
Toronto, ON, Canada

Nathalie Jetté
Department of Clinical Neurosciences,
University of Calgary,
Calgary, AB, Canada

Emily Johnson
Department of Neurology
Johns Hopkins School of Medicine
Baltimore, MD, USA

Suchitra Joshi
Department of Neurology
University of Virginia Health Sciences Center
Charlottesville, VA, USA

Jaideep Kapur
Departments of Neurology and Neuroscience
UVA Brain Institute
University of Virginia Health Sciences Center
Charlottesville, VA, USA

Alexa King
Department of Neurology
Feinberg School of Medicine
Northwestern University
Chicago, IL, USA

Dilip Koshy
Temerty Faculty of Medicine
Department of Psychiatry
University of Toronto
University Health Network Centre for

Mental Health
Toronto, ON, Canada

Véronique Latreille
Department of Neurology
Montreal Neurological Institute–Hospital
McGill University
Montreal, QC, Canada

Kristi McIntosh
Electroneurophysiology Program
British Columbia Institute
of Technology Burnaby,
BC, Canada

Ginette Moores
Division of Neurology and Department of Medicine
University of Toronto
Toronto, ON, Canada

Barbara Mostacci
IRCCS Istituto delle Scienze
Neurologiche di Bologna, European
Reference Network for Rare
and Complex Epilepsies (EpiCARE),
Bologna, Italy.

Katherine Muir
Children's Hospital of Eastern Ontario
CHEO Research Institute University of Ottawa
Ottawa, ON, Canada

Eugene Ng
Department of Newborn and
Developmental Paediatrics
Sunnybrook Health Sciences
Centre
Department of Paediatrics
University of Toronto
Toronto, ON, Canada

Alison M. Pack
Department of Neurology
Columbia University Irving Medical
Center
New York, NY, USA

Trudy D. Pang
Beth Israel Deaconess Medical Center
Harvard Medical School
Boston, MA, USA

Milena K. Pavlova
Department of Neurology
Brigham and Women's Hospital
Boston, MA, USA

Kalliopi A. Petropoulou
Radiology Department
State University of New York Upstate
Medical University
Syracuse, NY, USA

Mark Quigg
Department of Neurology
University of Virginia
Charlottesville, VA, USA

Arezoo Rezazadeh
The Ottawa Hospital
University of Ottawa
Ottawa Hospital Research Institute
Ottawa, ON, Canada

Natalia Rincon
Department of Neurology
University of Miami Miller School of
Medicine
Miami, FL, USA

Carlos I. Salazar
Division of Neurology
The Hospital for Sick Children
University of Toronto
Toronto, ON, Canada

Mona Sazgar
University of California–Irvine
Irvine, CA, USA

Anna Serafini
Department of Neurology and
Rehabilitation
University of Illinois–Chicago
Chicago, IL, USA

Mathew Sermer
Sinai Health System Department of Obstetrics and Gynaecology
University of Toronto
Toronto, ON, Canada

Stephanie Shatzman
University of Michigan Health,
Ann Arbor, MI

John W. Snelgrove
Sinai Health System Department of Obstetrics and Gynaecology
University of Toronto
Toronto, ON, Canada

Paula Teixeira Marques
Epilepsy Program
McMaster University
Hamilton, ON, Canada

Benjamin Tolchin
Department of Neurology
Yale School of Medicine
Center for Clinical Ethics
Yale New Haven Health
New Haven, CT, USA

Naymee J. Velez-Ruiz
Department of Neurology
University of Miami Miller School of Medicine
Miami, FL, USA

Janet F. R. Waters
Division of Women's Neurology
UPMC Magee Women's Hospital
Pittsburgh, PA, USA

Jonathan H. Waters
Department of Anesthesiology
University of Pittsburgh
Pittsburgh, PA, USA

Fatima Zahir
UPMC Passavant Hospital
Pittsburgh, PA, USA

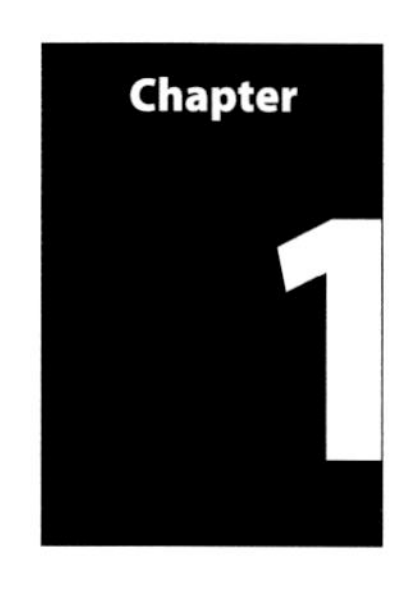

Epidemiology of Women with Epilepsy

Kristi McIntosh, Nathalie Jette, and Leah J. Blank

Introduction

Key Points

- Epilepsy is common with a prevalence of between 3 and 10 cases per 1,000.
- There is a similar overall prevalence between males and females, although rare studies report a slightly higher lifetime incidence in males (1 of every 21 males) as compared to females (1 of every 28 females).
- Female sex is associated with increased risk of depression and anxiety in those with epilepsy.
- We lack large, population-based studies for antiseizure medications' effects on sexual function and fertility.
- There is no association between oral contraceptive use and seizure frequency.
- Registry-based data on antiseizure medication in pregnancy continue to support the recommendation that valproic acid should be avoided in women of reproductive age and favor treating women considering pregnancy with lamotrigine or levetiracetam.
- Few population-level data remain on women with epilepsy in pregnancy, during lactation, and during the menopausal transition.

Epidemiology of Epilepsy

Almost 50 million individuals worldwide are estimated to have active epilepsy at any given time [1, 2]. The prevalence of epilepsy is defined as the number of persons with epilepsy in a defined population at one point in time, divided by the number of persons in that population and time. The incidence of epilepsy is defined as the number of new cases of epilepsy over a specified time period [1, 3]. The reported incidence and prevalence of epilepsy vary widely across studies. Reasons for these estimate differences may include variation in the case ascertainment methods, diagnostic criteria, or study location, or because of concealment by some individuals due to the stigma associated with epilepsy.

The overall prevalence of epilepsy is estimated to be between 3 and 10 cases per 1,000 persons, excluding febrile convulsions, single seizures, and inactive epilepsy [3–8], but the median lifetime prevalence of epilepsy has been reported to be as high as 15.4 per 1,000 (4.8–49.6) in rural areas and 10.3 per 1,000 (2.8–37.7) in urban areas of low-income countries [5]. The prevalence of epilepsy is slightly higher in males than females in many door-to-door and record-review studies. However, any sex difference in prevalence is slight

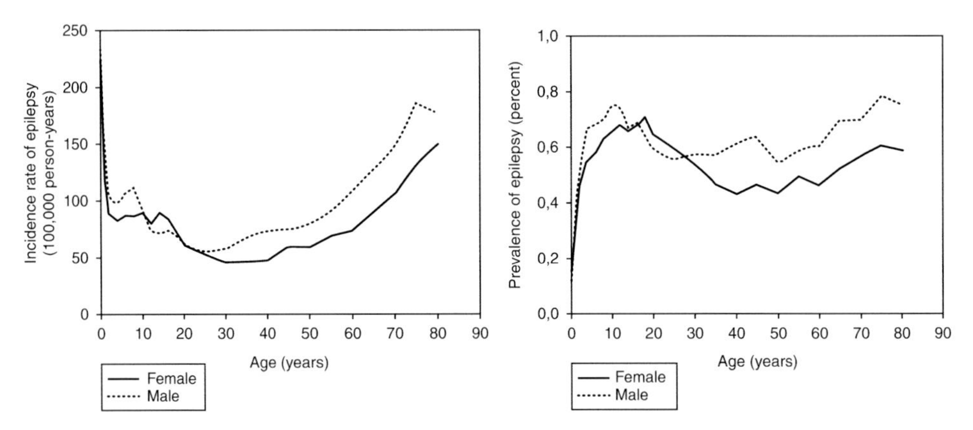

Figure 1.1 A. Left panel: Age- and gender-specific incidence of epilepsy in Denmark. Estimates were based on 5,491,652 people born in Denmark followed up for development of epilepsy between 1995 and 2002, including 33,140 who developed epilepsy. The incidence measures the number of new cases per 100,000 person-years at risk. B. Right panel: Five-year prevalence of epilepsy in Denmark. Estimates were based on 4,977,482 persons born in Denmark and resident in Denmark on December 31, 1999, including 28,303 diagnosed with epilepsy between 1995 and 1999. Modified with permission from Christensen et al. [4]

and usually not significant [1, 3, 9]. Some studies do continue to report a sex difference in epilepsy prevalence. For example, in a Danish study using population-based data from a national registry (Figure 1.1A), the prevalence of epilepsy was higher in men compared to women for most age groups, except for the 16–25 age group [4, 10]. In this study, men were also found to have higher incidence rates than women in all age categories, again with the exception of the 10–20 age group (Figure 1.1B) [4].

The overall incidence rate of epilepsy is usually reported to be about 40–70 cases per 100,000 person-years in high-income countries, and about 100–190 cases per 100,000 person-years in low-income countries [2, 3, 5, 9, 11]. In a recent systematic review and meta-analysis, the estimated incidence rate of epilepsy was reported to be 48.86 per 100,000 person-years for high-income countries and 138.99 per 100,000 person-years for low- and middle-income countries [3, 11]. The incidence of epilepsy is often reported to have a bimodal distribution (Figure 1.2). It is highest in early childhood, lowest in the early adult years, and then increases again after age 55 with the highest reported incidence in those older than 75 years of age [12]. A similar pattern is described in both males and females.

The lifetime risk of epilepsy is the probability that a person will develop epilepsy over their lifetime. Based on calculations in a population-based study, 1 in 26 people will develop epilepsy during their lifetime, and men have a higher risk of developing epilepsy (1 of every 21 males) than women (1 of every 28 females) [13]. There does not appear, however, to be a sex difference in the incidence of drug-resistant epilepsy [14].

The causes behind these potential sex differences have not been elucidated. One hypothesis of why epilepsy may be more common in men than in women is that men have a higher incidence of traumatic brain injury, which in turn is associated with epilepsy. Focal epilepsy has also been found to occur more frequently among men than women (Figure 1.3) [2, 3, 10, 12]. Notably, the higher incidence of epilepsy in men relative to women has not been reported in adolescents. This may be due to the higher incidence of idiopathic generalized epilepsy in women between the ages

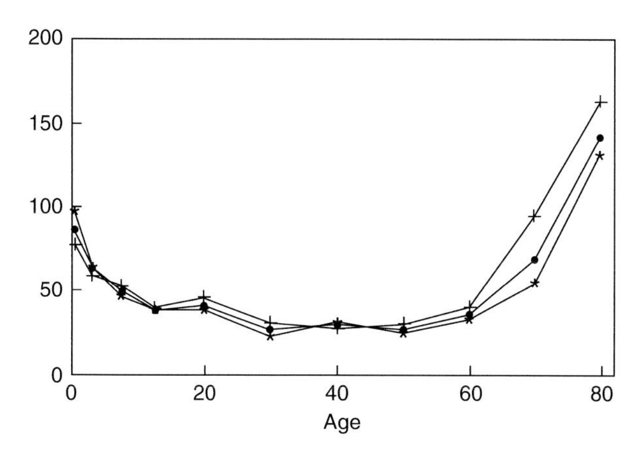

Figure 1.2 Age- and gender-specific incidence per 100,000 of epilepsy in Rochester, Minnesota, 1935–84. Total (solid circles), male (plus signs), female (stars). Reproduced with permission from Hauser et al. [12]

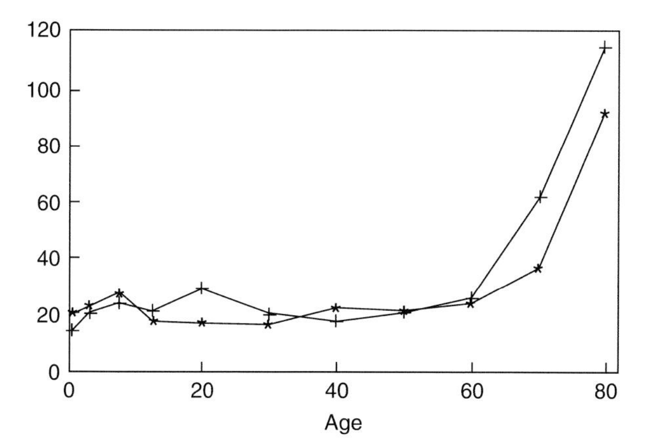

Figure 1.3 Age- and gender-specific incidence per 100,000 of focal epilepsy in Rochester, Minnesota, 1935–84. Male (plus signs), female (stars). Reproduced with permission from Hauser et al. [12]

of 12 and 20 years (Figure 1.4). The reason for increased incidence of generalized epilepsy in women relative to men in adolescence is not fully known but may be attributed to genetic or hormonal factors [10]. If female sex hormones contribute to the development of idiopathic generalized epilepsy in women, this difference would be more obvious before menopause and decline with age, which is demonstrated in the Danish study just discussed [10, 15]. It has also been suggested that the higher reported estimates in males compared to females may be due to a sex bias in reporting due to the concealment of symptoms by women in cultures where women might be considered "unmarriageable" if they have epilepsy [1, 3].

Comorbidities

A number of mental health conditions are increased in persons with epilepsy as compared to those without epilepsy [16, 17]. Studies have shown that major depression, anxiety, and

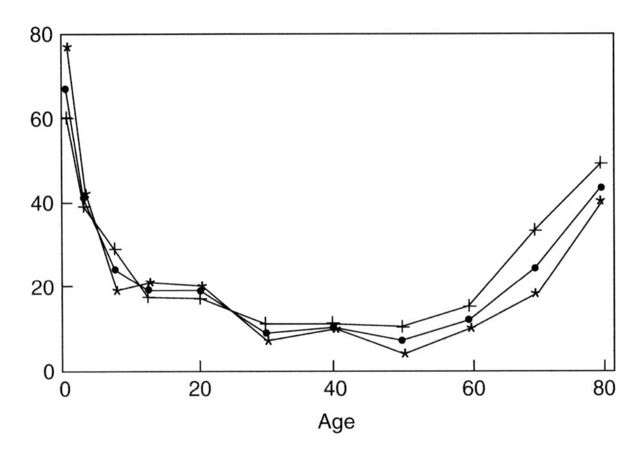

Figure 1.4 Age- and gender-specific incidence per 100,000 of generalized onset epilepsy in Rochester, Minnesota, 1935–84. Total (solid circles), male (plus signs), female (stars). Reproduced with permission from Hauser et al. [12]

psychosis are associated with an increased risk for developing epilepsy and vice versa [18, 19]. This bidirectional relationship suggests a possible shared pathogenetic origin [18]. Having epilepsy is also associated with a higher prevalence of somatic comorbidities as compared to the general population [8, 20, 21]. Here, we discuss sex differences in the epidemiology of mood and anxiety as well as sleep disorders in epilepsy.

Psychiatry

Mood Disorders in Epilepsy

Mood disorders are prevalent in those with epilepsy, with major depression the most common [22, 23]. Female sex is associated with depression in both those with and without epilepsy [22]. In those without epilepsy, the prevalence of depressive mood disorders has been reported to be approximately two times higher in women than in men. However, this sex difference is less pronounced in those with epilepsy [24–27].

In a nationally representative Canadian health survey using structured interviews for the assessment of major depressive disorder, depression was identified in 13% of those with epilepsy compared to 7% of those without epilepsy [22]. Women with epilepsy (WWE) had 2.6 times the odds (95% confidence interval [CI], 1.6–4.3) of depression as compared to men with epilepsy [22]. A meta-analysis found that the odds of active depression was higher in people with epilepsy compared to those without epilepsy (odds ratio [OR] 2.77; 95% CI, 2.09–3.67) [27, 28]. The lifetime prevalence of major depressive disorder in those with epilepsy was 17.4% (95% CI, 10.0–24.9), compared to 10.7% (95% CI, 10.2–11.2) in those without epilepsy, with an OR of 1.8 (95% CI, 1.0–3.1). Furthermore, the lifetime prevalence of major depressive disorders, while still increased for those with epilepsy, has been shown to decline with age in women while remaining relatively stable in men (Figure 1.5A) [16].

While there are fewer studies examining the incidence of postpartum depression (PPD) in WWE, smaller studies have reported an increased frequency of PPD in WWE compared to women without epilepsy (WWoE). Increased rates of depression in WWE have been confirmed in a Norwegian population-based study of mothers with a peripartum depression rate of 26.7% in WWE as compared to 18.9% in WWoE ($p < 0.001$) [29]. No specific

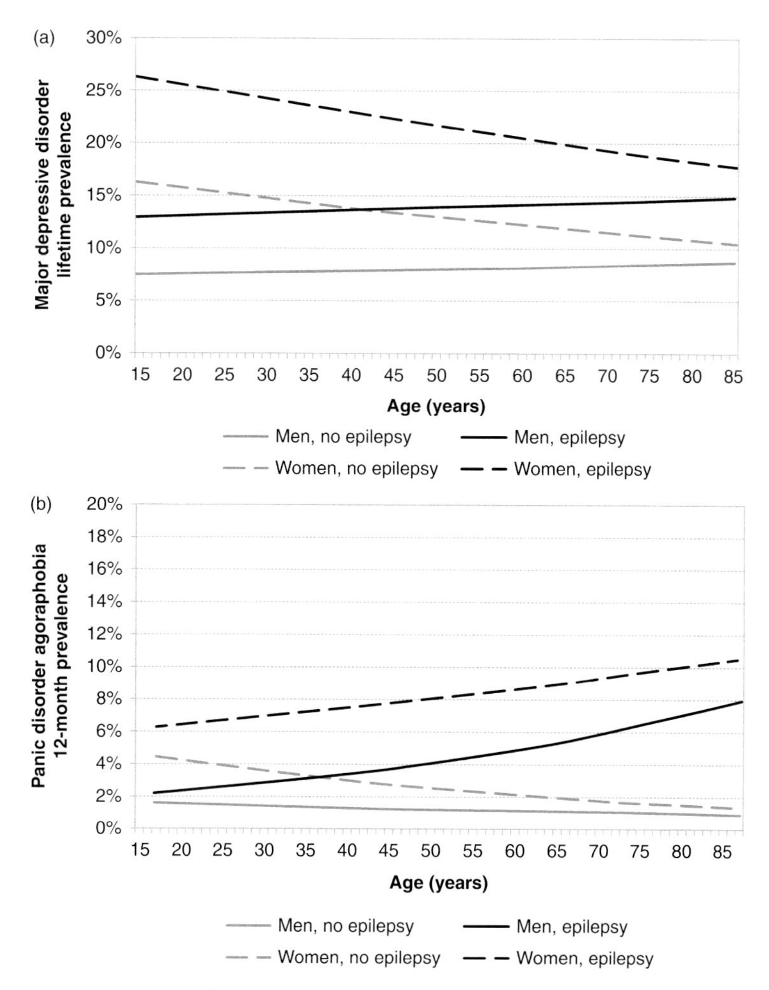

Figure 1.5 A. Logistic regression (fitted) models predicting the lifetime prevalence (proportion in percentage) of major depression disorder (on the y-axis) based on age (on the x-axis) and gender. Reproduced with permission from Tellez-Zenteno et al. [16]. B. Logistic regression (fitted) models predicting the 12-month prevalence (proportion in percentage) of panic disorder/agoraphobia (on the y-axis) based on age (on the x-axis) and gender. Reproduced with permission from Tellez-Zenteno et al. [16]

causative factor has been identified to explain this disparity although frequent seizures, polytherapy, previous psychiatric disease, and sexual or physical abuse are all associated with a higher risk of peripartum depression in WWE [30]. Similarly, a recent study of a nationally representative sample of admissions to US hospitals for childbirth showed increased rates of 30-day readmission for psychiatric illness among WWE (OR, 10.13; 95% CI, 5.48–18.72). The most common cause for psychiatric readmission in these women was mood disorder.

Anxiety Disorders

Anxiety is known to be a significant psychiatric comorbidity in epilepsy. A bidirectional association between anxiety and epilepsy has been described with an almost twofold increase in odds of developing anxiety in people with epilepsy as compared to those without [19].

In a cross-sectional, population-based study from the United Kingdom using diagnoses from primary care records, anxiety disorders were reported in 11% of 5,834 people who had epilepsy, compared to 5.6% of 831,163 who did not have epilepsy [31]. The risk of anxiety was higher in both men and women with epilepsy compared to control, but higher in WWE overall. For example, in the 16–64 year age group, anxiety was reported in 14.2% of 2,338 WWE compared to 7.5% of 410,851 WWoE (relative risk [RR], 1.95; 95% CI, 1.8–2.2). In the same age group, 9.4% of 2,321 men with epilepsy and 3.8% of 420,312 men without epilepsy (RR 2.6; 95% CI, 2.3–2.9) were found to have anxiety. In the 64 years and older age group, 9.0% of 642 WWE had anxiety compared to 7.8% of 118.516 WWoE (RR, 1.2; 95% CI, 0.9–1.5). In the same age group, anxiety occurred in 7.5% of 533 men with epilepsy, and only in 3.8% of 86,130 men without epilepsy (RR, 2.0; 95% CI, 1.5–2.7). Finally, in a population-based Canadian survey using structured interviews based on DSM-IV, both panic disorder and agoraphobia became more prevalent with age (and were found to be higher in women compared to men with epilepsy), but this was not found to occur in the general population (Figure 1.5B) [16]. A recent meta-analysis calculated a pooled prevalence of anxiety disorders at 20.2% (95% CI, 15.3–26.0%) [28] as compared to approximately 9.4% of people in the general population [32]. A similar meta-analysis in youth (<18) confirmed that youth with epilepsy had significantly higher anxiety symptoms than youth without epilepsy (moderator coefficient $d = 0.57$, 95% CI, 0.32–0.83, $p < .0005$) [26]. For a more detailed review, see Chapter 2.

Sleep

Sleep disturbances are reported more frequently in adults with than in adults without epilepsy. Obstructive sleep apnea (OSA), excessive daytime sleepiness (EDS), and sleep maintenance insomnia (difficulty staying asleep) are more commonly found in those with epilepsy than in those without [33–37]. Sleep disorders in people with epilepsy have also been associated with ongoing seizures and worse quality of life [38]. However, population-based studies on sleep disturbances in patients with epilepsy are lacking. Furthermore, there has been little attention to sex differences in those existing smaller studies.

In a mail survey of 1,183 Dutch outpatients, the 6-month prevalence of sleep disturbances in people with focal epilepsy was more than two times greater than that of healthy controls (38.6% vs. 18.0%) [39]. This was not due to any one particular type of sleep disturbance; all sleep disturbances were significantly more prevalent in patients with epilepsy. A prospective Swiss study of 100 adult epilepsy patients found sleep symptoms were three times as likely (30% vs. 10%) in a population of people with epilepsy compared with controls [35]. In small case series, OSA has been reported in 10% of adults with epilepsy, 20% of children with epilepsy, and approaching 30% in patients with drug-resistant epilepsy [33]. Furthermore, OSA occurs more frequently in those who are older, male, overweight, and with drug-resistant or late-onset epilepsy [33, 34]. Identification and treatment of sleep disorders may be important: a retrospective review of epilepsy patients with OSA treated at the Cleveland

Clinic showed improvement in seizure frequency with treatment of OSA using positive airway pressure [40].

Notably, more sleep problems are encountered by children with epilepsy than their healthy siblings and other healthy controls [34, 37]. Sex, however, does not contribute to the frequency of problems with sleep in children [34]. For a more detailed review, see Chapter 3.

Epilepsy in Childhood and Adolescence

Inheritance and Genetics

Genetic testing, although primarily used in children, is climbing as increasing numbers of known mutations are identified. Several factors have been found to be associated with a predisposition to epilepsy, particularly in a family where one member is already affected. Affected children have a greater risk of being born to a mother with epilepsy (8.7%) as compared to a father with epilepsy (2.4%) [41]. How early a parent developed epilepsy also predicts the likelihood of a child developing epilepsy [41]. The children of parents who develop epilepsy before age 20 have a 2.3–6% risk of epilepsy in their offspring as compared to 1.0–3.6% in the offspring of those who develop epilepsy after age 20 [41]. Furthermore, when the parent also has epilepsy, the risk of epilepsy in offspring with epilepsy increases from approximately 3% to 8% [41].

The epilepsy syndrome or seizure type also contributes to the likelihood of epilepsy developing in relatives. Occurrence of epilepsy in relatives is increased when the proband has idiopathic epilepsy with seizures such as myoclonic or absence seizures. In those with myoclonic seizures, a 4–8% risk of any epilepsy in offspring is seen, while in those with absence seizures, a 5–9% risk of any epilepsy is observed (Figure 1.6) [41]. The risk of epilepsy in those related to individuals with generalized epilepsies is greater than in those related to individuals with focal epilepsy in some studies; however, this has not been observed in all studies (Figure 1.6) [41, 42]. The pattern of inheritance in generalized epilepsies is unknown and the development of epilepsy is suspected to be complex: an interaction between genetic susceptibility and the environment [43]. A recent meta-analysis

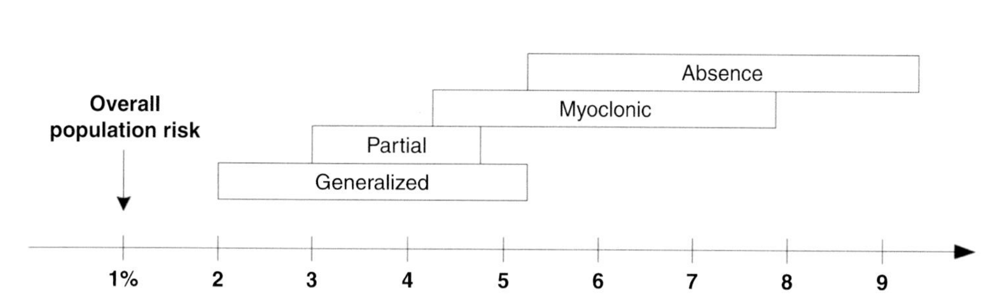

Figure 1.6 Percent of offspring affected with epilepsy. Reproduced with permission from Winawer and Shinnar [41]

of electroencephalograms (EEGs) of asymptomatic first-degree relatives of patients with juvenile myoclonic, childhood absence, and Rolandic epilepsies suggests that the susceptibility to seizures in some of these families may be compatible with Mendelian genetics [44]. For a more detailed review, see Chapter 6.

Sex Differences in Epilepsies in Children and Adolescents

Sex differences have been identified in various epilepsy syndromes. Idiopathic generalized epilepsy, which accounts for 15–20% of the epilepsies, can be found more frequently in females than in males [45]. Childhood absence epilepsy (CAE) was reported in 2.5% of boys compared to 11.4% of girls in a Norwegian population-based study [46]. Juvenile absence epilepsy (JAE) and juvenile myoclonic epilepsy (JME) were more common among females than males using data from 2,488 individuals with epilepsy from a Danish outpatient epilepsy clinic and the Danish Twin Registry [10]. Juvenile absence epilepsy was three times more common in females than males (76% vs. 24%), whereas JME was 1.5 times more common in females than males (61% vs. 39%) [10]. However, there has been less agreement as to whether sex differences exist in focal epilepsies. While one prospective study of 996 patients with suspected seizures conducted over a 4-year period in Australia reported an equal sex distribution of hippocampal sclerosis (81% in men vs. 79% in women) [47], another retrospective study of 153 patients presenting for presurgical evaluation in Germany found that the expression of focal epilepsy due to mesial temporal sclerosis is not the same in females and in males [48]. Females had higher odds of experiencing isolated auras than males (OR, 2.1; 95% CI, 1.1–4.2) and lower odds of having focal to bilateral tonic-clonic seizures (OR, 0.44; 95% CI, 0.21–0.92). Furthermore, they also found that electrographic findings were more likely to be on the same side of hippocampal sclerosis in females compared to males (98% vs. 84%). For a more detailed review, see Chapter 7.

Catamenial Epilepsy

Catamenial epilepsy is defined as a doubling in daily seizure frequency during specific phases of the menstrual cycle [49]. Three categories of catamenial seizure patterns have been described: perimenstrual, periovulatory, and entire luteal phase in anovulatory cycles [49]. Population-based studies exploring the prevalence of catamenial epilepsy are lacking. However, a catamenial pattern was found in 39% of women with localization-related epilepsy (LRE) in a prospective study of 87 women [50] and 31% of adolescent females in a prospective study of 42 WWE from an Egyptian pediatric neurology clinic [51]. The laterality and focality of epilepsy may play a role in the likelihood of cyclical hormonal fluctuations affecting the seizure pattern [52]. For a more detailed review, see Chapter 8.

Epilepsy in Women of Reproductive Potential

Fertility and Epilepsy

Sexual Dysfunction

There are no population-based studies examining sexual dysfunction in WWE. While sexual dysfunction has been documented in both men and women with epilepsy, very little research has been done to investigate gender differences in the rates of dysfunction. However, sexual dysfunction has been found to be increased in epilepsy patients of both sexes. Persons with epilepsy have reported reduced quality of life and most commonly report symptoms of depression, decreased sexual desire, and problems with orgasms. Women with epilepsy also often report vaginal dryness [53].

Smaller series show that WWE are more likely to suffer from sexual dysfunction than WWoE. The particular neural networks involved in epilepsy may affect the occurrence of sexual dysfunction. A US study explored sexual dysfunction in 57 reproductive-aged women on antiseizure medication (ASM) monotherapy recruited from tertiary epilepsy centers as compared to 17 WWoE. Increased sexual dysfunction was found in women with generalized epilepsies (20.0%) or focal epilepsies (20.7%) as compared to controls (9%) [54].

Furthermore, sexual dysfunction is seen more frequently in right as compared to left temporal lobe epilepsy (TLE) in both men and women [55]. A controlled prospective study of 36 women with TLE recruited from a neurology outpatient clinic and 12 controls recruited from the community found that sexual function scores were substantially worse with right TLE as compared to left TLE. Additionally, women with right TLE (50%) and women with left TLE (30%) had increased rates of sexual dysfunction as compared to WWoE (8.3%). However, these differences were only significant for those with right TLE [55].

Antiseizure medications have been believed to play a role in sexual dysfunction in epilepsy. In particular, some older, enzyme-inducing ASMs may contribute to sexual dysfunction due to central nervous system changes or through changes in the levels of hormones supporting sexual behavior. Enzyme-inducing ASMs increase sex hormone-binding globulin and thereby decrease bioavailable testosterone, which may contribute to the emergence of sexual dysfunction [55]. While not statistically significant, 40.7% of WWE receiving an ASM reported increased sexual dysfunction compared to 33.3% of those not receiving an ASM in the same study [55]. However, recent studies have also found no association between sexual dysfunction and enzyme-inducing ASMs after controlling for sex [53].

Reproductive Dysfunction and Fertility

In WWE, menstrual cycle irregularities, increased risk of infertility, and/or signs of polycystic ovary syndrome (PCOS) are frequently encountered. Both seizures and ASMs have been causally implicated [56]. Two of the greatest challenges in comparing the results from studies looking at menstrual disorders in WWE are the lack of menstrual disorder definition and the limited number of population-based studies. Most published studies report data from highly selective, biased populations (e.g., women referred to a neuroendocrine clinic).

In a retrospective, questionnaire-based study of 265 WWE and 142 matched WWoE from three different Norwegian hospitals, menstrual disorders were significantly higher in WWE (48.0%) than in controls (30.7%) [57]. In other studies, menstrual disorders were more common in WWE: for example, 32% in one retrospective US analysis of 100 women with focal epilepsy [58]. In a controlled study, 12 of 36 (33.3%) of WWE compared to 14 of 100 (14%) community-based WWoE ($p = 0.02$) had a menstrual disorder [59].

Menstrual cycle irregularities, anovulation, higher androgen levels, carbohydrate intolerance with obesity, and polycystic-appearing ovaries are all characteristics of PCOS. A lack of a standardized definition of PCOS may explain the varying reported rates in women both with and without epilepsy, although again, there is a lack of population-based studies of PCOS in WWE [60]. In a Finnish study examining reproductive endocrine function in 148 WWE, PCOS was found to occur in 28% of WWE, 52% of WWE on valproate (VPA), and 11% of controls. Women with epilepsy on VPA were significantly more likely to have PCOS when compared to controls (OR, 5.46; 95% CI, 2.23–13.03) [61]. A meta-analysis including 556 WWE treated with VPA, 593 women treated with other ASMs, 120 untreated WWE, and 329 healthy controls, found the odds of developing PCOS was 1.94 times greater (95% CI, 1.28–2.95) in VPA-treated WWE compared to other ASM-treated women [60]. The possibility of developing features of PCOS in those treated with VPA seems to be age-dependent [62]. In a prospective US study of 225 WWE taking VPA compared to 222 WWE taking lamotrigine (LTG), the occurrence of PCOS symptoms occurred more frequently in women started on VPA rather than LTG before the age of 26 years compared to WWE in whom VPA was started at the age of 26 years or older [62].

Valproate continues to show similar results in more recent studies. A US retrospective study investigated the risks of infertility and impaired fecundity of 1,000 WWE via the Epilepsy Birth Control Registry (EBCR) [63]. Of the 373 WWE, 724 pregnancies occurred with 445 births. While the rate of live births was similar among WWE on no ASM (71.3%), ASM monotherapy (71.8%), and polytherapy (69.7%), glucuronidated ASM (LTG) had the highest ratio of live birth/pregnancy compared to enzyme-inhibiting ASM (VPA), which had the lowest (89.1% vs. 63.3%; RR, 1.41; 95% CI, 1.05–1.88).

Another notable pattern of reproductive dysfunction described in patients with epilepsy is hypothalamic amenorrhea – a severe yet common pattern of hypogonadotropic hypogonadism. In one study, 50 women with TLE referred for neurologic evaluation were studied, with eight (16%) found to have amenorrhea. This is much higher than the expected frequency of 1.5% in the general population [64]. Furthermore, amenorrhea has been found to occur more commonly in women with right TLE than women with left TLE [59, 65]. Unfortunately, we do not believe that population-based estimates of amenorrhea in WWE have been published.

Overall fertility has also been examined in WWE. There are population-based data examining fertility rates in WWE from 1991 to 1995 compared to the 1993 fertility rates for England and Wales [66]. The fertility rate in WWE aged 15–44 was 47.1 live births per 1,000 women per year (95% CI, 42.3–52.2), compared with a national rate of 62.6. The most significant decrease in fertility rates was among WWE in the 25–39 year age groups ($p < 0.001$). Reassuringly, a US study of women with and without epilepsy seeking pregnancy found no differences in pregnancy rates or time to pregnancy [67]. This may suggest that the lower birth rates seen in WWE may be less due to reproductive dysfunction as compared to lower marriage rates, fear of birth defects, and/or concern for an increased risk of epilepsy in the offspring [68]. In a population-based study of 19 US states, 55.5% (95% CI, 51.3–59.7) of those with epilepsy were married or in a common-law relationship compared to 64.1% (95% CI, 63.6–64.7) of those without epilepsy. Of those with epilepsy, 22.9% (95% CI, 20.0–26.2) were formerly married compared to 18.0% (95% CI, 17.6–18.3) of those without epilepsy. Finally, 21.5% (95% CI, 17.7–26.0) of those with epilepsy were never married compared to 17.9% (95% CI, 17.4–18.4) of those without epilepsy [8]. Similar findings were reported in an Indian study of 300 epilepsy patients. Among those with epilepsy, 55.5% of men and 44.6% of women were never married compared to 43.3% of men and 22.3% of women in the general population (n = 4,687). Indeed, only 44.5% of men and 51.1% of women with epilepsy were currently married compared to 56.2% of men and 75.7%

of women in the general population. No men with epilepsy and 4.3% of WWE were divorced compared to 0.5% of men and 2% of women in the general population [69].

As in the general population, pregnancies in WWE are often unplanned. In the EBCR study, 78.9% of WWE reported having at least one unintended pregnancy with 65.0% of all 804 pregnancies being unintended. This is significantly greater than the 45–51% range of the general US population of childbearing women having unintended pregnancies [70]. However, according to a survey administered by the Centers for Disease Control and Prevention that randomly sampled 73,619 postpartum women from 13 US states and adjusted for covariates including age, race, ethnicity, and socioeconomic status (SES), the 541 (0.7%) WWE did not have a higher rate of unintended pregnancy when compared to WWoE [71].

More population-based studies about reproductive dysfunction in WWE are needed. For a more detailed review, see Chapter 9.

Hormonal Contraceptives and Epilepsy

As just described, pregnancies are often unplanned. Contraceptive management in WWE is paramount due to the possible maternal and fetal complications if contraception fails. Furthermore, the use of enzyme-inducing ASMs can result in the failure of common oral contraceptives (OCs) and may contribute to the relatively high number of unplanned pregnancies in WWE [72, 73]. Prepregnancy counseling for all WWE of childbearing age is necessary.

The prevalence of contraceptive use in 1,630 Dutch women of childbearing age on ASMs was calculated in a study using a population-based pharmaceutical dispensing database [74]. The authors found that only 34.3% of ASM users were prescribed highly effective contraceptives as compared with 41.2% of the general population of women of childbearing age ($p < 0.001$). They also found that of WWE who used enzyme-inducing ASMs in combination with a highly effective contraceptive method, 43.5% were on an OC containing less than the recommended 50 μg of estrogen. These findings are consistent with a large, population-based study of childbearing WWE on ASMs in the United Kingdom. This latter study found that 16.7% of WWE were on OC, and of those on both an enzyme-inducing ASM and an OC, 56% were on OC with an estrogen content less than 50 μg [75].

Importantly, despite the well-known effects of estrogen on lowering seizure threshold, an association between estrogen-containing OC and seizure exacerbation in WWE has not been seen. A large UK cohort study of 17,032 WWE followed for up to 26 years examined whether there was a relationship between OC use and an increase in the incidence of epilepsy or seizures [76]. No association was found between OC use and the development of epilepsy in WWoE or between OC use and seizure frequency in WWE.

Preconception Counseling

There are no studies examining how commonly preconception counseling occurs in WWE. However, the evidence for the use of preconceptual folic acid by WWE was reviewed by a committee assembled by the American Academy of Neurology (AAN) and American Epilepsy Society (AES), and is discussed later in this section [77]. A prospective study of 970 pregnancies and 979 offspring in WWE reported a significant correlation between serum folic acid concentrations less than 4.4 nmol/L and malformations in newborns (adjusted OR, 5.8; 95% CI, 1.3–27) [78]. However, several other studies reviewed did not show a relationship between folic acid and major congenital malformations (MCMs) but were insufficiently powered to exclude a significant risk reduction from folic acid supplementation.

The effectiveness of preconceptual folic acid supplementation was prospectively examined in an observational study by looking at the rate of MCMs in a group of women on ASM monotherapy in the United Kingdom [79]. In the 1,935 cases that received preconceptual folic acid, 76 MCMs (3.9%; 95% CI, 3.1–4.9) and eight neural tube defects (NTDs) (0.4%; 95% CI, 0.2–0.8) were observed. There were 53 occurrences of an MCM (2.2%; 95% CI, 1.7–2.9) and eight NTDs (0.34%; 95% CI, 0.2–0.7) in the 2,375 women who obtained folic acid but did not start taking it until later in the pregnancy (n = 1,825) or not at all (n = 550). Folic acid supplementation in this population of WWE was not associated with a reduction in the frequency of MCMs or NTDs. This study suggests that extrapolating findings from population-based studies of all pregnant women who took folate to groups of selected WWE enrolled in registries may be inappropriate. The higher risk of MCMs in WWE may be multifactorial and may also be explained by mechanisms other than those related to folic acid metabolism.

The prophylactic effect of folic acid supplementation on the likelihood of spontaneous abortion and preterm delivery was examined prospectively in pregnant WWE on ASMs. These WWE were all registered in the International Registry of ASM and Pregnancy (EURAP) at a single center, with 388 pregnancies in 244 patients investigated [80]. Women with epilepsy who did not supplement with folic acid were more likely to have a spontaneous abortion than those who did supplement (OR, 2.6; 95% CI, 1.2–5.6). Consequently, pregnancies with folic acid supplementation were associated with a significant reduction of spontaneous abortion.

As epilepsy is more prevalent among those with decreased SES, which is itself associated with unintended pregnancy [7, 71], it is important to examine whether WWE of childbearing age are being counseled appropriately preconceptually about folate and ASM selection, including the risks of fetal malformations. In a 2013 prospective study of 1,526 pregnancies in Scottish WWE, significantly different rates of preconceptual folic acid supplementation existed when the highest and lowest socioeconomic quintiles were compared (56.8% vs. 14.0%; RR, 4.1; 95% CI, 3.1–5.2), yet no associated difference in the rate of major malformations was found (4.4% compared to 4.7%, p = 0.84) [81].

The evidence regarding the effectiveness of preconception counseling for WWE, calculated by a decrease in adverse pregnancy outcomes, was published in a Cochrane review [82]. No studies met all study eligibility criteria. There is thus no strong evidence regarding the effectiveness of preconception counseling to decrease adverse pregnancy outcomes for WWE and their offspring [83]. More population-based studies are required. For a more detailed review, see Chapter 10.

Antiseizure Medications and Fetal Effects

The occurrence of fetal malformations is associated with the use of ASMs in pregnancy. Different ASMs are associated with different types of malformations in the offspring. Data on fetal effects of ASMs generally come from epilepsy and pregnancy registries, as randomized clinical trials are not possible in pregnancy. Registries are found in many countries and differ in methodology and outcomes. Pharmaceutical companies may collect pregnancy data related to their product while other registries are driven by independent research groups who may collect and publish data on more than one ASM for comparison [84]. Here, we primarily discuss population-based studies reporting on ASM and the risk of MCMs.

A Finnish retrospective, population-based study of WWE using data from the National Medical Birth Registry showed a higher risk of MCMs in the newborns of WWE exposed to any ASM in utero (OR, 1.7; 95% CI, 1.1, 2.8) compared to the newborns of WWE not exposed to ASM. The odds of MCMs in infants exposed to in utero VPA monotherapy (OR, 4.2; 95% CI, 2.3–7.6) or polytherapy (OR, 3.5; 95% CI, 1.4–8.1) were also increased [85].

A systematic review and meta-analysis of international published registries examined the incidence of congenital malformations and other pregnancy outcomes after in utero ASM exposure [86]. Fifty-nine studies involving 65,533 pregnancies in WWE and 1,817,024 pregnancies in WWoE were included. The incidence of congenital malformations in offspring born to WWE was greater (7.1%; 95% CI, 5.6–8.5) compared to offspring born to WWoE (2.3%; 95% CI, 1.5, 3.1). The incidence was greatest for ASM polytherapy [16.8%; 95% CI, 0.5–33.1). The highest CM incidence rate belonged to VPA, at 10.7% (95% CI, 8.2–13.3) for monotherapy. Valproate monotherapy and polytherapy drugs that included phenobarbital (PB), phenytoin (PHT), or VPA significantly increased the risk of CM in offspring exposed in utero.

Data on newer-generation ASMs are emerging. A population-based cohort study of 837,795 infants born in Denmark investigated the relationship between in utero exposure to newer-generation ASMs during the first trimester of pregnancy and the likelihood of developing MCMs [87]. Of the 1,532 infants exposed to LTG, oxcarbazepine (OXC), topiramate (TPM), gabapentin (GBP), or levetiracetam (LEV) during the first trimester, 3.2% were diagnosed with an MCM compared with 2.4% who were not exposed to an ASM with an adjusted OR of 1.0 (95% CI, 0.7–1.4). Of 1,019 ASM-exposed newborns, an MCM was discovered in 38 (3.7%) exposed to LTG during the first trimester (OR, 1.2; 95% CI, 0.8–1.7), in 11 of 393 (2.8%) exposed to OXC (OR, 0.9; 95% CI, 0.5–1.6), and in 5 of 108 (4.6%) exposed to TPM (OR, 1.4; 95% CI, 0.6–3.6). Only 1 (1.7%) infant exposed to GBP (n = 59) and no infants exposed to LEV (n = 58) were diagnosed with MCMs, but the use of these ASMs is still less common in pregnancy.

A prospective, non-population-based, cohort study using data from the North American AED Pregnancy Registry (NAAPR) investigated 7,370 pregnancies among women taking ASM in the United States and Canada between 1997 and 2011. Pregnant women (n = 1,562) exposed to LTG were the main comparison group [88, 89]. The risk of major malformations was as follows: 9.3% (95% CI, 6.4–13.0%) for VPA; 5.5% (95% CI, 2.8–9.7%) for PB; 4.2% (95% CI, 2.4–6.8%) for TPM; 3.0% (95% CI, 2.1–4.2%) for carbamazepine (CBZ); 2.9% (95% CI, 1.5–5.0%) for PHT; 2.4% (95% CI, 1.2–4.3%) for LEV; 2.2% (95% CI, 0.6–5.5%) for OXC; 0.7% (0.02–3.8) for GBP; and 3.1% (0.4–10.8%) for clonazepam (CZP). In comparison, the risk of malformations in the infants exposed to LTG was 2.0% (95% CI, 1.4–2.8%) and 1.1% (95% CI, 0.4–2.6%) in the unexposed hospital population. The ASMs with significantly elevated unadjusted RRs when compared to LTG exposure included VPA (RR, 5.1; 95% CI, 3.0–8.5), phenobarbital (RR, 2.9; 95% CI, 1.4–5.8), and TPM (RR, 2.2; 95% CI, 1.2–4.0). Notably, prevalence of oral clefts was 1.4% (95% CI, 0.51–3.1%) in the TPM-exposed pregnancies, which was higher than in the study comparison group [88] or other reference populations [87, 90].

In 2014, the Australian Pregnancy Register published a prospective, cohort study of 1,572 pregnancies of both treated and untreated WWE aimed at determining the rate of major malformations after exposure to three newer ASMs (LTG, LEV, and TPM) [91].

Malformations were seen in 3.3% of infants of 153 untreated WWE. The proportion and risk of major malformations for those exposed to monotherapy were as follows: LTG, 4.6% (RR, 1.40; 95% CI, 0.51–3.80); TPM, 2.4% (RR, 0.73; 95% CI, 0.09–6.07); and LEV, 2.4% (RR, 0.75; 95% CI, 0.15–3.76). For those exposed to polytherapy ASM treatment, the proportion of major malformations were as follows: LTG, 5.5% (RR, 1.67; 95% CI, 0.61–4.59); TPM, 14.1% (RR, 4.32; 95% CI, 1.57–11.05); and LEV, 8.7% (RR, 2.25; 95% CI, 0.76–6.69).

Other adverse pregnancy outcomes reported in the offspring of ASM-treated WWE include small-for-gestational age (SGA) infants, decreased head circumference, and microcephaly, but many of these studies involved older-generation drugs with limited information on the contribution of newer-generation ASMs [92–95].

In a 2014 cohort study from the Medical Birth Registry of Norway, the risks of fetal growth restriction in 2,600 infants exposed in utero to newer or older ASM were investigated [96]. Comparisons were made to 771,412 unexposed infants of WWoE. The overall risk of SGA outcomes was significantly increased in infants exposed to an ASM (10.7%; OR, 1.17; 95% CI, 1.03–1.33), especially for TPM exposure (25.0%; OR 3.29; 95% CI, 1.70–6.39) compared to unexposed infants (8.9%). The overall risk of head circumference less than the 10th percentile was increased in infants prenatally exposed to an ASM (10.8%; OR, 1.24; 95% CI, 1.09–1.40) compared to unexposed infants (8.7%). The overall risk of decreased head circumference (less than 2.5th percentile) was increased in infants exposed in utero to ASM (3.4%; OR, 1.39; 95% CI, 1.12–1.72) and significantly increased for those exposed to TPM (14.9%; OR 7.21; 95% CI, 3.23–16.1) compared to unexposed infants (2.4%). An increased rate of SGA outcomes (10.3%; adjusted OR 1.15; 95% CI, 1.03–1.27) was found in the 3,773 infants born to untreated WWE compared to unexposed infants of WWoE (8.9%). However, when comparing the rate of head circumference less than the 10th percentile to the reference group of unexposed infants, no difference was found.

There have also been studies examining the association between ASM use and cognitive outcomes in children. A prospective, observational (non-population-based) study from the NAAPR examined the cognitive effects of fetal exposure to ASM in 309 children at 3 years of age [97]. A nonexposed control group was not included. Pregnant WWE were enrolled who were taking ASM monotherapy (CBZ, LTG, PHT, or VPA). Lower intelligence quotient (IQ) scores were found in 3-year-old children who had been exposed in utero to VPA compared to children exposed to any other ASM. A dose-dependent relationship between VPA use and IQ was noted. These findings persisted to 4.5 years of age [98]. The mean IQ after adjustment at age 4.5 years was 106 (95% CI, 102–109) for those exposed in utero to CBZ, 106 (95% CI, 102–109) for LTG, 105 (95% CI, 102–109) for PHT, and 96 (95% CI, 91–100) for VPA. Frequency of marked intellectual impairment decreased with age in children exposed to LTG, PHT, and CBZ, but not for children whose mothers took VPA. Verbal abilities were found to be impaired compared to nonverbal skills in all four groups studied. As expected, maternal IQ correlated with children's IQ, except for those children with in utero exposure to VPA where the authors found IQs to be significantly lower. Right-handedness was seen less frequently in children exposed to ASM overall when compared to a normative sample of 187 unexposed children (86% vs. 93%; $p = 0.0404$), especially in the VPA (79%, $p = 0.0089$) and LTG groups (83%; $p = 0.0287$). In addition, the exposed children in this study had relatively decreased verbal abilities compared to nonverbal abilities for children whose mothers had taken LTG ($p = 0.028$) or VPA ($p = 0.0063$) during pregnancy.

In utero VPA exposure was again associated with several reduced cognitive abilities (e.g., IQ, verbal, nonverbal, memory, and executive function) at 6 years of age.

Recent studies have also demonstrated a link between maternal use of VPA and an elevated risk of autism spectrum disorder (ASD) and attention-deficit/hyperactivity disorder (ADHD) in the offspring. A 2020 Swedish study of 14,614 children born between 1996 and 2011 and maternal use of VPA, LTG, and CBZ in WWE found that only VPA was associated with either ASD and ADHD ICD-10 outcomes [99]. In addition, a 2019 Danish population-based study of 913,302 singletons exposed to ASM in utero demonstrated a 48% increased risk of ADHD (adjusted hazard ratio, 1.48; 95% CI, 1.09–2.00) in children exposed compared to those unexposed to valproic acid [100].

An observational (non-population-based) study of WWE and their children was conducted through the Australian Pregnancy Register for WWE and Allied Disorders [101]. Researchers investigated the language skills of 102 school-aged kids exposed prenatally to ASM. Children exposed to VPA monotherapy or polytherapy were significantly more likely to have below normal language scores compared to children exposed to CBZ or LTG monotherapy, or polytherapy without VPA. For a more detailed review, see Chapter 11.

Seizure Control during Pregnancy

No population-based studies, to our knowledge, have examined seizure control during pregnancy. However, some of the pregnancy registries have studied this in selected WWE. The International Registry of ASM and Pregnancy reported prospectively documented seizure control and treatment in 1,956 pregnancies of 1,882 WWE [102]. Of all pregnant WWE, 58.3% were seizure free throughout pregnancy. Focal epilepsy (OR, 2.5; 95% CI, 1.7–3.9), polytherapy (OR, 9.0; 95% CI, 5.6–14.8), and OXC monotherapy (for tonic-clonic seizures only) (OR, 5.4; 95% CI, 1.6–17.1) predicted the occurrence of seizures. Seizure control stayed constant during pregnancy in 63.6% of WWE pregnancies. Of those, 92.7% remained seizure free during the complete pregnancy. In pregnant WWE, 17.3% had an increase in the frequency of seizures while 15.9% of pregnant WWE had a decrease. The same ASM treatment continued in 62.7% of the pregnancies.

The risk of seizing during pregnancy has been reported to be significantly decreased if there has been no seizures for a year before pregnancy, according to an Australian registry-based study of 841 ASM-treated pregnancies [103]. Of all ASM-treated WWE, 49.7% had seizures while pregnant. The risk of having seizures during pregnancy was 24.9%, with a minimum of 1 year of freedom from seizures before pregnancy, 22.8% with a minimum of 2 years of freedom from seizures, 20.5% with a minimum of 3 years of freedom from seizures, and 20% with 4 or more years of freedom from seizures. The association between the length of time of freedom from seizures prior to becoming pregnant and the chances of being seizure free during and after pregnancy was the most relevant finding of this study. With 1 year of freedom from seizures before pregnancy, the likelihood of seizures in pregnancy was decreased by 50–70% [103]. For a more detailed review, see Chapter 12.

Pregnancy and Epilepsy

Women with epilepsy have been found to have a higher risk of pregnancy and delivery complications. However, it is not clear if this is due to epilepsy or the use of ASMs during pregnancy. A population-based study examined whether pregnant WWE had a greater likelihood of complications during pregnancy and also explored the effects of ASM use via databases on all births in Norway from 1999 to 2005 [104]. The outcomes included preeclampsia, gestational hypertension, eclampsia, vaginal bleeding, and prematurity. Women with epilepsy had greater odds of mild preeclampsia (OR, 1.3; 95% CI, 1.1–1.5) and delivery before week 34 (OR, 1.2; 95% CI, 1.0–1.5). Women with epilepsy on ASMs had higher odds of mild preeclampsia (OR, 1.8; 95% CI, 1.3–2.4), gestational hypertension (OR, 1.5; 95% CI, 1.0–2.2), vaginal bleeding late in pregnancy (OR, 1.9; 95% CI 1.1–3.2), and delivery before 34 weeks of gestation (OR, 1.5; 95% CI, 1.1–2.0) when compared to WWoE. However, these increased risks of complications were not seen in WWE not using ASMs.

A population-based study using the same databases, including all births in Norway, looked at whether WWE have greater odds of complications during labor and investigated the impact of ASMs [105]. Outcomes included induction, caesarean section, use of forceps and vacuum, abnormal presentation, placental abruption, mechanical disproportion, postpartum hemorrhage, atony, and decreased Apgar scores after 5 minutes. Elevated odds of induction (OR, 1.3; 95% CI, 1.1–1.4), caesarean section (OR, 1.4; 95% CI, 1.3–1.6) and postpartum hemorrhage (OR, 1.2; 95% CI, 1.1–1.4) were seen in WWE (on or off ASMs) compared with WWoE. However, even higher estimates were obtained in WWE on ASMs with ORs (95% CIs) of 1.6 (1.4–1.9), 1.6 (1.4–1.9), and 1.5 (1.3–1.9), respectively. The odds of an Apgar score less than 7 was higher in WWE on ASM (OR, 1.6; 95% CI, 1.1–2.4) compared to WWoE. Only a mildly increased likelihood of caesarean delivery was found among WWE without ASMs compared to WWoE (OR, 1.3; 95% CI, 1.2–1.5).

A retrospective study from 2011 examined complications during pregnancy and delivery in 205 WWE and compared them to a control group of WWoE matched for age and parity [106]. After adjustment for age, parity, education, smoking, medical conditions and body mass index, WWE treated with ASMs had increased odds of severe preeclampsia (adjusted odds ratio [AOR], 5.0; 95% CI, 1.3–19.9), bleeding in early pregnancy (AOR, 6.4; 95% CI, 2.7–15.2); induction (AOR, 2.3; 955 CI, 1.2–4.3); and caesarean section (AOR, 2.5; 95% CI, 1.4–4.7) when compared to WWoE. While WWE using ASMs had greater odds for pregnancy and delivery complications, WWoE not using ASMs had few complications. Increased risks of pregnancy complications were not observed among WWE with no ASM use as compared to WWoE. However, not all studies found an increased risk for pregnancy and perinatal complications among WWE using ASMs. In a Swedish population-based cohort study of 1,429,652 singleton births, out of which 5,373 were born to 3,586 WWE [107], with the exception of an increased rate of labor induction (adjusted relative risk [ARR], 1.30; 95% CI, 1.10–1.55), the risks of pregnancy and perinatal complications among WWE using ASMs were not increased when compared to WWE not using ASMs [107]. For a more detailed review, see Chapter 13.

Postpartum Monitoring

Lactation

Few population-based studies of breastfeeding WWE have been conducted. Pregnant WWE taking a single ASM (CBZ, LTG, PHT, or VPA) were enrolled between 1999 and 2004 in an observational prospective study from epilepsy centers in the United States and the United Kingdom. The implications of breastfeeding during ASM therapy on cognitive outcomes in

3-year-old children were investigated [108]. Of the 199 children studied, 42% were breastfed. There were no differences in IQs for breastfed children compared to non-breastfed children for all ASMs combined and for each of the four individual ASM groups. The mean adjusted IQ score (95% CIs) across all ASM-exposed infants who were breastfed was 99 (96–103) while for non-breastfed it was 98 (95–101). This investigation does not show adverse effects of breastfeeding during ASM therapy on cognitive outcomes in children exposed in utero to four common ASMs.

A prospective cohort study from Norway of children born to 78,744 mothers provided detailed information on motor skills, social skills, language, and behavior at 6 months, 18 months, and 36 months of age [109]. The children of WWE using ASMs were compared to a reference group of children born to parents without epilepsy. In children of women using ASMs, continuous breastfeeding was associated with less impaired development at both 6 and 18 months when compared with those with no breastfeeding or breastfeeding for less than 6 months. However, adverse development was associated with prenatal ASM exposure at 36 months regardless of breastfeeding status during the first year. Compared to the reference population, continuous breastfeeding during the first year occurred less frequently among women using ASMs, particularly with LTG monotherapy and polytherapy. For a more detailed review, see Chapter 18.

Epilepsy in Menopause

Menopause, Hormone Replacement Therapy

Treatment of epilepsy may disrupt the effects of hormone replacement therapy (HRT) and conversely HRT may influence the occurrence of seizures. During the menopausal transition, catamenial seizures may increase in frequency due to hyperestrogenism and then decrease afterward. Sexual dysfunction may be exacerbated due to the lack of estrogen in menopause and epilepsy itself [110, 111]. Menopause tends to occur about 3 years earlier with a history of one or more seizures per month for much of the duration of epilepsy and lifetime use of multiple enzyme-inducing ASMs [112]. Premature ovarian failure (POF) in WWE has been noted in some studies, but no predisposing factors such as epilepsy duration, seizure severity, or use of enzyme-inducing ASMs have been identified [65, 113].

Menopause may also affect ASM metabolism. Hormone replacement therapy may lower LTG levels [114], and although the evidence is mixed, ASM clearance may also be affected by menopause [115, 116]. No population-based studies of menopause in WWE have, to our knowledge, been conducted.

Bone Health

Osteoporosis is associated with both menopause and the use of ASMs. The occurrence of menopause and the use of ASMs in WWE concurrently may combine to exacerbate this risk. Osteoporosis and fractures may increase in menopausal WWE because of hypoestrogenism in menopause and the use of cytochrome P450-inducing ASMs [110].

A Danish, population-based, case-control study investigated fracture risk associated with various ASMs (124,655 fracture cases and 373,962 controls) using the National Hospital Discharge Register and the National Pharmacological Database [117]. After adjustment, a significant association was found between CBZ (OR, 1.18; 95% CI, 1.10–1.26), OXC (OR, 1.14; 95% CI, 1.03–1.26), CZP (OR, 1.27; 95% CI, 1.15–1.41), PB (OR, 1.79;

95% CI, 1.64–1.95), and VPA (OR, 1.15; 95% CI, 1.05–1.26) and the likelihood of fracture. This association was not seen in ethosuximide (ETX), LTG, PHT, PR, tiagabine (TGB), TPM, or vigabatrin (VGB). Age and sex did not impact the risk of fracture [117].

A 2020 population-based study of epilepsy patients enrolled in Taiwan's National Health Insurance between 1998 and 2011 examined the risk of fracture and cost associated with fracture comparing enzyme-inducing ASMs to non-enzyme-inducing ASMs [118]. This study found 6,995 fractures (3,686 in the enzyme-inducing group). The non-enzyme-inducing ASMs were less likely to be associated with fracture (hazard ratio [HR] of 0.70, 95% CI, 0.50–0.97). In multivariate analysis, female sex was associated with risk of fracture (adjusted HR 1.80; 95% CI, 1.09–2.97).

Women with epilepsy of reproductive age are also at risk of experiencing bone loss while on ASMs, as shown in a prospective US study of WWE in taking ASM monotherapy (CBZ, LTG, PHT, or VPA) [119]. Of note, no control group of WWoE was included for comparison. In the PHT group, a significant decrease (2.6%) was found at the femoral neck over 1 year, unlike those treated with CBZ, LTG, and VPA who did not have evidence of bone turnover. For a more detailed review, see Chapter 19.

Summary

Epilepsy is one of the most common neurological conditions affecting women and men of all ages. Women with epilepsy encounter particular issues throughout their life span, and we have only begun to collect the population-level data that allow us to make counseling recommendations in this population. There unfortunately remain few population-level data on WWE during hormonal transitions, including in pregnancy, during lactation, and during the menopausal transition.

References

1. Banerjee PN, Filippi D, Hauser WA. The descriptive epidemiology of epilepsy: A review. *Epilepsy Research.* 2009;**85**(1):31–45.
2. Collaborators, GBDE. Global, regional, and national burden of epilepsy, 1990–2016: A systematic analysis for the Global Burden of Disease Study 2016. *Lancet Neurol.* 2019;**18**(4):357–75.
3. Fiest KM, Sauro KM, Wiebe, S, et al. Prevalence and incidence of epilepsy: A systematic review and meta-analysis of international studies. *Neurology.* 2017;**88**(3):296–303.
4. Christensen J, Vestergaard, M, Pedersen, MG, et al. Incidence and prevalence of epilepsy in Denmark. *Epilepsy Res.* 2007;**76**(1):60–5.
5. Ngugi AK, Bottomley C, Kleinschmidt I, et al. Estimation of the burden of active and life-time epilepsy: A meta-analytic approach. *Epilepsia.* 2010;**51**(5):883–90.
6. Forsgren L, Beghi E, Oun A, Sillanpaa M. The epidemiology of epilepsy in Europe: A systematic review. *Eur J Neurol.* 2005;**12**(4):245–53.
7. Tellez-Zenteno JF, Pondal-Sordo M, Matijevic S, Wiebe S. National and regional prevalence of self-reported epilepsy in Canada. *Epilepsia.* 2004;**45**(12):1623–9.
8. Kobau R, Zahran H, Thurman DJ, et al. Epilepsy surveillance among adults: 19 states, Behavioral Risk Factor Surveillance System, 2005. *MMWR Surveill Summ.* 2008;**57**(6):1–20.
9. Kotsopoulos IA, Van Merode T, Kessels FG, de Krom MC, Knottnerus JA. Systematic review and meta-analysis of incidence

studies of epilepsy and unprovoked seizures. *Epilepsia*. 2002;**43**(11):1402–9.

10. Christensen J M.J. Kjeldsen, H Andersen, M.L. Friis, and P Sidenius Gender differences in epilepsy. *Epilepsia*. 2005;**46**(6):956–60.
11. Ngugi AK, Kariuki SM, Bottomley C, et al. Incidence of epilepsy: A systematic review and meta-analysis. *Neurology*. 2011;77(10):1005–12.
12. Hauser WA, Annegers JF, Kurland LT. Incidence of epilepsy and unprovoked seizures in Rochester, Minnesota: 1935–1984. *Epilepsia*. 1993;**34**(3):453–68.
13. Hesdorffer DC, Logroscino G, Benn, EKT et al. Estimating risk for developing epilepsy: A population-based study in Rochester, Minnesota. *Neurology*. 2010;**76**(1):23–7.
14. Kalilani L, Sun X, Pelgrims, B, Noack-Rink M, Villanueva V. The epidemiology of drug-resistant epilepsy: A systematic review and meta-analysis. *Epilepsia*. 2018;**59**(12):2179–93.
15. Reddy DS, Thompson W, Calderara G. Molecular mechanisms of sex differences in epilepsy and seizure susceptibility in chemical, genetic and acquired epileptogenesis. *Neurosci Lett*. 2021;**750**:135753.
16. Tellez-Zenteno JF, Patten SB, Jette N, Williams J, Wiebe S, Psychiatric comorbidity in epilepsy: A population-based analysis. *Epilepsia*. 2007;**48**(12):2336–44.
17. Wilner AN, Sharma BK, Soucy A, Thompson A, Krueger A. Common comorbidities in women and men with epilepsy and the relationship between number of comorbidities and health plan paid costs in 2010. *Epilepsy Behav*. 2014;**32**:15–20.
18. Hesdorffer DC, Hauser WA, Olafsson E, Ludvigsson P, Kjartansson O. Depression and suicide attempt as risk factors for incident unprovoked seizures. *Ann Neurol*. 2006;**59**(1):35–41.
19. Hesdorffer DC, Ishihara L, Mynepalli, L, et al. Epilepsy, suicidality, and psychiatric disorders: A bidirectional association. *Ann Neurol*. 2012;**72**(2):184–91.
20. Tellez-Zenteno JF, Matijevic S, Wiebe S. Somatic comorbidity of epilepsy in the general population in Canada. *Epilepsia*. 2005;**46**(12):1955–62.
21. Centers for Disease Control and Prevention. Comorbidity in adults with epilepsy: United States, 2010. *MMWR Morb Mortal Wkly Rep*. 2013;**62**(43):849–53.
22. Fuller-Thomson E, Brennenstuhl S. The association between depression and epilepsy in a nationally representative sample. *Epilepsia*. 2009;**50**(5):1051–8.
23. Ajinkya S, Fox J, Lekoubou A. Trends in prevalence and treatment of depressive symptoms in adult patients with epilepsy in the United States. *Epilepsy Behav*. 2020;**105**:106973.
24. Kanner AM. Depression in epilepsy: Prevalence, clinical semiology, pathogenic mechanisms, and treatment. *Biological Psychiatry*. 2003;**54**(3):388–98.
25. Gaus V, Kiep H, Holtkamp M, Burkert S, Kendel F. Gender differences in depression, but not in anxiety in people with epilepsy. *Seizure*. 2015;**32**:37–42.
26. Scott AJ, Sharpe L, Loomes M, Gandy M. Systematic review and meta-analysis of anxiety and depression in youth with epilepsy. *J Pediatr Psychol*. 2020;**45**(2):133–44.
27. Fiest KM, Dykeman J, Patten, SB, et al. Depression in epilepsy: A systematic review and meta-analysis. *Neurology*. 2013;**80**(6):590–9.
28. Scott AJ, Sharpe L, Hunt C, Gandy M. Anxiety and depressive disorders in people with epilepsy: A meta-analysis. *Epilepsia*. 2017;**58**(6):973–82.
29. Bjork MH, Veiby G, Reiter SC, et al. Depression and anxiety in women with epilepsy during pregnancy and after delivery: A prospective population-based cohort study on frequency, risk factors, medication, and prognosis. *Epilepsia*. 2015;**56**(1):28–39.

30. Bjork MH, Veiby G, Engelsen BA, Gilhus NE. Depression and anxiety during pregnancy and the postpartum period in women with epilepsy: A review of frequency, risks and recommendations for treatment. *Seizure.* 2015;**28**:39–45.
31. Gaitatzis A, Carroll K, Majeed A, Sander JW. The epidemiology of the comorbidity of epilepsy in the general population. *Epilepsia.* 2004;**45**(12):1613–22.
32. Kessler RC, Chiu WT, Demler O, Merikangas KR, Walters EE. Prevalence, severity, and comorbidity of 12-month DSM-IV disorders in the National Comorbidity Survey Replication. *Arch Gen Psychiatry.* 2005;**62**(6):617–27.
33. Manni R, Terzaghi M. Comorbidity between epilepsy and sleep disorders. *Epilepsy Research.* 2010;**90**(3):171–7.
34. Van Golde EGA, Gutter T, de Weerd AW. Sleep disturbances in people with epilepsy: Prevalence, impact and treatment. *Sleep Medicine Reviews.* 2011;**15**(6):357–68.
35. Khatami R, Zutter D, Siegel A. Sleep-wake habits and disorders in a series of 100 adult epilepsy patients: A prospective study. *Seizure.* 2006;**15**(5):299–306.
36. Safarpour Lima B, Zokaei A, Assarzadegan F, Hesami O, Zareh Shahamati S. Prevalence of sleep disorders in patients with epilepsy: A questionnaire-based cross-sectional study. *Epilepsy Behav.* 2021;**114**(Pt A):107635.
37. Gogou M, Haidopoulou K, Eboriadou M, Pavlou E. Sleep apneas and epilepsy comorbidity in childhood: A systematic review of the literature. *Sleep Breath.* 2015;**19**(2):421–32.
38. Quigg M, Gharai S, Ruland J, et al. Insomnia in epilepsy is associated with continuing seizures and worse quality of life. *Epilepsy Res.* 2016;**122**:91–6.
39. de Weerd A, de Haas S, Otte A, et al. Subjective sleep disturbance in patients with partial epilepsy: A questionnaire-based study on prevalence and impact on quality of life. *Epilepsia.* 2004;**45**(11):1397–1404.
40. Pornsriniyom D, Kim H, Bena J, et al. Effect of positive airway pressure therapy on seizure control in patients with epilepsy and obstructive sleep apnea. *Epilepsy Behav.* 2014;**37**:270–5.
41. Winawer MR, Shinnar S. Genetic epidemiology of epilepsy or what do we tell families? *Epilepsia.* 2005;**46** Suppl 10:24–30.
42. Vadlamudi L, Milne RL, Lawrence K, et al. Genetics of epilepsy: The testimony of twins in the molecular era. *Neurology.* 2014;**83**(12):1042–8.
43. Thomas RH, Berkovic SF. The hidden genetics of epilepsy: A clinically important new paradigm. *Nat Rev Neurol.* 2014;**10**(5):283–92.
44. Tashkandi M, Baarma D, Tricco, AC et al. EEG of asymptomatic first-degree relatives of patients with juvenile myoclonic, childhood absence and rolandic epilepsy: A systematic review and meta-analysis. *Epileptic Disord.* 2019;**21**(1):30–41.
45. McHugh JC, Delanty N. Chapter 2 Epidemiology and classification of epilepsy: Gender comparisons. *International Review of Neurobiology.* 2008;**83**:11–26.
46. Waaler PE, Blom BH, Skeidsvoll H, Mykletun A. Prevalence, classification, and severity of epilepsy in children in western Norway. *Epilepsia.* 2000;**41**(7):802–10.
47. Briellmann RS, Jackson GD, Mitchell LA, et al. Occurrence of hippocampal sclerosis: Is one hemisphere or gender more vulnerable? *Epilepsia.* 1999;**40**(12):1816–20.
48. Janszky J. Medial temporal lobe epilepsy: Gender differences. *Journal of Neurology, Neurosurgery & Psychiatry.* 2004;**75**(5):773–5.
49. Herzog AG. Catamenial epilepsy: Definition, prevalence pathophysiology and treatment. *Seizure.* 2008;**17**(2):151–9.
50. Herzog AG, Harden CL, Liporace J, et al. Frequency of catamenial seizure exacerbation in women with localization-related epilepsy. *Annals of Neurology.* 2004;**56**(3):431–4.

51. el-Khayat HA, Soliman NA, Tomoum HY, et al. Reproductive hormonal changes and catamenial pattern in adolescent females with epilepsy. *Epilepsia.* 2008;**49**(9):1619–26.

52. Quigg M, Smithson SD, Fowler KM, Sursal T, Herzog AG. Laterality and location influence catamenial seizure expression in women with partial epilepsy. *Neurology*, 2009;**73**(3):223–7.

53. Henning OJ, Nakken KO, Traeen B, Mowinckel P, Lossius M. Sexual problems in people with refractory epilepsy. *Epilepsy Behav.* 2016;**61**:174–9.

54. Morrell MJ, Flynn KL, Doñe S, et al. Sexual dysfunction, sex steroid hormone abnormalities, and depression in women with epilepsy treated with antiepileptic drugs. *Epilepsy Behav.* 2005;**6**(3):360–5.

55. Herzog AG, Coleman AE, Jacobs AR, et al. Relationship of sexual dysfunction to epilepsy laterality and reproductive hormone levels in women. *Epilepsy Behav.* 2003;**4**(4):407–13.

56. Pack AM. Implications of hormonal and neuroendocrine changes associated with seizures and antiepileptic drugs: A clinical perspective. *Epilepsia.* 2010;**51**:150–3.

57. Svalheim S, Taubøll E, Bjørnenak T, et al. Do women with epilepsy have increased frequency of menstrual disturbances? *Seizure.* 2003;**12**(8):529–33.

58. Herzog AG, Friedman MN. Menstrual cycle interval and ovulation in women with localization-related epilepsy. *Neurology.* 2001;**57**(11):2133–5.

59. Herzog AG, Coleman AE, Jacobs AR, et al. Interictal EEG discharges, reproductive hormones, and menstrual disorders in epilepsy. *Ann Neurol.* 2003;**54**(5):625–37.

60. Hu X, Wang J, Dong W, et al. A meta-analysis of polycystic ovary syndrome in women taking valproate for epilepsy. *Epilepsy Research.* 2011;**97**(1–2):73–82.

61. Lofgren E, Mikkonen K, Tolonen U, et al. Reproductive endocrine function in women with epilepsy: The role of epilepsy type and medication. *Epilepsy Behav.* 2007;**10**(1):77–83.

62. Morrell MJ, Hayes FJ, Sluss PM, et al. Hyperandrogenism, ovulatory dysfunction, and polycystic ovary syndrome with valproate versus lamotrigine. *Ann Neurol.* 2008;**64**(2):200–11.

63. MacEachern DB, Mandle HB, Herzog AG. Infertility, impaired fecundity, and live birth/pregnancy ratio in women with epilepsy in the USA: Findings of the Epilepsy Birth Control Registry. *Epilepsia.* 2019;**60**(9):1993–8.

64. Herzog AG, Seibel MM, Schomer DL, Vaitukaitis JL, Geschwind N. Reproductive endocrine disorders in men with partial seizures of temporal lobe origin. *Arch Neurol.* 1986;**43**(4):347–50.

65. Herzog AG, Seibel MM, Schomer DL, Vaitukaitis JL, Geschwind N. Reproductive endocrine disorders in women with partial seizures of temporal lobe origin. *Arch Neurol.* 1986;**43**(4):341–6.

66. Wallace H, Shorvon S, Tallis R. Age-specific incidence and prevalence rates of treated epilepsy in an unselected population of 2 052 922 and age-specific fertility rates of women with epilepsy. *Lancet.* 1998;**352**(9145):1970–3.

67. Pennell PB, French JA, Harden CL, et al. Fertility and birth outcomes in women with epilepsy seeking pregnancy. *JAMA Neurol.* 2018;**75**(8):962–9.

68. Pack AM. Infertility in women with epilepsy: What's the risk and why? *Neurology.* 2010;**75**(15):1316–17.

69. Gopinath M, Sarma PS, Thomas SV. Gender-specific psychosocial outcome for women with epilepsy. *Epilepsy Behav.* 2011;**20**(1):44–7.

70. Herzog AG, Mandle HB, Cahill KE, Fowler KM, Hauser WA. Predictors of unintended pregnancy in women with epilepsy. *Neurology.* 2017;**88**(8):728–33.

71. Johnson EL, Burke E, Wang A, Pennell PB. Unintended pregnancy, prenatal care, newborn outcomes, and breastfeeding in

women with epilepsy. *Neurology*. 2018;**91**(11):e1031–e1039.

72. Pack AM, Davis AR, Kritzer J, Yoon A, Camus A. Antiepileptic drugs: Are women aware of interactions with oral contraceptives and potential teratogenicity? *Epilepsy Behav*. 2009;**14**(4):640–4.
73. Pennell PB. Hormonal aspects of epilepsy. *Neurologic Clinics*. 2009;**27**(4):941–65.
74. Wang H, Bos JH, de Jong–van den Berg LT. Co-prescription of antiepileptic drugs and contraceptives. *Contraception*. 2012;**85**(1):28–31.
75. Shorvon SD, Tallis RC, Wallace HK. Antiepileptic drugs: Coprescription of proconvulsant drugs and oral contraceptives: A national study of antiepileptic drug prescribing practice. *J Neurol Neurosurg Psychiatry*. 2002;**72**(1):114–15.
76. Vessey M, Painter R, Yeates D. Oral contraception and epilepsy: Findings in a large cohort study. *Contraception*. 2002;**66**(2):77–9.
77. Harden CL, Pennell PB, Koppel BS, et al. Management issues for women with epilepsy: Focus on pregnancy (an evidence-based review) III. Vitamin K, folic acid, blood levels, and breast-feeding. Report of the Quality Standards Subcommittee and Therapeutics and Technology Assessment Subcommittee of the American Academy of Neurology and the American Epilepsy Society. *Epilepsia*. 2009;**50**(5):1247–55.
78. Kaaja E, Kaaja R, Hiilesmaa V. Major malformations in offspring of women with epilepsy. *Neurology*. 2003;**60**(4):575–9.
79. Morrow JI, Hunt SJ, Russell AJ, et al. Folic acid use and major congenital malformations in offspring of women with epilepsy: A prospective study from the UK Epilepsy and Pregnancy Register. *Journal of Neurology, Neurosurgery & Psychiatry*. 2009;**80**(5):506–11.
80. Pittschieler S, Brezinka C, Jahn B, et al. Spontaneous abortion and the prophylactic effect of folic acid supplementation in epileptic women undergoing antiepileptic therapy. *J Neurol*. 2008;**255**(12):1926–31.
81. Campbell E, Hunt S, Kinney MO, et al. The effect of socioeconomic status on treatment and pregnancy outcomes in women with epilepsy in Scotland. *Epilepsy Behav*. 2013;**28**(3):354–7.
82. Winterbottom JB, Smyth RM, Jacoby A, Baker GA. Preconception counselling for women with epilepsy to reduce adverse pregnancy outcome. *Cochrane Database Syst Rev*. 2008(3):CD006645.
83. Winterbottom J, Smyth R, Jacoby A, Baker G. The effectiveness of preconception counseling to reduce adverse pregnancy outcome in women with epilepsy: What's the evidence? *Epilepsy Behav*. 2009;**14**(2):273–9.
84. Tomson T, Battino D, French J, et al. Antiepileptic drug exposure and major congenital malformations: The role of pregnancy registries. *Epilepsy Behav*. 2007;**11**(3):277–82.
85. Artama M, Auvinen A, Raudaskoski T, Isojarvi I, Isojarvi J. Antiepileptic drug use of women with epilepsy and congenital malformations in offspring. *Neurology*. 2005;**64**(11):1874–8.
86. Meador K, Reynolds MW, Crean S, Fahrbach K, Probst C. Pregnancy outcomes in women with epilepsy: A systematic review and meta-analysis of published pregnancy registries and cohorts. *Epilepsy Research*. 2008;**81**(1):1–13.
87. Molgaard-Nielsen D, Hviid A. Newer-generation antiepileptic drugs and the risk of major birth defects. *JAMA*. 2011;**305**(19):1996–2002.
88. Hernandez-Diaz S, Smith CR, Shen A, et al. Comparative safety of antiepileptic drugs during pregnancy. *Neurology*. 2012;**78**(21):1692–9.
89. Holmes LB, Hernandez-Diaz S. Newer anticonvulsants: Lamotrigine, topiramate and gabapentin. *Birth Defects Res A Clin Mol Teratol*. 2012;**94**(8):599–606.
90. Hunt S, Russell A, Smithson WH, et al. Topiramate in pregnancy: Preliminary

experience from the UK Epilepsy and Pregnancy Register. *Neurology*. 2008;**71**(4):272–6.

91. Vajda FJ, O'Brien TJ, Lander CM, Graham J, Eadie MJ. The teratogenicity of the newer antiepileptic drugs: An update. *Acta Neurol Scand*. 2014;**130**(4):234–8.
92. Hvas CL, Henriksen TB, Ostergaard JR, Dam M. Epilepsy and pregnancy: Wffect of antiepileptic drugs and lifestyle on birthweight. *BJOG*. 2000;**107**(7):896–902.
93. Viinikainen K, Heinonen S, Eriksson K, Kalviainen R. Community-based, prospective, controlled study of obstetric and neonatal outcome of 179 pregnancies in women with epilepsy. *Epilepsia*. 2006;**47**(1):186–92.
94. Tomson T, Battino D. Teratogenic effects of antiepileptic drugs. *Lancet Neurol*. 2012;**11**(9):803–13.
95. Ashwal S, Michelson D, Plawner L, Dobyns WB. Practice parameter: Evaluation of the child with microcephaly (an evidence-based review). Report of the Quality Standards Subcommittee of the American Academy of Neurology and the Practice Committee of the Child Neurology Society. *Neurology*. 2009;**73**(11):887–97.
96. Veiby G, Daltveit AK, Engelsen BA, Gilhus NE. Fetal growth restriction and birth defects with newer and older antiepileptic drugs during pregnancy. *J Neurol*. 2014;**261**(3):579–88.
97. Meador KJ, Baker GA, Browning N, et al. Cognitive function at 3 years of age after fetal exposure to antiepileptic drugs. *N Engl J Med*. 2009;**360**(16):1597–1605.
98. Meador KJ, Baker GA, Browning N, et al. Effects of fetal antiepileptic drug exposure: Outcomes at age 4.5 years. *Neurology*. 2012;**78**(16):1207–14.
99. Wiggs KK, Rickert ME, Sujan AC, et al. Antiseizure medication use during pregnancy and risk of ASD and ADHD in children. *Neurology*. 2020;**95**(24):e3232–e3240.
100. Christensen J, Pedersen L, Sun Y, et al. Association of prenatal exposure to valproate and other antiepileptic drugs with risk for attention-deficit/hyperactivity disorder in offspring. *JAMA Netw Open*. 2019;**2**(1):e186606.
101. Nadebaum C, Anderson VA, Vajda F, et al. Language skills of school-aged children prenatally exposed to antiepileptic drugs. *Neurology*. 2011;**76**(8):719–26.
102. EURAP Study Group. Seizure control and treatment in pregnancy: Observations from the EURAP Epilepsy Pregnancy Registry. *Neurology*. 2006;**66**(3):354–60.
103. Vajda FJE, Hitchcock A, Graham J, et al. Seizure control in antiepileptic drug-treated pregnancy. *Epilepsia*. 2008;**49**(1):172–6.
104. Borthen I, Eide MG, Veiby G, Daltveit AK, Gilhus NE. Complications during pregnancy in women with epilepsy: Population-based cohort study. *BJOG*. 2009;**116**(13):1736–42.
105. Borthen I, Eide MG, Daltveit AK, Gilhus NE. Delivery outcome of women with epilepsy: A population-based cohort study. *BJOG*. 2010;**117**(12):1537–43.
106. Borthen I, Eide MG, Daltveit AK, Gilhus NE. Obstetric outcome in women with epilepsy: A hospital-based, retrospective study. *BJOG*. 2011;**118**(8):956–65.
107. Razaz N, Tomson T, Wikstrom AK, Cnattingius S. Association between pregnancy and perinatal outcomes among women with epilepsy. *JAMA Neurol*. 2017;**74**(8):983–91.
108. Meador KJ, Baker GA, Browning N, et al. Effects of breastfeeding in children of women taking antiepileptic drugs. *Neurology*. 2010;**75**(22):1954–60.
109. Veiby G, Engelsen BA, Gilhus NE. Early child development and exposure to antiepileptic drugs prenatally and through breastfeeding: A prospective cohort study on children of women with epilepsy. *JAMA Neurol*. 2013;**70**(11):1367–74.
110. Erel T, Guralp O. Epilepsy and menopause. *Archives of Gynecology and Obstetrics*. 2011;**284**(3):749–55.

111. Harden CL, Pulver MC, Ravdin L, Jacobs AR. The effect of menopause and perimenopause on the course of epilepsy. *Epilepsia*. 1999;**40**(10):1402–7.

112. Harden CL, Koppel BS, Herzog AG, Nikolov BG, Hauser WA. Seizure frequency is associated with age at menopause in women with epilepsy. *Neurology*. 2003;**61**(4):451–5.

113. Klein P, Serje A, Pezzullo JC. Premature ovarian failure in women with epilepsy. *Epilepsia*. 2001;**42**(12):1584–9.

114. Reimers A. Hormone replacement therapy with estrogens may reduce lamotrigine serum concentrations: A matched case-control study. *Epilepsia*. 2017;**58**(1):e6–e9.

115. Tomson T, Lukic S, Ohman I. Are lamotrigine kinetics altered in menopause? Observations from a drug monitoring database. *Epilepsy Behav*. 2010;**19**(1):86–8.

116. Wegner I, Wilhelm AJ, Sander JW, Lindhout D. The impact of age on lamotrigine and oxcarbazepine kinetics: A historical cohort study. *Epilepsy Behav*. 2013;**29**(1):217–21.

117. Vestergaard P, Rejnmark L, Mosekilde L. Fracture risk associated with use of antiepileptic drugs. *Epilepsia*. 2004;**45**(11):1330–7.

118. Cheng HH, Kung PT, Wang BR, Chiu LT, Tsai WC. Cost-benefit analysis, cost-effectiveness analysis, and impact of antiepileptic drugs on the risk of fracture in patients with epilepsy: A nationwide cohort study. *Epilepsy Behav*. 2020;**103**(Pt A):106851.

119. Pack AM, Morrell MJ, Randall A, McMahon DJ, Shane E. Bone health in young women with epilepsy after one year of antiepileptic drug monotherapy. *Neurology*. 2008;**70**(18):1586–93.

Chapter 2

Neuropsychiatric Issues for Women with Epilepsy

Dilip Koshy and Benjamin Tolchin

Key Points

- There is up to a 50% prevalence of neuropsychiatric issues in women with epilepsy, including a high rate of depression and anxiety.
- The peripartum and perimenopause periods are higher risk for experiencing depression, due in part to the impact of sex hormones.
- Up to 75% of people with psychogenic non-epileptic seizures (PNES) are women, and PNES can confer mortality like that of treatment-resistant epilepsy.
- Antiseizure medications (ASMs) can contribute to or produce neuropsychiatric issues such as low mood, anxiety, irritability, cognitive concerns, and even psychosis.
- While there are safe pharmacological options for treating neuropsychiatric issues in women with epilepsy, there are important considerations for impact on seizure threshold, breastfeeding safety, and teratogenicity.

Introduction

The link between epileptic and psychiatric phenomena has been recognized since the era of Hippocrates. The overall prevalence of neuropsychiatric comorbidities in people with epilepsy is estimated at 30–50% [1] and a bidirectional etiological relationship has been proposed between epilepsy and several psychiatric disorders, including depression, anxiety, psychosis, and suicidality, evidenced in part by the increased incidence of these disorders both before and after epilepsy onset [2]. Comorbid psychiatric disorders in people with epilepsy also impact prognosis, conferring negative effects on overall quality of life and premature mortality, and increased rates of drug-related adverse events and poorer adherence to epilepsy treatment [3].

Women with epilepsy are at higher risk than their male counterparts for developing neuropsychiatric disorders such as depression and anxiety, and particularly so in the peripartum and perimenopausal periods. Additionally, special treatment considerations must be made when treating these conditions pharmacologically at various reproductive stages.

Psychiatric comorbidities in people with epilepsy are often complex in both their diagnosis and management and highlight the importance of a multidisciplinary and multimodal biological, psychological, and social treatment approach that brings together psychiatrists, neurologists, social workers, psychotherapists, and other allied health professionals.

Mood Disorders: Depression

Major Depressive Disorder

Major depressive disorder (MDD) is the prototypical depressive disorder, consisting of major depressive episodes (MDEs) characterized by weeks of either persistently low mood or anhedonia (the loss of ability to experience pleasure), in addition to several neurovegetative and negative cognitions about oneself or the world [4].

The point prevalence of MDD in patients in epilepsy clinics is estimated at 22% [5]. People with epilepsy are about 2.8 times more likely to have depression compared with healthy controls [6] and women with epilepsy are 1.8 times as likely to be depressed as men with epilepsy [5]. Risks factors for depression in people with epilepsy include epilepsy-related disability, impaired social support, and perceived stigma associated with epilepsy. Admission to the hospital for epilepsy also predicts subsequent admissions for depression or bipolar disorder [5] and highlights the need to screen carefully for mood during or after an epilepsy admission. Not only are people with epilepsy at greater risk of developing depression, but having an incident episode of depression also confers 2.5 times greater risk of developing epilepsy thereafter [7]. Depression severity may also modulate prognosis in terms of subsequent freedom from seizures [7]. In recent years, the evidence of this bidirectional relationship has been a topic of increased study, and pathophysiological mechanisms proposed have included shared propensities toward a hyperactive hypothalamic-pituitary-adrenal (HPA) axis; aberrancies in serotonergic, noradrenergic, GABAergic, and glutamatergic transmission; and decreased frontal lobe and hippocampal volumes [8].

There is an overall susceptibility toward depression in women as compared with men, and fluctuation of sex hormones in reproductive stages in a woman's life may influence both mood and seizures. It has long been observed that there is a marked increase in depression risk in girls versus boys in the pubertal transition occurring in adolescence, increasing from approximately equal rates in young children to about a twofold rate in adolescent girls, and the relative preponderance in rates of depression among women continue throughout the life span into old age. A prevailing conceptual theory of depression is the diathesis-stress model whereby genetic and biological predisposition combine with life stressors that can precipitate depression. From a biological perspective, gene-environment studies have found variability in serotonin receptor expression that may explain some sex difference in depression. So too may the direct impact of hormonal fluctuation. For example, increasing estrogen concentrations in adolescence correlate with negative emotional states. Exactly how hormonal fluctuations impact emotional states remains uncertain, but there are several mechanisms whereby estradiol can modulate serotonergic transmission. Estradiol, for example, facilitates serotonin transmission by inhibiting monoamine oxidases (MAOs), increasing tryptophan hydroxylase expression, and increasing gene expression of the serotonin reuptake transporter [9]. Psychosocial factors associated with different reproductive life stages can also contribute to depression in some women. Examples include the impact of negative self-evaluation during pubertal body changes and the social and occupational impacts of transitioning to motherhood. In keeping with the impact of stressors on depression, one hypothesis is that estrogen-mediated dampening of HPA physiological reactivity to stress – a proposed evolutionary benefit in protecting the fetus from maternal stress sequelae – can increase risk of depression in women [9]. Another mediator in stress response appears to be allopregnanolone, a major metabolite of progesterone, which

Table 2.1 Neurological Disorders Depression Inventory for Epilepsy (NDDI-E) [9]
For the statements below, please circle the number that best describes you over the past 2 weeks, including today.

	Always or often	Sometimes	Rarely	Never
Everything is a struggle	4	3	2	1
Nothing I do is right	4	3	2	1
Feel guilty	4	3	2	1
I'd be better off dead	4	3	2	1
Frustrated	4	3	2	1
Difficulty finding pleasure	4	3	2	1

provides a sedative and antiseizure effect via allosterically enhancing GABAergic transmission [9]. In its pharmaceutical form of brexanolone, allopregnanolone has proven effective and is approved by the US Food and Drug Administration (FDA) in treating postpartum depression. Interestingly, women with premenstrual dysphoric disorder (PMDD) show a lower than typical allopregnanolone increase during acute stress [9].

In considering depression in women with epilepsy, it is important to note that the characteristic neurovegetative symptoms of depression, including disruptions in sleep, weight, appetite, concentration, and psychomotor retardation or agitation, can overlap with those found in epilepsy or with antiseizure medication (ASM) side effects. For this reason, negative cognitions and suicidality can often aid in distinguishing true clinical depression, and the most validated scale for depression in epilepsy, the Neurological Disorders Depression Inventory for Epilepsy (NDDI-E) [10], focuses on these characteristic features (Table 2.1).

Perinatal Depression, Perimenopausal Depression, and Premenstrual Dysphoric Disorder (PMDD)

Major depressive episodes with onset during pregnancy or during the first year postpartum are considered perinatal depression [11, 12]. This is an extremely high-risk period for the development of depression with an estimated 7.5% of women having an MDE during pregnancy, and 6.5% in the first 3 months postpartum. Of note, up to 40% of postpartum MDEs have onset during the pregnancy itself. Psychosocial factors to consider that can contribute to precipitating and perpetuating depression in the perinatal period include unintended or unwanted pregnancy, past negative pregnancy experiences including miscarriage, body image concerns, and job and career disruption.

The perimenopausal period confers risk of a first-time onset of depression as well as recurrence of depression. Vasomotor symptoms of perimenopause, including hot flashes and night sweats, have been shown to be independently correlated with perimenopausal depression, and additional menopausal symptoms such as decreased libido, vaginal dryness, sleep disturbance, and subjective cognitive concerns can also negatively impact mood.

It has been reported that up to 85% of women experience a premenstrual syndrome (PMS) as defined by at least one emotional symptom, such as anxiety or irritability, and one physical symptom, such as abdominal bloating or headache. Premenstrual dysphoric disorder (PMDD) can be conceptualized as a more pervasive premenstrual mood disturbance, the severity of which results in significant distress or interference with social or vocational activities, or with relationships. The prevalence of PMDD is estimated at around 5% in North American and European populations. The symptoms are present in the majority of menstrual cycles in the week before the onset of menses and subside in the week post menses. These symptoms include affective lability, irritability, depressed mood, hopelessness, and anxiety, as well as changes in appetite, sleep, and concentration.

Bipolar Disorder and Mania

The characteristic feature of bipolar disorders is varying degrees and lengths of mood fluctuation, lasting persistently for at least several days, alternating between depression and mania or hypomania. A manic episode is characterized by persistently elevated, expansive, or irritable mood along with increased activity or energy concurrent with a significant change in behavior represented by several symptoms, including grandiosity, decreased need for sleep, logorrhea, racing thoughts/flight of ideas, distractibility, increase in goal-directed activity or psychomotor agitation, and engagement in high-risk activities such as buying sprees or sexual indiscretions [4]. Hypomania involves the same symptoms but to a lesser degree of severity or level of impairment [4].

Bipolar symptoms have been estimated to be present in about 15% of people with epilepsy, and about half of these had a formal diagnosis of bipolar disorder, whereas bipolar spectrum illness (including bipolar 1 or 2 disorder, or cyclothymia) is seen in only 2–5% of the general population [13]. Some have estimated that bipolar disorder is more than 20 times more likely in people with epilepsy than in the general population [14], but in population-based studies using measures such as insurance claims, it is uncertain how many have true bipolar disorder versus a cluster of symptoms with phenotypic overlap with interictal, ictal, and peri-ictal mood and behavior disturbance phenomena. One study found that female sex was a protective factor for bipolar symptoms among people with epilepsy, although this finding has not been confirmed in other studies [15].

Temporal and frontal seizure foci can cause "secondary" hypomania or mania. The limbic system is important in the regulation of mood, and this secondary mood disorder may not be a comorbidity so much as a psychiatric and behavioral expression of the underlying illness. Rates of bipolar disorder diagnoses are as high as 10% among those with temporal lobe epilepsy (TLE) [13]. In preictal states, irritability, aggression, depression, dysphoria, and emotional lability often occur. Ictally, patients can display or experience inappropriate laughter, anxiety, confusion, aggression, dysphoria, paranoia, hallucinations, delusions, and grandiosity. Postictally, even more fulsome clusters of hypomanic, manic, and psychotic symptoms can be seen above and beyond the more usual postictal symptoms of isolated confusion, agitation, or aggression. The definitive treatment of these types of "secondary" phenomena is of course to treat the underlying seizures.

The period following epilepsy surgery, particularly after temporal lobectomy, has also been noted to be a higher-risk interval for the development of mania. Manic episodes in this period typically follow a transient course with episodes occurring within the first few weeks after surgery, resolving within days to weeks, especially with treatment using antimanic agents, and not progressing to a relapsing and remitting course of manic and depressive states as in bipolar disorder.

Interictal dysphoric disorder is a controversial concept but stemmed from experts noting an atypical profile in a number of people with epilepsy with chronic depression, with symptoms of fluctuating dysthymia, irritability, alternation with occasional euphoric periods, fear, anxiety, anergia, pain, and insomnia. There has been no agreement on whether this forms a distinctive neuropsychiatric diagnostic entity in people with epilepsy.

Anxiety

The term "anxiety" is often used colloquially in broad terms to define any sort of psychological distress; however, anxiety disorders can be more specifically conceptualized as a heightened fear response, in cognitive, physical, and behavioral spheres, out of keeping with real threat and presenting in a way that causes significant distress or impairment in life. Generalized anxiety disorder (GAD), for example, includes excessive and difficult-to-control worry and physical symptoms such as restlessness, muscle tension, and sleep disturbance.

It is estimated that 20% of people with epilepsy suffer from an anxiety disorder [16], and anxiety disorders in the general population are about twice as likely to affect women, with the pregnancy and postpartum periods incurring even higher risk. Similar to depression, modulation of the HPA axis, GABAergic, and serotonergic transmission by the impacts of estradiol, progesterone, and allopregnanolone play a role in the propensity of women toward anxiety and fluctuations in this propensity across reproductive life stages [17]. For example, premenstrual worsening can occur in panic disorder, obsessive compulsive disorder, and GAD.

The rates of anxiety appear to be equally elevated in focal and generalized epilepsy, although some early studies showed specifically elevated rates in focal epilepsy, TLE, and even specifically in left TLE. As with other neuropsychiatric syndromes in people with epilepsy, it is important to consider preictal, ictal, and postictal anxiety, especially in seizures with limbic onset that can induce anxiety, agoraphobia, panic, compulsions, and other dysphoric symptoms. It is important to note that these symptoms can last up to 24 hours after seizure offset.

As with other neuropsychiatric syndromes, there has been study of common neural substrates that may make patients more prone to both anxiety and epilepsy. More clinically useful to consider in terms of etiology, however, is the impact of seizure control, ASMs (described later in the chapter), and the psychological impact of epilepsy. This psychological impact is related not only to coping with a chronic neurological condition, but particularly one that produces unexpected and unpredictable attacks, which of itself can precipitate and perpetuate anxiety. For example, a patient diagnosed with epilepsy may become prone to anxiety with a newfound perception that their own body is unpredictable and so may develop illness anxiety or somatic symptoms. Another example would be that if a person with epilepsy experienced a seizure while alone shopping, they might begin to avoid being without friends or family, especially in crowded places, further reinforcing their anxiety in such situations.

Psychosis

Psychosis is characterized by delusions, hallucinations, and grossly disorganized behavior or thought form, and in people with epilepsy, it may be due to a primary psychotic disorder such as schizophrenia, or more directly caused by epilepsy such as in ictal or postictal psychosis. All forms of psychosis considered, there is an estimated prevalence of about 5%, with eightfold higher odds of psychosis in people with epilepsy compared to those without epilepsy [18].

In evaluating people with epilepsy suffering from psychosis, it is important to consider disorders that may produce both seizures and psychosis: neurodegenerative dementia syndromes, alcohol or drug intoxication and withdrawal, thiamine or B12 deficiency, systemic illness such as infection or metabolic derangement, and infectious or autoimmune encephalitides. However, these represent the minority of people with epilepsy with psychosis and diagnostic workup should not delay appropriate treatment.

Preictal and ictal psychotic symptoms can include visual, olfactory, or gustatory hallucinations, as well as depersonalization, derealization, or a feeling of presence (a vivid sensation that somebody is nearby). These are generally very short-lived, typically lasting on the order of minutes, and are generally not associated with gross thought form or behavioral disorganization.

Postictal psychosis accounts for up to 25% of psychosis in people with epilepsy. The classical description is that of psychosis onset after a lucid interval of a few days following a cluster of seizures, more common in those with complex partial seizures with secondary generalization. The duration of symptoms is typically several days up to 2 weeks and they include visual and auditory hallucinations, and delusions (often religious). When an affective component is present, especially with grandiose delusions, a postictal mania should be suspected.

Interictal psychosis classically has an onset 10 to 15 years after the onset of epilepsy and is associated with delusions and visual or auditory hallucinations. In general, interictal psychosis may be differentiated from schizophrenia by a later age of onset, absence of the typical schizophrenic prodrome, absence of negative symptoms, and less frequent command auditory hallucinations. Schizophrenia typically has onset in early adulthood (early 20s), progressive negative symptoms including blunted affect, avolition, and social withdrawal, and frequently includes command auditory hallucinations. The terms "interictal psychosis" and "schizophrenia-like psychosis" are sometimes used interchangeably in the literature, given that if epilepsy were not present, then many patients with interictal psychosis would indeed meet the categorical DSM-V diagnostic criteria for schizophrenia. It is unclear, however, what proportion of these truly have a shared pathophysiological etiology with what would be considered a "primary" psychotic disorder such as schizophrenia. The pathophysiological and genetic underpinnings of psychotic disorders as a whole are multifactorial and still poorly understood. Nonetheless, there appears to be a bidirectional relationship between schizophrenia and epilepsy, with the chance of developing epilepsy after schizophrenia diagnosis 5 times higher and the chance of developing schizophrenia after epilepsy diagnosis 6.5 times higher [19].

The concept of forced normalization or alternative psychosis describes, opposite to the epilepsy-associated psychosis, an inverse correlation between seizure control and development of psychosis. The classic description has been of a patient with chronic epilepsy achieving seizure freedom and thereafter developing a paranoid psychosis that persists until adjustment of ASMs allows recurrence of seizures. While this pattern can be seen, it is rare and has not been consistently elucidated in observational studies, and it has been argued that it may represent adverse psychiatric symptoms of ASMs rather than being a distinct entity. The mechanism is also unknown, but a limbic kindling effect has been posited.

Postpartum psychosis occurs in about 1 in 1,000 childbirths and occurs on average about 2 weeks following birth but can begin within days or up to 8 weeks following. It is extremely important to identify postpartum psychosis and to refer urgently to a psychiatrist for management given the significant risks posed to both the mother and the newborn. The course of postpartum psychosis typically begins with the mother experiencing insomnia, restlessness, and emotional lability, followed by confusion, suspiciousness, delusions about herself or her baby, and auditory hallucinations. Both infanticidal and suicidal thoughts as well as command auditory hallucinations are common, highlighting the need for urgent care and observation. Of note, these women often have a personal or family history of mood disorders such as depression or bipolar disorder and are at risk of developing these conditions if they experience postpartum psychosis.

Neurocognitive and Behavioral Problems

Comorbid neurodevelopmental disorders as well as other subtle cognitive impairments are often seen in people with epilepsy. Subtle impairments can occur in memory, executive function, attention, and processing speed, even before treatment with ASMs. The prevalence of these impairments is quite high, about 50%, but is under-recognized by patients, with only about half that number subjectively endorsing cognitive issues. It may be that a significant proportion of these patients do not have impairments severe enough to cause functional difficulties [20]. In focal epilepsies, location of the seizure focus can predict cognitive deficits to some extent. For example, verbal memory deficits commonly occur in mesial temporal epilepsies. However, broader deficits are also seen in localized epilepsies, likely due to network dysfunction. There is limited evidence of sex differences in the neurocognitive impact of focal epilepsies; for example, in early-onset TLE, women show greater functional plasticity for verbal memory compared to men [21].

Attention deficit hyperactivity disorder (ADHD) is a very common comorbidity and there is again some evidence of possible common etiology, with children with ADHD 2.7 times more likely to subsequently develop epilepsy [22] and a high degree of hereditary influence with 40% of the overlap between patients with ADHD and epilepsy accounted for by genetic correlation [23]. Inattention is a common consequence of having frequent seizures and being on ASMs, but ADHD often precedes or is present at the time of epilepsy onset. There has traditionally been some concern about the treatment of ADHD in people with epilepsy with psychostimulants; however, large studies have not shown an increase in seizures and there is even evidence toward a reduced rate of seizures [24]. In adults, women are about 40% less likely to be diagnosed with ADHD than men and there are important gender differences in terms of its clinical presentation and its psychiatric comorbidities. In girls and women, ADHD is more likely to present with inattention alone, while men are more likely to present with hyperactivity and impulsivity. Women are more likely to present with comorbid "internalizing" disorders such as depression, anxiety, somatization, and bulimia nervosa, whereas in men, there is a predilection toward "externalizing" disorders such as substance use, antisocial personality, or conduct disorder. This difference and the bias toward presentations with less "acting out" to be diagnosed may lead to misdiagnosis and underdiagnosis in women and may account for some of the gender difference in prevalence [25]. In women with epilepsy, ADHD should be treated using the regular treatment guidelines, which generally recommend treatment with long-acting psychostimulants as first-line agents.

Autism spectrum disorder (ASD) is characterized by impairments in social communication or interaction and restricted or repetitive patterns of behaviors, interests, or activities [4]. It is disproportionately common in people with epilepsy especially in children, but also occurs in 8% of adults with epilepsy. Autism spectrum disorder is less prevalent in women versus men in a 1:3 ratio. A number of biological and genetic theories have been put forward to explain this difference. Genetic observations, for example, have shown a higher rate of ASD in the offspring of autistic females compared to males, and girls with ASD have a higher rate of genetic mutations. It has therefore been posited that there is a higher biological threshold for phenotypic females to present with ASD and as such that female sex is protective. However, there is also suggestion of a "camouflaging" effect wherein girls with ASD display higher intellectual and adaptive functioning, and so are missed on typical diagnostic tools or have delayed diagnosis [26]. Intellectual disability is also common in childhood-onset epilepsy, and less so in cases with adult-onset epilepsy. The prevalence of intellectual disability is 25% in children with epilepsy [27]. Intellectual disability frequently coexists with ASD, and in ASD, having intellectual disability is the major risk factor for epilepsy [28]. Specific epilepsy syndromes like West syndrome and Lennox–Gastaut syndrome raise the risk of ASD, and risk also increases with epilepsy severity, earlier age of onset, and drug resistance. Of note, epileptiform discharges seen in ASD are of unclear significance, but do not require antiepileptic treatment unless associated with clinical seizures [29]. The treatment of ASD is highly complex and requires intensive multidisciplinary care, which is beyond the scope of this chapter.

Suicidality

As may be expected with the high psychiatric comorbidity in people with epilepsy, suicidality (suicidal ideation or behavior) is more than three times higher in people with epilepsy, and more than six times higher in people with TLE, compared with control subjects [30]. Women are known to be 1.5 times more likely to attempt suicide, while men are twice as likely to die from completed suicide. Some data point toward a difference in suicidal intent while other evidence suggests that these differences may result from greater aversion and less access to high lethality means such as guns in the North American context [31]. For example, in China, where a common high-lethality suicide method is agricultural or other poisons, there is far less of a gender difference in suicide completion. Importantly, no such gender difference in completed suicide has been found in relevant studies in people with epilepsy.

Of note, the US FDA has issued an alert regarding an increased risk of suicidal ideation and behavior in people treated with ASMs. A number of observational studies have been completed since this alert was issued in 2008, with mixed results but large cohort studies showing no significant association [32]. Expert consensus in this regard, including from the International League Against Epilepsy (ILAE), has been to treat epilepsy regardless because the harms and risks associated with untreated epilepsy greatly outweigh a potential small risk of suicidality directly associated with ASM treatment.

Suicide risk should be screened for regularly. The NDDI-E item 4 "I'd be better off dead" (see Table 2.1), although not specifically asking about suicidality but rather about passive death wishes, has been validated, with a score of 3 or 4 on that question having high sensitivity and specificity for suicidal risk [33]. The Patient Health Questionnaire-9 (PHQ-9), which assesses depression, is also validated in people with epilepsy and can help predict suicide given that depression has been the factor most consistently found to predict suicidality risk in people with epilepsy.

Psychogenic Non-epileptic Seizures

Psychogenic non-epileptic seizures, also known as functional or dissociative seizures, are characterized by episodes resembling epileptic seizures with involuntary movements or sensory symptoms with or without altered consciousness, but that – unlike epileptic seizures – are not caused by epileptiform cortical electrical activity. In terms of semiology, PNES can have a wide variety of presentations. For example, it can appear as hyperkinetic movements resembling generalized tonic clonic or frontal lobe seizures, as focal movements or automatisms, as alterations in consciousness including lack of responsiveness, behavioral arrest, immobility, or with somatic sensations or perceptual disturbances resembling complex partial epileptic seizures. The gold standard for PNES diagnosis is video electroencephalogram (EEG) and requires capturing all typical episodes without epileptiform activity and an experienced clinician discerning semiology consistent with PNES. Some clinical features helpful in differentiating PNES from epilepsy are described in Table 2.2.

By DSM-V classification, PNES is considered a functional neurologic disorder (FND) or conversion disorder with seizures [4]. The term "pseudoseizure" was commonly used in the past but has fallen out of favor because the term "pseudo" can imply the patient's symptoms are not genuine, which can be experienced as pejorative or invalidating. Unlike in factitious disorders or malingering, the signs and symptoms of PNES are not consciously produced.

One in four patients being evaluated for seizures in epilepsy-monitoring units are ultimately found to have PNES [35] and a large majority of PNES patients, about 75%, are women [36]. These patients have a high rate of having had psychologically traumatic experiences [37] and a large preponderance of PNES patients have at least one psychiatric comorbidity such as depression or anxiety [38]. There is also a close association with other functional and somatic symptom disorders, or medically unexplained symptoms [36]. The rates of all these associated factors are higher in women, including, for example, that in Canada, women are five times as likely as men to have experienced sexual assault, a trend that is similar across various sociocultural contexts. A prevailing observation in gender differences in stress response following traumatic experiences or other more minor stressors, which may apply to the development of PNES, is that women have a greater propensity to internalize emotions resulting in depression, anxiety, and somatization, whereas men

Table 2.2 Clinical features differentiating PNES from epilepsy [34]

Favoring PNES	Favoring ES
Long duration	Occurring from sleep
Fluctuating course	Postictal confusion
Asynchronous movements	Stertorous breathing
Pelvic thrusting	
Side to side head or body movements	
Closed eyes	
Ictal crying	
Memory recall	

Table 2.3 Antiseizure medications categorized by psychiatric effects [41, 42]

ASMs with positive psychiatric effect	Mixed, minimal, or no psychiatric adverse effects	ASMS with common psychiatric adverse effects
Lamotrigine, Valproic acid, Carbamazepine, Oxcarbazepine, Eslicarbazepine	Clobazam, Rufinamide, Lacosamide, Gabapentin, Pregabalin, Topiramate	Perampanel, Levetiracetam, Zonisamide, Vigabatrin, Tiagabine, Phenobarbital

tend toward externalizing their emotions via behavioral impulsivity, including substance use and aggression. Psychogenic non-epileptic seizures are associated with significant impacts on healthcare costs and quality of life, and quite strikingly, there is recent evidence indicating a mortality rate in PNES like that of drug-resistant epilepsy at 2.5 times the general population [39].

A significant comorbidity exists between epilepsy and PNES, with pooled estimates in studies from the 1990s onward indicating the frequency of epilepsy in PNES at 22% and PNES in epilepsy at 12% [40]. However, in more recent studies utilizing the more accurate method of video EEG rather than clinical diagnosis, these numbers appear closer to 10% and 5%, respectively.

Neuropsychiatric Effects of Antiseizure Medications

Some ASMs have positive psychiatric effects and indeed some are used for psychiatric indications alone, including lamotrigine and valproate for bipolar disorders. Notably, gabapentin and pregabalin, which have indications for treatment in anxiety disorders, have been found to have mild or mixed adverse psychological or behavioral effects at the higher doses used to treat epilepsy. A number of ASMs are indeed known to produce adverse psychiatric effects, and this is summarized in Tables 2.3 and 2.4.

A few ASMs are also associated with cognitive side effects, summarized in Table 2.5. Of these, topiramate is by far the agent with the greatest negative impact on cognition, with as high as 18.5% of people with epilepsy treated with topiramate monotherapy finding it intolerable and the vast majority of these choosing to discontinue it rather than adjust the dose [43]. The most common cognitive adverse side effect seen with ASMs is cognitive slowing, but decreased concentration and memory, disorientation, and word-finding difficulties are also seen at significant rates.

Treatment of Psychiatric Conditions in People with Epilepsy and Special Considerations for Women

Psychotropic Medications and Risk of Seizures

A risk of seizures has been reported with several psychotropic medications, and these have been studied to various degrees. Table 2.6 shows the risk stratification of psychotropics based on the available data. Those classified as low and intermediate risk are considered safe to use, especially with concomitant ASM treatment, whereas high-risk psychotropics should

Table 2.4 Antiseizure medications commonly producing psychiatric and behavioral adverse effects [41, 42]

ASM	Psychiatric and behavioral adverse effects (rates where available)	
Perampanel	Irritability Depressed mood Anxiety	
Levetiracetam	Irritability (12.5%) Aggression (1.4%) Depressed mood (7.3%) Anxiety (2.5%) Psychosis (0.6%)	**Overall 22.1%**
Zonisamide	Depressed mood (4.3%) Mania (0.8%)	**Overall 9.7%**
Vigabatrin	Psychosis (2.7%)	
Tiagabine	Irritability (10.9%) Psychosis (2.2%) Anxiety (4.4%)	**Overall 15.2%**
Phenobarbital	Depression	
Topiramate	Depression Mania Psychosis	

Table 2.5 Antiseizure medications and impact on cognition [43]

ASMs with minimal or mixed effects on cognition	ASMs with greatest negative effect on cognition
Gabapentin, Pregabalin, Lamotrigine, Levetiracetam, Brivaracetam, Carbamazepine, Oxcarbazepine, Eslicarbazepine, Perampanel, Rufinamide, Lacosamide, Valproic acid, Tiagabine	Topiramate, Zonisamide, Phenobarbital

be avoided or used cautiously when other treatment options are untenable, along with careful monitoring and with consideration for slow dose titrations given their dose-dependent risk of producing seizures.

Psychotropic Medications in Pregnancy and Breastfeeding

Clinicians should always use the currently available data, including through the FDA pregnancy and lactation labeling in collaboration with patients and their families when coming to treatment decisions in the perinatal period [47]. Considerations for psychotropic medications that are also used as ASMs, including agents such as valproate or carbamazepine, are discussed in Chapter 18 and so will not be discussed here.

Both pregnancy and postpartum are a high-risk phase for several mental health disorders and involving a psychiatrist, especially one with expertise in perinatal disease, is

Table 2.6 Psychotropic medications and impact on seizure threshold [44, 45, 46]

	High risk (all dose-dependent increase)	Intermediate risk	Low risk
Antipsychotics	Clozapine Chlorpromazine	Haloperidol	Fluphenazine Trifluoperazine Risperidone Paliperidone Iloperidone Quetiapine Olanzapine Aripiprazole Ziprasidone Asenapine
Antidepressants	Bupropion Clomipramine Maprotiline	Venlafaxine	Paroxetine Sertraline Fluoxetine Fluvoxamine Citalopram Escitalopram Amitriptyline Trazodone Monoamine oxidase inhibitors
Others	Lithium		Methylphenidate

recommended. The rate of relapse in depression, for example, is up to 70% in women discontinuing antidepressants in pregnancy. There are major negative consequences of untreated mental illness for the mother, her family, and the fetus or newborn. For example, in maternal depression, amotivation can lead to low self-care and poor diet, risk of receiving inadequate perinatal care, as well as being a risk for paternal depression. For the newborn, it results in lower birth weight, prematurity, and lasting increased risk in childhood of several affective and behavioral disorders, including ADHD. These risks must of course be weighed against the risk to the fetus of adverse effects related to psychotropic medications, including birth defects. An overarching consideration is that there is a shift in the risk–benefit ratio for treating mental health disorders with psychotropics in pregnancy and breastfeeding. In many cases, there can be a greater priority for consideration of psychotherapies over psychotropic medications, but psychotropics continue to have an important role in more severe or impairing illness.

Research on the use of psychotropics in pregnancy has been fraught with limitations in elucidating the impact of these medications independent of the psychiatric conditions they are used to treat. In fact, a number of initially described adverse effects have since been found to be either of much smaller magnitude or indeed nonexistent after controlling for psychiatric disorder–related confounders such as disease severity, comorbidities such as substance use, or medical comorbidities such as metabolic syndrome. A few early studies on the safety of antipsychotic medications in pregnancy raised concerns for an increased risk of cardiac malformations, for example, but these failed to control for factors such as women treated with antipsychotics being more likely at baseline to be obese, have diabetes and hypertension, smoke, drink alcohol, and use illicit substances compared with the general population. A more recent large-cohort study controlling for a number of important confounders found no meaningfully increased risk of congenital malformations in newborns exposed to antipsychotics in gestation [48]. A summary of considerations for psychotropics in pregnancy and breastfeeding can be found in Table 2.7.

Treatment of Major Depressive Disorders

Psychotherapy

Offering evidence-supported psychotherapeutic interventions, where available, is strongly encouraged and can also be combined with pharmacotherapy. Psychotherapy in combination with antidepressant medication is more effective than psychotherapy alone, but with small-to-moderate effect size, this approach is best reserved for patients with moderate-to-severe depression considering the possible benefit versus burden of treatment. Psychotherapy can be used at any degree of depression severity, but since the time course of improvement is generally faster with pharmacological or neurostimulation modalities, these are preferred over psychotherapy in severe and high-risk cases where there is a greater degree of urgency. Cognitive behavior therapy (CBT), interpersonal therapy (IPT), and behavioral activation are all considered first-line treatments for acute depression, and CBT and mindfulness-based cognitive behavior therapy (MBCT) are considered the first line in maintenance. Cognitive behavior therapy has been well studied for depression in people with epilepsy [49] and found to be effective, and it has similar effectiveness in terms of rates of and time to remission compared with an antidepressant such as sertraline [50].

Psychotropic Medications

First-line antidepressant medications can be effectively initiated and titrated, and the patient's mood can be monitored by their neurologist. In this regard, depression does not always necessitate referral to a psychiatrist. However, it is of paramount importance when initiating antidepressants to rule out the possibility of a bipolar illness for risk of precipitating a hypomanic or manic episode. Apart from current or past symptoms of hypomania or mania (discussed in the bipolar section of this chapter), features of the patient's history may suggest bipolarity, including hypersomnia, hyperphagia, psychomotor retardation or agitation, leaden paralysis, psychotic features, pathological guilt, mood lability, irritability, racing thoughts, early onset of first depression (<25 years old), multiple previous episodes (>4), or a positive family history of bipolar disorder in first-degree blood relatives. If there is significant concern of bipolarity on history, then the patient's depression is best treated by a psychiatrist and a referral should be made. Similarly, depression refractory to first- and second-line treatments, depression complicated by psychosis, and patients considered to be at risk for suicide should be referred for expert psychiatric treatment.

Selective serotonin reuptake inhibitors (SSRIs), serotonin-norepinephrine reuptake inhibitors (SNRIs), and medications from other antidepressant classes, including agomelatine, mirtazapine, and vortioxetine, are considered first line. Both patient and medication factors should be considered. Of these, escitalopram, mirtazapine, sertraline, and

Table 2.7 Psychotropics and considerations in pregnancy and breastfeeding [47]

Drug/Drug class	Pregnancy	Breastfeeding
SSRI/SNRI (no major difference between the two classes)	• Paroxetine: risk of cardiac malformations reported, so avoid in pregnancy. • Others SSRIs: no major risk of teratogenicity. • Transient neonatal adaptation syndrome may present. • PPHN absolute risk increases by 0.1%.	• Considered safe. • Sertraline has the lowest known transfer to infant.
Bupropion and mirtazapine	• No known teratogenic risks. Limited data available.	• No known adverse effects. Limited data available.
TCAs	• No major risk of teratogenicity. • Transient neonatal adaptation syndrome may present.	• Considered safe.
Antipsychotics (no major difference between FGA and SGA)	• No major risk of teratogenicity. Absolute risk increase of up to 1.3% for cardiac malformations, but mixed results and major limitations in data. • Late pregnancy exposure: neonatal signs including tremor, sedation, agitation, and feeding and breathing difficulties.	• Clozapine contraindicated due to risk of infant agranulocytosis and seizures. • Up to 10% RID. Can cause drowsiness, poor feeding, irritability. Close monitoring of infant especially if premature or low birth weight.
Lithium	• Mixed data regarding risk of Ebstein's anomaly (cardiac). Estimated absolute risk increase of approximately 0.05%. • "Floppy baby" syndrome may present: hypotonicity, cyanosis.	• Infant serum levels up to 50% of the mother's can cause hypotonicity, cyanosis, and thyroid dysfunction. Avoid in breastfeeding.

FGA: First-generation antipsychotics. PPHN: Persistent pulmonary hypertension of newborn. RID: Relative infant dose. SGA: Second-generation antipsychotics. SNRI: Serotonin-norepinephrine reuptake inhibitor. SSRI: Selective serotonin reuptake inhibitor. TCA: Tricyclic antidepressants venlafaxine have evidence of superior efficacy. A first-line SSRI should be trialed at effective doses for 4–6 weeks prior to considering a switch to another one of the first-line options, or if there is some response, then augmenting with antipsychotics that are considered first line: aripiprazole, quetiapine, or risperidone. In epilepsy, however, careful consideration should be given to augmentation strategies due to the lowering of seizure threshold with antipsychotic agents and so switching to another antidepressant may be preferable to augmentation in this population.

Neurostimulation

Repetitive transcranial magnetic stimulation (rTMS) is generally considered a useful treatment for patients without epilepsy who have failed one adequate antidepressant trial. However, in people with epilepsy, other strategies should be considered preferentially due to considerations of safety given potential seizure induction. Electroconvulsive therapy (ECT) is considered for treatment of refractory depression but is first line for certain indications, including acute suicidality, psychotic features, catatonic features, repeated medication intolerance, and rapidly deteriorating physical status.

There have been concerns among clinicians regarding neurostimulation as psychiatric treatment in people with epilepsy given the intuitive notion that either producing therapeutic seizures, as in ECT, or localized cortical electrical stimulation, as in rTMS, may exacerbate epilepsy. Studies, however, have found both to be relatively safe [51].

Electroconvulsive therapy involves eliciting a therapeutic seizure under general anesthetic by scalp electrical stimulation, most commonly in the right temporal region. The original theoretical underpinnings when ECT was introduced in the 1930s were of "biological antagonism" between neurological and psychiatric disorders, as is the case with the concept of forced normalization discussed previously. The indications for the use of ECT include for severe or refractory depression, for psychosis, and for catatonia, and the current evidence indicates that people with epilepsy can safely receive and should be offered ECT. When a patient is undergoing ECT, ASMs are typically held the night prior to the scheduled treatment in order to achieve a therapeutic seizure without stimulating at unnecessarily suprathreshold levels, which would increase the risk of adverse cognitive effects such as amnesia and delirium. Interestingly, there is evidence that ECT increases seizure threshold for epileptic seizures during the treatment course, and there is also some evidence that ECT can be used in refractory status epilepticus, but the mechanism for this is unclear.

Repetitive transcranial magnetic stimulation is indicated in depression after at least one medication trial, whereas ECT is used in more severe or refractory cases. There are various treatment protocols in terms of anatomical area of stimulation and pulse frequency, but the dorsolateral prefrontal cortex is a common target. The risk of seizure induction in a non-epilepsy population is approximately 1 in 30,000 treatment sessions or fewer than 1 in 1,000 patients in high-pulse frequency protocols of 10 Hz. In a systematic review of people with epilepsy receiving rTMS under various protocols and for various indications, the risk of seizure was estimated at 2.9% per patient, much higher than in the non-epilepsy population [52]. However, importantly, no seizures were noted as adverse events in low-frequency < 1 Hz stimulation. It is unclear, however, whether rTMS even confers any additional risk of seizure above the baseline risk in those epilepsy patients and has not yet been studied. Overall, there appears to be a reasonable safety profile to justify treating depression in epilepsy with rTMS.

Complementary and Alternative Medicine

Exercise monotherapy is a first-line option for mild-to-moderate depression, and useful as an adjunct in more severe depression. Light therapy is first line in seasonal winter depression and for mild-to-moderate nonseasonal MDD. Bright-light therapy is tested and effective for anxiety and depression in epilepsy [53]. The best natural health product evidence is for St. John's wort in mild-to-moderate depression as monotherapy, and it can be used as an adjunct in moderate-to-severe depression. Of note, St. John's wort is a moderate inducer of cytochrome P450 enzymes 1A2, 2C19, 2C9, and 3A4, as well as intestinal P-glycoprotein/multidrug efflux pump (MDR)-1 drug transporters. As such, coadministration of St. John's wort with carbamazepine requires monitoring [54]. Omega-3 fatty acids and S-adenosylmethionine (SAM-e) have also shown some degree of benefit.

Treatment of Perinatal Depression

If available in your practice setting, it is beneficial to seek the assistance of a psychiatrist with expertise in the perinatal period, but this should not act as a barrier to initiating treatment. When choosing a course of therapy, consideration should be given to known risks of infant exposure to pharmacological treatments during pregnancy and breastfeeding (discussed later in this chapter) weighed against the risk posed by untreated depression in both the mother and fetus or newborn. Risks of untreated depression include a negative impact on childhood development, and future risk of depression and poor family and vocational functioning for the mother [47].

First-line treatment for mild-to-moderate depression both in pregnancy and postpartum is psychotherapy with CBT or IPT, either individually or in groups, whereas pharmacotherapy is second line, followed by structured exercise, acupuncture, and bright-light therapy [14]. The preferred pharmacotherapies are citalopram, escitalopram, and sertraline and are to be used as first-line agents in severe cases of depression [11].

Treatment of Perimenopausal Depression

Given an overall paucity of evidence, the expert consensus is to follow the same approach as in general adult MDD [11]. Pharmacotherapy with desvenlafaxine has been the best studied in this population and has been shown to also have benefit in treating hot flashes, and for this reason it is a good treatment option, although it is not necessarily to be chosen preferentially compared to other antidepressants that have a greater evidence base in the adult MDD population as a whole. Cognitive behavior therapy has specific evidence in the perimenopausal period and, as in all adults, should be offered. Transdermal estradiol is considered second line, but it should be noted that women with an intact uterus should be prescribed concomitant progesterone to reduce risk of endometrial cancer.

Treatment of Premenstrual Dysphoric Disorder

A stepwise approach to treatment includes beginning with psychoeducation, namely that this is a hormonal phenomenon due to the menstrual cycle that some women are prone to, and that lifestyle modification can be helpful, including healthy eating, regular exercise, good sleep hygiene, limit-setting and stress management, and reducing alcohol intake if present [12]. Psychoeducation can also include a focus on positive reframing of perceptions of the menstrual cycle. Dietary supplementation with 1,200 mg of calcium daily reduces symptoms of PMS, including depression, and takes two or three menstrual cycles to take effect. Evidence also supports vitamin B6 supplementation at 80 mg daily. Cognitive behavior therapy is effective, but the effect size appears to be lower than that of pharmacotherapy, so it should be considered in women who have a preference against pharmacotherapy or in combination for women amenable to pharmacotherapy. Unlike in MDD, both SSRI and SNRI antidepressants can work quickly and have efficacy not only when dosed continuously but also when dosed only in the luteal (premenstrual) phase of each cycle. Of note, SSRI discontinuation symptoms are rarely seen in luteal phase dosing. Hormonal treatments have been studied but few ovulation suppressants have been found to be effective and carry with them risks of venous thromboembolism with oral contraceptive pills (OCPs), and osteoporosis and androgenization with gonadotropin-releasing hormone (GnRH) agonists. Of those studies, OCPs, particularly combined ethinyl estradiol and drospirenone, have a reasonable safety profile and can be used effectively, especially in women who wish to use these as a means of contraception.

Treatment of Bipolar Disorder

Bipolar disorder, even in those without epilepsy, is a complex condition given its multiphasic nature, and it requires specialized psychiatric care preferably within a multidisciplinary team. A referral to psychiatry is certainly recommended and management of bipolar disorder is outside the scope of practice for most neurologists.

The mainstay of treatment are mood stabilizers, several of which are antiepileptics, in addition to antipsychotic medications, and in some cases antidepressants. The treatment of bipolar is too nuanced to be discussed in detail here, but one may wish to refer to relevant consensus guidelines such as CANMAT/ISBD [55].

Treatment of Anxiety

In terms of treatment, studies in specific anxiety disorders in epilepsy are absent. The mainstay of treatment for anxiety disorders is CBT or antidepressant medications, or a combination of both [56]. The focus of CBT is often around graded exposure to feared situations, such as the avoidance of being alone as described in the example just provided. Specific pharmacological considerations in epilepsy may be to preferentially use anticonvulsants and benzodiazepines among first- and second-line evidence-based options. Pregabalin is a good choice in this regard for social anxiety disorder (SAD) and GAD, and clonazepam is a good option in panic disorder.

Treatment of Psychosis

Since peri-ictal and ictal psychoses are most often self-limiting, they can frequently be managed conservatively with close clinical observation, reassurance, and general supportive care. Benzodiazepines can be helpful to reduce overall distress. For more persistent or worsening cases, or where there are severe and distressing symptoms or acute safety concerns, treatment with antipsychotics can be used. In interictal psychosis, antipsychotics are the mainstay of treatment. In more severe cases or where psychosis lasts for more than several days, referral to a psychiatrist is recommended.

Treatment of Psychogenic Non-epileptic Seizures

Following the diagnosis of PNES, psychotherapy is the treatment of choice and ASMs do not provide benefit. Of the psychotherapies, CBT has been the best studied, including in large, randomized, controlled trials, and has been shown to have significant benefit, so should be offered to all PNES patients where available [57]. An early component of CBT is psychoeducation, including communicating to the patient a psychological explanatory model for their symptoms, which can and should be done even before referral to CBT by the diagnosing clinician. Psychoeducation alone often results in a significant symptomatic improvement and psychological relief in many patients. Emphasis must be placed on a multidisciplinary approach with close collaboration between neurologists, psychiatrists, and psychotherapists. Additional evidence-supported psychotherapies can also be considered, including mindfulness and brief psychodynamic therapy.

References

1. Lin JJ, Mula M, Hermann BP. Uncovering the neurobehavioural comorbidities of epilepsy over the lifespan. *Lancet.* 2012;**380**(9848):1180–92. http://dx.doi.org/10.1016/S0140-6736(12)61455-X
2. Hesdorffer DC, Ishihara L, Mynepalli L, Webb DJ, Weil J, Hauser WA. Epilepsy, suicidality, and psychiatric disorders: A bidirectional association. *Ann Neurol.* 2012;**72**(2):184–91.
3. Fazel S, Wolf A, Långström N, Newton CR, Lichtenstein P. Premature mortality in epilepsy and the role of psychiatric comorbidity: A total population study. *Lancet.* 2013;**382**(9905):1646–54.
4. American Psychiatric Association. *Diagnostic and statistical manual of mental disorders.* 5th edition. Arlington, VA: American Psychiatric Publishing; 2013.
5. Kim AM, Rossi KC, Jetté N, Yoo JY, Hung K, Dhamoon MS. Increased risk of hospital admission for mood disorders following admission for epilepsy. *Neurology.* 2018;**91**(9):e800–10.
6. Fiest KM, Dykeman J, Patten SB, Wiebe S, Kaplan GG, Maxwell CJ, et al. Depression in epilepsy: A systematic review and meta-analysis. *Neurology.* 2013;**80**(6):590–9.
7. Josephson CB, Lowerison M, Vallerand I, Sajobi TT, Patten S, Jette N, et al. Association of depression and treated depression with epilepsy and seizure outcomes: A multicohort analysis. *JAMA Neurol.* 2017;**74**(5):533–9.
8. Kanner AM. Depression and epilepsy: A bidirectional relation? *Epilepsia.* 2011;**52** (Suppl. 1):21–7.
9. Kuehner C. Why is depression more common among women than among men? *Lancet Psychiatry.* 2017;**4**(2):146–58. http://dx.doi.org/10.1016/S2215-0366(16)30263-2.
10. Friedman DE, Kung DH, Laowattana S, Kass JS, Hrachovy RA, Levin HS. Identifying depression in epilepsy in a busy clinical setting is enhanced with systematic screening. *Seizure.* 2009;**18**(6):429–33.
11. MacQueen GM, Frey BN, Ismail Z, Jaworska N, Steiner M, Lieshout RJV, et al. Canadian Network for Mood and Anxiety Treatments (CANMAT) 2016 clinical guidelines for the management of adults with major depressive disorder: Section 6. Special populations: Youth, women, and the elderly. *Can J Psychiatry.* 2016;**61**(9):588–603.
12. Vigod SN, Frey BN, Soares CN, Steiner M. Approach to premenstrual dysphoria for the mental health practitioner. *Psychiatr Clin North Am.* 2010;**33**(2):257–72.
13. Knott S, Forty L, Craddock N, Thomas RH. Epilepsy and bipolar disorder. *Epilepsy Behav.* 2015;**52**:267–74. http://dx.doi.org/10.1016/j.yebeh.2015.07.003

14. Chang HJ, Liao CC, Hu CJ, Shen WW, Chen TL. Psychiatric disorders after epilepsy diagnosis: A population-based retrospective cohort study. *PLoS One*. 2013;**8**(4):2–8.
15. Ettinger AB, Reed ML, Goldberg JF, Hirschfeld RM. Prevalence of bipolar symptoms in epilepsy vs. other chronic health disorders. *Neurology*. 2005 Aug 23;**65**(4):535–40. https://doi.org/10.1212/01.wnl.0000172917.70752.05. PMID: 16116112.
16. Scott AJ, Sharpe L, Hunt C, Gandy M. Anxiety and depressive disorders in people with epilepsy: A meta-analysis. *Epilepsia*. 2017;**58**(6):973–82.
17. Li SH, Graham BM. Why are women so vulnerable to anxiety, trauma-related and stress-related disorders? The potential role of sex hormones. *Lancet Psychiatry*. 2017;**4**(1):73–82. http://dx.doi.org/10.1016/S2215-0366(16)30358-3.
18. Clancy MJ, Clarke MC, Connor DJ, Cannon M, Cotter DR. The prevalence of psychosis in epilepsy: A systematic review and meta-analysis. *BMC Psychiatry*. 2014;**14**(1):75.
19. Chang YT, Chen PC, Tsai IJ, Sung FC, Chin ZN, Kuo HT, et al. Bidirectional relation between schizophrenia and epilepsy: A population-based retrospective cohort study. *Epilepsia*. 2011;**52**(11):2036–42.
20. Witt JA, Helmstaedter C. Should cognition be screened in new-onset epilepsies? A study in 247 untreated patients. *J Neurol*. 2012;**259**(8):1727–31.
21. Reddy DS. The neuroendocrine basis of sex differences in epilepsy. *Pharmacology Biochemistry and Behavior*. 2017;**152**:97–104.
22. Davis SM, Katusic SK, Barbaresi WJ, Killian J, Weaver AL, Ottman R, et al. Epilepsy in children with attention-deficit/hyperactivity disorder. *Pediatr Neurol*. 2010;**42**(5):325–30. http://dx.doi.org/10.1016/j.pediatrneurol.2010.01.005.
23. Brikell I, Ghirardi L, D'Onofrio BM, Dunn DW, Almqvist C, Dalsgaard S, et al. Familial liability to epilepsy and attention-deficit/hyperactivity disorder: A nationwide cohort study. *Biol Psychiatry*. 2018 Jan;**83**(2):173–80. https://linkinghub.elsevier.com/retrieve/pii/S0006322317318589.
24. Brikell I, Chen Q, Kuja-Halkola R, D'Onofrio BM, Wiggs KK, Lichtenstein P, et al. Medication treatment for attention-deficit/hyperactivity disorder and the risk of acute seizures in individuals with epilepsy. *Epilepsia*. 2019;**60**(2):284–93.
25. Nussbaum NL. ADHD and female specific concerns: A review of the literature and clinical implications. *J Atten Disord*. 2012;**16**(2):87–100.
26. Ratto AB, Kenworthy L, Yerys BE, Bascom J, Wieckowski AT, White SW, et al. What about the girls? Sex-based differences in autistic traits and adaptive skills. *J Autism Dev Disord*. 2018;**48**(5):1698–1711. http://dx.doi.org/10.1007/s10803-017-3413-9.
27. Berg AT, Langfitt JT, Testa FM, Levy SR, DiMario F, Westerveld M, et al. Global cognitive function in children with epilepsy: A community-based study. *Epilepsia*. 2008;**49**(4):608–14.
28. el-Achkar CM, Spence SJ. Clinical characteristics of children and young adults with co-occurring autism spectrum disorder and epilepsy. *Epilepsy Behav*. 2015;**47**:183–90. http://dx.doi.org/10.1016/j.yebeh.2014.12.022.
29. Ghacibeh GA, Fields C. Interictal epileptiform activity and autism. *Epilepsy Behav*. 2015;**47**:158–62. http://dx.doi.org/10.1016/j.yebeh.2015.02.025.
30. Bell GS, Gaitatzis A, Bell CL, Johnson AL, Sander JW. Suicide in people with epilepsy: How great is the risk? *Epilepsia*. 2009;**50**(8):1933–42.
31. Freeman A, Mergl R, Kohls E, Székely A, Gusmao R, Arensman E, et al. A cross-national study on gender differences in suicide intent. *BMC Psychiatry*. 2017;**17**(1):1–11.
32. Arana A, Arellano F, Suissa S. Suicide-related events in patients treated with antiepileptic drugs: Not an example of

time-window bias. *Epidemiology*. 2011;**22**(6):876–7.

33. Mula M, McGonigal A, Micoulaud-Franchi JA, May TW, Labudda K, Brandt C. Validation of rapid suicidality screening in epilepsy using the NDDIE. *Epilepsia*. 2016;**57**(6):949–55.

34. Avbersek A, Sisodiya S. Does the primary literature provide support for clinical signs used to distinguish psychogenic nonepileptic seizures from epileptic seizures? *J Neurol Neurosurg Psychiatry*. 2010;**81**(7):719–25.

35. Salinsky M, Spencer D, Boudreau E, Ferguson F. Psychogenic nonepileptic seizures in US veterans. *Neurology*. 2011 Sep 6;**77**(10):945–50. www.neurology.org/cgi/doi/10.1212/WNL.0b013e31822cfc46.

36. Dixit R, Popescu A, Bagić A, Ghearing G, Hendrickson R. Medical comorbidities in patients with psychogenic nonepileptic spells (PNES) referred for video-EEG monitoring. *Epilepsy Behav*. 2013;**28**(2):137–40.

37. Myers L, Perrine K, Lancman M, Fleming M, Lancman M. Psychological trauma in patients with psychogenic nonepileptic seizures: Trauma characteristics and those who develop PTSD. *Epilepsy Behav*. 2013;**28**(1):121–6. http://dx.doi.org/10.1016/j.yebeh.2013.03.033.

38. Tolchin B, Dworetzky BA, Martino S, Blumenfeld H, Hirsch LJ, Baslet G. Adherence with psychotherapy and treatment outcomes for psychogenic nonepileptic seizures. *Neurology*. 2019;**92**(7):E675–9.

39. Nightscales R, McCartney L, Auvrez C, Tao G, Barnard S, Malpas CB, et al. Mortality in patients with psychogenic nonepileptic seizures. *Neurology*. 2020;**95**(6):e643–52.

40. Kutlubaev MA, Xu Y, Hackett ML, Stone J. Dual diagnosis of epilepsy and psychogenic nonepileptic seizures: Systematic review and meta-analysis of frequency, correlates, and outcomes. *Epilepsy Behav*. 2018;**89**:70–8. https://doi.org/10.1016/j.yebeh.2018.10.010.

41. Chen B, Choi H, Hirsch LJ, Katz A, Legge A, Buchsbaum R, et al. Psychiatric and behavioral side effects of antiepileptic drugs in adults with epilepsy. *Epilepsy Behav*. 2017;**76**:24–31. http://dx.doi.org/10.1016/j.yebeh.2017.08.039.

42. Stephen LJ, Wishart A, Brodie MJ. Psychiatric side effects and antiepileptic drugs: Observations from prospective audits. *Epilepsy Behav*. 2017;**71**:73–8. http://dx.doi.org/10.1016/j.yebeh.2017.04.003

43. Javed A, Cohen B, Detyniecki K, Hirsch LJ, Legge A, Chen B, et al. Rates and predictors of patient-reported cognitive side effects of antiepileptic drugs: An extended follow-up. *Seizure*. 2015;**29**:34–40. http://dx.doi.org/10.1016/j.seizure.2015.03.013.

44. Alper K, Schwartz KA, Kolts RL, Khan A. Seizure incidence in psychopharmacological clinical trials: An analysis of Food and Drug Administration (FDA) Summary Basis of Approval Reports. *Biol Psychiatry*. 2007;**62**(4):345–54.

45. Kanner AM. Most antidepressant drugs are safe for patients with epilepsy at therapeutic doses: A review of the evidence. *Epilepsy Behav*. 2016;**61**:282–6. http://dx.doi.org/10.1016/j.yebeh.2016.03.022.

46. Okazaki M, Adachi N, Akanuma N, Hara K, Ito M, Kato M, et al. Do antipsychotic drugs increase seizure frequency in epilepsy patients? *Eur Neuropsychopharmacol*. 2014;**24**(11):1738–44. http://dx.doi.org/10.1016/j.euroneuro.2014.09.012.

47. Mcallister-Williams RH, Baldwin DS, Cantwell R, Easter A, Gilvarry E, Glover V, et al. British Association for Psychopharmacology consensus guidance on the use of psychotropic medication preconception, in pregnancy and postpartum 2017. *J Psychopharmacol*. 2017;**31**(5):519–52.

48. Huybrechts KF, Hernández-Díaz S, Patorno E, Desai RJ, Mogun H, Dejene SZ, et al. Antipsychotic use in pregnancy and the risk for congenital malformations. *JAMA Psychiatry*. 2016;**73**(9):938–46.

49. Mehndiratta P, Sajatovic M. Treatments for patients with comorbid epilepsy and depression: A systematic literature review. *Epilepsy Behav.* 2013;**28**(1):36–40. http://dx.doi.org/10.1016/j.yebeh.2013.03.029.

50. Gilliam FG, Black KJ, Carter J, Freedland KE, Sheline YI, Tsai WY, et al. A trial of sertraline or cognitive behavior therapy for depression in epilepsy. *Ann Neurol.* 2019;**86**(4):552–60.

51. Conway CR, Udaiyar A, Schachter SC. Neurostimulation for depression in epilepsy. *Epilepsy Behav.* 2018;**88**:25–32. https://doi.org/10.1016/j.yebeh.2018.06.007.

52. Pereira LS, Müller VT, da Mota Gomes M, Rotenberg A, Fregni F. Safety of repetitive transcranial magnetic stimulation in patients with epilepsy: A systematic review. *Epilepsy Behav.* 2016;**57**:167–76. http://dx.doi.org/10.1016/j.yebeh.2016.01.015.

53. Baxendale S, O'Sullivan J, Heaney D. Bright light therapy for symptoms of anxiety and depression in focal epilepsy: Randomised controlled trial. *Br J Psychiatry.* 2013;**202**(5):352–6.

54. Mills E, Montori VM, Wu P, Gallicano K, Clarke M, Guyatt G. Interaction of St John's wort with conventional drugs: Systemic review of clinical trials. *BMJ.* 2004;**329**(July):27–30.

55. Yatham LN, Kennedy SH, Parikh SV, Schaffer A, Bond DJ, Frey BN, et al. Canadian Network for Mood and Anxiety Treatments (CANMAT) and International Society for Bipolar Disorders (ISBD) 2018 guidelines for the management of patients with bipolar disorder. *Bipolar Disord.* 2018;**20**(2):97–170.

56. Katzman MA, Bleau P, Blier P, Chokka P, Kjernisted K, Van Ameringen M, et al. Canadian clinical practice guidelines for the management of anxiety, posttraumatic stress and obsessive-compulsive disorders. *BMC Psychiatry.* 2014;**14**(Suppl. 1):1–83.

57. Goldstein LH, Robinson EJ, Mellers JDC, Stone J, Carson A, Reuber M, et al. Cognitive behavioural therapy for adults with dissociative seizures (CODES): A pragmatic, multicentre, randomised controlled trial. *Lancet Psychiatry.* 2020;7(6):491–505.

Chapter 3

Sleep-Related Comorbidities in Women with Epilepsy

Milena K. Pavlova and Véronique Latreille

Key Points

- Seizures can aggravate sleep quality, and poor-quality sleep can aggravate seizure disorders.
- Antiseizure medications can alter sleep architecture and aggravate daytime sleepiness; timing of therapy can have significant effects on this profile.
- Hormonal, reproductive, and life-cycle events alter sleep and consequently have effects on sleep disorders that may be present in women.
- Sleep disorders such as insomnia, sleep-disordered breathing, and restless legs syndrome are common in women.
- Simple sleep interventions can often have significant impact on seizure management and quality of life for women.

Introduction

The interactions between sleep and epilepsy are numerous, yet much remains to be elucidated. Little is known about the combination of epilepsy, sleep, sleep disorders, and women's health. Therefore, much has to be extrapolated from work that has been done about sleep disorders in women and sleep disorders in epilepsy.

Sleep and epilepsy have a bidirectional influence on one another. Sleep itself, as well as sleep deprivation and fragmentation, influences electrographic features, seizures, cognitive function, and quality of life in patients with epilepsy. Sleep disorders can exacerbate a person's seizures. Some seizure types and occurrence of interictal discharges seem to be facilitated in certain stages of sleep. A common perception is that the relationship between seizures and sleep is governed by the sleep state itself, though time of day or circadian factors are also important. Both interictal discharges and seizures during sleep can disrupt sleep and decrease its restorative effect. Good seizure control, therefore, is of importance in promoting good sleep. One must also be cognizant of the effect of antiseizure medications (ASMs) on sleep architecture and daytime function.

Sleep Physiology

Sleep can be defined as a state of reversible alteration in the state of consciousness characterized by decreased responsiveness to the external environment, reduction in movement, typical posture, and eye closure. The sleep state is associated with predictable changes in physiology. These include alterations in autonomic and endocrine functions, decreases in muscle tone, and characteristic electroencephalographic (EEG) changes. Sleep is actively regulated by neural processes, and in humans it occurs in a circadian pattern.

Sleep is objectively assessed by using polysomnography (PSG), which utilizes EEG, electrooculography, electromyography, electrocardiography, and pulse oximetry, as well as airflow and respiratory effort. Polysomnography is the gold standard for diagnosis of sleep disorders and evaluation of sleep architecture. In the context of epilepsy and to assist in diagnosing paroxysmal nocturnal events and differentiate between the presence of sleep disorders and/or seizure activity, use of PSG with extended 10–20 EEG montage is recommended [1].

Sleep is divided into non–rapid eye movement (NREM) sleep and rapid-eye-movement (REM) sleep. The EEG shows evidence of progressively more synchronized activity during NREM sleep, with increased amplitude and lower frequencies as sleep progresses. Non–rapid eye movement sleep is further subdivided into N1, N2, and N3 stages. Stage N1 represents light transitional sleep and is characterized by replacement of alpha in the posterior dominant rhythm by low-amplitude, mixed-frequency theta, as well as slow, roving eye movements and vertex sharp waves. Stage N2 represents consolidated sleep and is characterized by sleep spindles and K-complexes on the EEG. Stage N3 is fundamentally a homeostatic restorative component of sleep and is synonymous with slow-wave, delta, or deep sleep. Stage N3 is scored when more than 20% of the 30-second epoch comprises generalized 0.5–2 Hz, high-amplitude waves. Rapid-eye-movement sleep, also known as stage R or paradoxical sleep, is characterized by a desynchronized EEG pattern with low-amplitude, mixed frequencies, and sawtooth waves, as well as rapid eye movements and skeletal muscle atonia.

Interactions between Sleep and Epilepsy

Circadian Influences of Epileptic Activity

Clinical observations of a relationship between sleep and epilepsy date back to antiquity [2]. For more than 100 years, physicians have looked at the sleep-wake timing of seizures in institutionalized patients and outpatients and distinguished three groups of epilepsy syndromes, described as "diurnal," "nocturnal," and "diffuse." Observations of periodicity in seizure activity suggest that the sleep-wake cycle and endogenous circadian factors influence seizure susceptibility.

Some epilepsy syndromes are significantly associated with sleep, and those include the self-limited focal epilepsies (e.g., self-limited focal epilepsy with centrotemporal spikes), the epileptic encephalopathies (e.g., Lennox–Gastaut syndrome or epileptic encephalopathy with continuous spike-and-wave during sleep), the epilepsies associated with awakening (e.g., juvenile myoclonic epilepsy), and sleep-related hypermotor epilepsy (SHE, formerly named nocturnal frontal lobe epilepsy). For focal seizures, the circadian influence of seizures varies according to the localization of epilepsy: extra-temporal seizures, especially frontal lobe seizures, predominantly occur during sleep, whereas temporal seizures are more likely to occur during wakefulness. Multiple studies reveal a 24-hour pattern in seizure frequency that depends on the epileptogenic zone, with frontal lobe seizures occurring predominantly at night or early morning and temporal lobe seizures in the late afternoon, or in a bimodal pattern with a smaller peak in the morning [3, 4]. Intracranial data from the NeuroPace RNS System trials showed that epileptiform activity also displays a strong 24-hour periodicity, as well as other cyclical patterns that were not 24 hours [5, 6]. Few data are available regarding the influence of gender on circadian epileptic activity distribution; one study found gender variations in seizure occurrence, with women with epilepsy having fewer seizures in the early morning and fewer seizures during sleep than men [7]. However, data from the NeuroPace trial reported a similar distribution of epileptic activity in men and women [8]. While the direct effect of the endogenous circadian system on the frequency of seizures has not been thoroughly investigated to date, a circadian protocol is feasible and has been tested in patients with generalized epilepsy [9]. Furthermore, there are 24-hour intracranial variations in glutamate measured in animal models of epilepsy, indicating a likely endogenous chronobiological effect [10].

Research over the past decades revealed a strong association between sleep and the risk of sudden unexpected death in epilepsy (SUDEP). The causes and mechanisms underlying SUDEP are poorly understood. Risk factors of SUDEP related to sleep should be considered, including sleeping in a prone position, occurrence of generalized tonic-clonic seizures, and postictal apnea [11]. Men have a 1.4-fold increase in the risk of SUDEP [11]. Measures to reduce the risk of SUDEP should be encouraged, and these consist first in educating patients and their family members about SUDEP and the importance of good compliance with ASM, maintaining a healthy lifestyle, and allowing adequate sleep opportunity. Nocturnal convulsions are a strong risk factor for sleep-related disorders, and intervention may be helpful in many of these patients [12].

Effect of Seizures and Interictal Discharges on Sleep

It is well recognized that seizures produce postictal somnolence. However, the consequences of ictal and interictal epileptic activity on sleep have been less well studied. Regarding sleep macro architecture, sleep-related seizures have been found to increase sleep-stage shifts and wakefulness after sleep onset. One recent study found that the vast majority (~80%) of sleep-related seizures are followed by intracranial arousals or awakenings [13]. Interictal epileptic activity during N2 sleep also decreased arousal thresholds, resulting in greater sleep fragmentation. Finally, the occurrence of sleep-related seizures is associated with increased risk of postictal generalized EEG suppression and respiratory disturbances [14].

Conversely, improved seizure control with pharmacological or non-pharmacological treatment likely improves sleep parameters. Although detailed data are still lacking, it is thought that interictal discharges can cause repeated arousals and sleep fragmentation, resulting in excessive daytime sleepiness (EDS). Adequate treatment with ASMs can decrease the frequency of these discharges and potentially improve sleep quality. Surgical treatment of epilepsy that results in improved seizure control has been shown to raise sleep quality and lower EDS. The vagal nerve stimulator has been used for the treatment of refractory epilepsy, is sometimes successful in treating the seizures, and may help with daytime alertness. Unfortunately, in some patients, it has caused or aggravated sleep apnea syndrome, and patients should be monitored for this possible complication [15].

Sleep Influences on Seizures and Interictal Discharges

Non–rapid eye movement sleep facilitates ictal events and interictal epileptiform discharges both in number and in spatial extent, while REM sleep inhibits interictal discharges. Results from a meta-analysis revealed that relative to REM sleep, focal seizure rates were respectively 68 and 51 times higher during N2 and N3 sleep, and focal interictal discharge rates during N2 and N3 sleep were respectively 1.7 and 2.5 times higher relative to REM sleep [16]. Although discharges are rarer during REM sleep, they tend to be locally restricted and may help localize the epileptogenic zone.

In a high percentage of patients with sleep-related epilepsies, the daytime EEG remains normal, emphasizing the importance of obtaining a sleep-deprived EEG with sleep if a routine EEG during wakefulness is normal and clinical suspicion of epilepsy persists. Sleep deprivation increases interictal discharges and seizures beyond the effect of sleep alone, but the exact mechanisms remain elusive. A sleep-deprived EEG increases the diagnostic yield when a diagnosis of epilepsy is considered [17].

Theoretical mechanisms that have been proposed to explain the interaction between sleep and epilepsy can be divided into the following categories: (i) shared neuronal circuits, (ii) hypersynchronization, (iii) hyperexcitability, (iv) failure of normal inhibitory mechanisms, and (v) chemical mediators [18, 19]. The most well-known example of a shared neuronal substrate for sleep and epilepsy is the thalamic reticular neurons [19]. These gamma-aminobutyric acid or GABAergic neurons inhibit the thalamocortical neurons in the dorsal thalamus, which have glutamatergic projections to the cortex. Through the intrinsic oscillatory properties of the reticular neurons, sleep spindles are generated. However, if $GABA_A$ receptor–mediated inhibition is reduced, 3 Hz spike-and-wave discharges characteristic of absence seizures can be produced.

As sleep progressively deepens, more sleep spindles and delta waves are seen on the EEG, reflecting synchronization activity as a feature of NREM sleep. Delta waves are mediated by a combination of the thalamocortical circuits just described and the cortex itself. Hypersynchronization is also a key feature of epilepsy. The NREM synchronization can create an opportunity for an already hyperexcitable cortex to produce epileptic activity. Related, intracranial recordings of adults with drug-resistant focal epilepsy revealed that interictal discharges preferentially occurred during the highly synchronous NREM sleep epochs, when high-amplitude, slow waves predominate [20].

Cortical hyperexcitability is likely mediated by genetic factors and/or by acquired, often injury-related mechanisms. Sleep arousals and micro arousals may also increase cortical hyperexcitability, consistent with the observation that many seizures occur in this context, as demonstrated using depth electrode recordings that seizures often precede (and therefore may cause) an arousal [18]. In addition, sleep deprivation enhances cortical hyperexcitability. For example, Scalise and colleagues used trans-magnetic stimulation to demonstrate a reduction of intracortical inhibition after total sleep deprivation in seven normal subjects [21].

Failure of normal inhibitory mechanisms likely allows the propagation of seizure activity and may even result in status epilepticus. Inhibitory mechanisms are less effective during NREM sleep. In contrast, REM sleep is characterized by inhibition of thalamocortical synchronization and a reduction in interhemispheric impulses across the corpus callosum, resulting in an anticonvulsant effect with an overall reduction in interictal discharges and seizures [19].

Alterations in chemical mediators, including neurotransmitters and neuropeptides, in various sleep states are also important. Neurotransmitters and hormones change dramatically based on stage of normal sleep and circadian patterns. As such, they may influence cortical excitability.

Effect of Antiseizure Medications on Sleep

The exact effect of an individual ASM on sleep can be difficult to determine, especially because the precise mechanisms of action are only partially understood. A recent meta-analysis indicated that ASMs can significantly alter sleep architecture, although the effects differ between the medications [22].

In general, most ASMs are sedating. This is more notable with the barbiturates and benzodiazepines but can also be seen with phenytoin, phenobarbital, and valproic acid and higher-dose levetiracetam. Certain ASMs, including carbamazepine, gabapentin, tiagabine, pregabalin, and clobazam, can improve sleep quality by reducing sleep latency and/or enhancing sleep efficiency in epilepsy patients. Withdrawal of sedating ASMs may also lead to insomnia. Sedating ASMs, especially benzodiazepines and barbiturates, have to be used with care in patients with untreated obstructive sleep apnea (OSA), as it can worsen the problem. Some medications, such as topiramate, can assist sleep apnea by associated weight loss and are even theoretically beneficial in central sleep apnea given their carbonic anhydrase inhibition.

Hormonal Influences on Sleep

Women sleep differently than men. They spend more time in bed, sleep longer, and have less light sleep and more slow-wave sleep than men at any given age. Women complain of poorer subjective sleep quality although this perception is not necessarily supported by objective PSG measures. Women are at 40% increased risk for developing insomnia and at twice the risk for restless legs syndrome (RLS) compared with men (see Section 5.5, "Restless Legs Syndrome"). Psychosocial issues also impact sleep quality in women much more than men and women respond differently to sleep deprivation, in general with greater levels of anxiety in response to sleep loss. Pregnancy and the postpartum period are also associated with significant changes in sleep quantity and quality (discussed in Section 6, "Pregnancy and Sleep"). Human studies of hormonal effects on women's sleep are scarce, partly due to significant barriers to study design [23].

Prenatal gonadal hormones alter brain development, with effects on receptor expression and neuronal networks that ultimately result in a phenotypically male or female brain. Animal data have suggested that sex-dependent differences in sleep are mediated by both hormone-dependent and hormone-independent mechanisms, and that the effects of sex steroids on sleep are gender-specific.

Reproductive hormones have neuroactive functions that are mediated through intracellular steroid receptors [24]. Many different cellular functions may be modulated, from neuronal excitability to neuroplasticity, and are discussed in greater detail in Chapter 4.

Estrogen

Estrogen seems to have a mainly neuroexcitatory role via inhibition of GABA and potentiation of glutamatergic conductance. Estrogen receptors are widely distributed throughout the brain, including many sleep-wake regulatory structures such as the basal forebrain, hypothalamus, locus coeruleus, and the dorsal raphe nucleus. Estrogen also has effects on sleep architecture, mainly in decreasing REM sleep duration.

Several lines of evidence reviewed by Mong suggest estradiol modulates adenosine and prostaglandin, known somnogens, at the level of the ventrolateral preoptic hypothalamus [25]. It may help consolidate wakefulness and thereby improve sleep, which is one of several possible mechanisms for the improvements in sleep quality in women taking hormone replacement therapy (HRT). Estradiol probably also plays a role in sleep-wake regulation via its effects on the suprachiasmatic nucleus (SCN). The SCN is the "master clock" that regulates all circadian aspects of physiology and behavior. At a basic physiological level, estrogen also contributes to nasal congestion and airway edema, particularly during pregnancy, by increasing blood flow to the nose and upper airway and can precipitate frank obstructive apnea, which can further affect sleep.

Progesterone

Progesterone exerts a mainly neuroinhibitory effect in the brain by promoting GABA and inhibiting glutamatergic conductance. It has anxiolytic and anticonvulsant properties, but in excess may cause sedation and depression. Many brain areas have progesterone receptors, and there is significant overlap with the estrogen receptors.

Progesterone improves sleep duration and quality, mainly by enhancing slow-wave sleep, possibly through an interaction between progesterone metabolites and $GABA_A$ receptors, which are found in the thalamocortical circuits. It is a potent respiratory stimulant and therefore can improve ventilation during sleep. It also increases tone in the genioglossus muscle, a key upper airway dilator, which may reduce upper airway collapsibility during sleep. In premenopausal women, the lowest rate of sleep-related respiratory events is seen during the luteal phase, when progesterone levels are highest [26]. Theoretically, this means that OSA can be falsely ruled out by a PSG done at this point in the menstrual cycle. Postmenopausally, when progesterone levels are low, women are at increased risk of sleep apnea. The withdrawal of progesterone, which may be as neuroactively potent as a sleeping medication, can lead to rebound insomnia perimenstrually.

Testosterone

Testosterone has been shown to affect sleep in men, and it may also play a role in sleep in women, specifically in mediating menopausal sleep complaints and OSA. However, studies of the effects of testosterone on women's sleep are rare, and this remains a complicated area because of conflicting results.

Support for the role of testosterone in mediating sleep in women comes from the effects on sleep-disordered breathing (SDB). Testosterone is known to downregulate estrogen and progesterone receptors, which may weaken the progesterone respiratory stimulant effect. This becomes relevant in polycystic ovarian syndrome, which is associated with endogenous overproduction of testosterone and a higher apnea–hypopnea index (AHI), although insulin resistance may also play a role in the significantly increased prevalence of OSA in this population. Testosterone has been shown to alter respiratory functions in women during wakefulness and may contribute to the increased risk of OSA in menopause [23].

The Menstrual Cycle and Sleep

About one-third of women report subjective changes in sleep quality, as well as hypersomnia or insomnia at the time of menses or during the premenstrual week. Women attribute sleep disruption during menses to physical discomforts such as cramps, bloating, breast tenderness, and headaches. While most studies show an effect of the menstrual phase on perceived sleep quality, consistent, objective PSG evidence of sleep architecture changes across the menstrual cycle is lacking.

Modest effects of oral contraceptive medications on sleep have been reported, including increased temperature, increased melatonin levels, and less stage N3 sleep, as well as a reduced REM latency. These studies are limited by the heterogeneity of oral contraceptive preparations [27]. Certain sleep disorders have been noted to have a catamenial pattern. In the third edition of the *International Classification of Sleep Disorders* (ICSD-3), menstrual-related hypersomnia is considered as a subtype of Kleine–Levin syndrome [28]. Menstrual-related hypersomnia may be more common in the few months following menarche. Hormonal contraceptives may also have a role in managing these conditions.

Upper airway resistance is usually more severe during the follicular phase, and theoretically a diagnosis of SDB can be missed if the PSG is performed during the luteal phase. The menstrual variability in the severity of sleep apnea may even necessitate varying the pressure of continuous positive airway pressure (CPAP) according to the patient's menstrual cycle.

Common Sleep Comorbidities in Women with Epilepsy

Among both men and women, patients with epilepsy are more likely to self-report poor sleep quality than healthy people. Sleep architecture is frequently disrupted in patients with epilepsy. Epilepsy itself impairs quality of life, and comorbid sleep disturbances compound this effect [29]. Factors associated with sleep disturbances in this population include use of first-generation ASMs and poor seizure control. Common complaints in patients with epilepsy are EDS, insomnia, SDB, and nocturnal behaviors [30]. Women probably accumulate a sleep debt more quickly than men and take longer to recover from it [25]. However, they are also more likely to have sleep-state misperception, which manifests as believing they have less sleep or poorer-quality sleep than what is objectively seen on PSG.

Excessive Daytime Sleepiness

In general, sleep deprivation is the most common cause of EDS. Much of this sleep deprivation is voluntary and there are limited data on gender differences in EDS. Most adults require approximately 8 hours of sleep, but many adults, including patients with epilepsy, routinely sleep less than this. When assessed objectively using the multiple sleep latency test (MSLT), EDS is found in about half of patients with epilepsy [31]. A recent meta-analysis found no influence of age and sex on subjective EDS in patients with epilepsy compared to controls [32]. Nevertheless, a heightened time of sleep deprivation is in the postpartum period, attributed to the care of a newborn. Education about adequate sleep time and good sleep hygiene is the first step in correcting this problem and avoiding a common trigger for seizures. Other causes of EDS in patients with epilepsy include seizures, frequent epileptiform discharges on EEG, comorbid sleep disorders (i.e., sleep apnea, RLS, periodic limb movement in sleep), and the effect of ASMs.

The effects of sleep deprivation go beyond sleepiness to affect quality of life and cognitive and neurobehavioral functions in normal individuals [29]. For example, a full night of sleep deprivation has been shown to result in cognitive impairment comparable to being legally intoxicated with alcohol [33]. Anxiety and depression are common in people with epilepsy, and this may reflect the high prevalence of sleep problems [29]. Sleep loss is a significant contributor to the psychosocial comorbidity of epilepsy.

Insomnia

Among the general population, about one-third of adults will experience transient insomnia at some point in their life. Insomnia is more common in women than in men across the life span independent of other factors. In epilepsy patients, the prevalence of clinical insomnia ranges from 36% to 74% depending on the criteria used [34]. A small number of studies found a higher occurrence of insomnia disorder in women with epilepsy. Presence of insomnia in epilepsy is associated with depressive symptoms, poorer quality of life, and lack of seizure freedom [30, 35].

Insomnia is sometimes divided by the predominant character of the symptoms to sleep onset and sleep maintenance insomnia. Both sleep onset and sleep maintenance insomnia can co-occur in the same individual, but it is a useful distinction for planning treatment strategies. It is particularly important to rule out RLS in patients with sleep initiation difficulties and SDB in those with sleep maintenance problems. After secondary causes of insomnia have been ruled out, including other primary sleep disorders that may require specific treatments and medication side effects, therapeutic options can be considered.

Non-pharmacological strategies are usually the mainstay of treatment because of better long-term efficacy and none of the potential complications associated with medications. For patients with chronic insomnia, cognitive behavioral therapy (CBT) should be the first-line treatment option. In addition to sleep hygiene counseling, CBT utilizes mindfulness principles to reduce negative thoughts about sleep; relaxation strategies such as progressive muscle relaxation, deep breathing, and imagery; and sleep-restriction strategies such as limiting time in bed with progressive monitoring of sleep diaries, gradually increasing allowed time in bed as patients begin to achieve improved sleep efficiency. In epilepsy patients, sleep restriction should be used with extreme caution, if at all, due to concern for seizure exacerbation. Other behavioral interventions include meditation, hypnosis, and biofeedback. Among the general population, multiple studies have shown that CBT for insomnia has equal or greater effect than pharmacological treatment, and even a longer-term impact. In epilepsy, a recent clinical trial testing the usefulness of an app-based (online) CBT intervention over 6 weeks in patients with moderate to severe insomnia showed significant improvements in sleep quality and sleep onset latency, as well as in mood and behavior (e.g., insomnia severity, sleep hygiene behavior, anxiety, depression, and quality of life) at 1, 3, and 6 months post intervention relative to a control group [36].

All patients can be educated about good sleep hygiene. Patients are counseled on the importance of maintaining a regular sleep-wake schedule; alcohol intake; avoiding caffeine, nicotine, bright light, and excessive fluid intake in the evenings; and ensuring the bedroom environment is conducive to sleep (quiet, cool, and dark).

Good Sleep Rules

- Determine time in bed: *most need 7–9 hours of sleep; do not stay in bed longer.*
- Use the bed for sleep/intimacy only.
- Turn the clock so it is not visible from the bed.
- Naps, if taken at all, should be brief (<30 minutes) and taken in the early afternoon at the latest.
- Schedule regular wake times.
- Allow an ample amount of light during the day.

- Allow dimmer light in the evening.
- Limit caffeine intake: *last intake at noon.*
- Moderate alcohol: *it is best not to have alcohol close to bedtime.*

The role of pharmacotherapy is best reserved for the treatment of acute insomnia or as an adjunct to non-pharmacological treatments. If a sedating ASM is to be used, it should be used at night to help with sleep initiation. Off-label use of antidepressants for insomnia is common in clinical practice. This may be particularly helpful in patients with epilepsy where comorbid depression may be more frequent. Many hypnotics are indicated for short-term use only (e.g., most benzodiazepines, zolpidem). Melatonin agonists, including ramelteon, are approved for insomnia, including for chronic use. Melatonin is a relatively weak and ineffective hypnotic for most adults; however, it may be more effective for use in children and adolescents. Orexin antagonists (suvorexant, lemborexant) are a novel class of hypnotics that do not use the GABA/benzodiazepine system and are thus attractive for use in older individuals or when benzodiazepines need to be avoided. Suvorexant has a sufficiently long half-life that it is approved for sleep-maintenance insomnia. Common side effects of orexin antagonists include nightmares. Non-benzodiazepine hypnotics (such as zolpidem) have been associated with risk of complex sleep behaviors and should be avoided in patients with any history of sleepwalking.

In general, most, if not all, of the nonspecific prescription medications used in the treatment of insomnia are associated with some degree of tolerance over time. Psychological dependence is not uncommon with chronic daily use. Besides side effects and interactions, counseling should include the potential for rebound insomnia (i.e., worse insomnia when a medication is stopped than before treatment started) and pregnancy/lactation considerations for women with epilepsy. Benzodiazepines are contraindicated during pregnancy, while some other medications may be used with caution [37].

Sleep-Disordered Breathing

Sleep-disordered breathing is a collective term that includes OSA, but also upper airway resistance syndrome, central apnea, and obesity-hypoventilation syndrome. Obstructive sleep apnea is caused by upper airway obstruction during sleep. This results in inadequate ventilation and relative hypercapnia and hypoxemia, which can rouse the patient from sleep in order to restore ventilation. Obstructive sleep apnea is more prevalent in men than women. The presentation of OSA symptoms also differs according to sex: women are more likely to report nonspecific symptoms of SDB, including unrefreshing sleep, fatigue, anxiety, depression, and insomnia, while men frequently report snoring, snorting, gasping, and daytime sleepiness. Anatomical differences of the upper airway may also contribute to the gender differences. The gender gap narrows in postmenopausal women because of the increased prevalence in this population. Upper airway resistance syndrome is a less overt form of OSA where the airflow limitations do not result in oxygen desaturation but cause arousals and therefore sleep fragmentation and daytime sleepiness. Risk factors include older age, obesity, especially central adiposity, enlarged neck circumference (>16 inches in a woman, >17 inches in a man), and genetic and anatomical reasons for upper airway narrowing. Most risk factors for OSA identified in the general population also apply to adults with epilepsy. Polysomnography is used to diagnose OSA and to distinguish it from other sleep and sleep-breathing disorders.

In epilepsy, OSA is the most common sleep comorbidity, with estimates approximating 33% of patients [38]. The risk of mild-to-severe OSA in women with epilepsy is about three times lower than that of men, though the continuum of SDB may be much more common than realized and is certainly more common in women with epilepsy.

It is important to note that ASMs can worsen OSA. For example, valproate, vigabatrin, and gabapentin promote weight gain, which is a well-known risk factor for sleep apnea. Similarly, benzodiazepines and barbiturates can also be problematic because they cause decreased sensitivity to carbon dioxide and therefore oxygen desaturation, as well as relaxation of the upper airway musculature.

Presence of OSA in the general population is associated with significant morbidity because it is an independent risk factor for several cardiovascular and cerebrovascular diseases, including hypertension, coronary heart disease, and stroke. When left untreated, OSA can negatively impact cognitive function in patients with epilepsy [39]. Treatment with CPAP helps reduce cardiovascular risk, and it has also been suggested in meta-analyses to decrease seizure frequency and improve seizure control [38]. Other alternatives include surgical correction of airway anatomy and use of a dental appliance to advance the tongue or mandible and improve airway patency. In pregnancy, sleep apnea may lead to adverse outcomes, as discussed later in the chapter (see Section 6.1, "Sleep-Disordered Breathing in Pregnancy").

Restless Legs Syndrome and Periodic Limb Movement Disorder

Restless legs syndrome is a clinical diagnosis characterized by unpleasant leg sensations that occur at rest and are associated with a strong urge to move. These symptoms are worse toward the end of the day and are relieved with movement. Restless legs syndrome is more common in women than men, and particularly more frequent in relation to pregnancy, as discussed later in this chapter. Most patients with RLS also have repetitive flexion movements of the toes, ankles, and hips during sleep, called periodic limb movement in sleep (PLMS). In epilepsy patients, RLS and PLMS prevalence is highly variable across the few available studies but seems to be slightly superior to the general population, occurring in 5–20% of patients.

Secondary causes of RLS such as iron deficiency, B12 deficiency, or neuropathy should be sought and corrected. Iron deficiency is particularly common in women given menstruation and pregnancy. In the setting of iron deficiency, iron supplementation is an effective treatment. The morbidity associated with RLS can be tremendous. Studies have found a reduction in quality of life related to RLS on par with suffering from a chronic medical condition like diabetes or heart disease [40]. Restless legs syndrome is associated with sleep initiation difficulties and can reduce total sleep time. As sleep loss can aggravate epilepsy, this may have significant consequences.

Therapeutic options for RLS include gabapentin, pregabalin, and benzodiazepines, which are particularly good avenues in the context of epilepsy. Treatment with dopamine agonists such as pramipexole, ropinirole, or rotigotine is usually effective. The medication is taken an hour before bedtime. Minimal effective doses should be used to avoid sedating side effects or impulse control problems. Furthermore, symptoms of RLS may occur earlier and earlier in the day and this phenomenon, called augmentation, is aggravated by use of dopaminergic agents, especially at higher doses. The typical therapeutic strategy for augmentation is to change medication, ideally avoiding dopaminergic agents.

In periodic limb movement disorder (PLMD), patients do not experience unpleasant leg sensations but rather develop involuntary limb movements during sleep associated with a clinical sleep disturbance or a complaint of daytime sleepiness. It is important to ensure that upper airway resistance is not present on the PSG, as it can cause excessive daytime sleepiness and can mimic isolated limb movements if signs of airflow limitation are missed. Treating the patient's SDB (e.g., CPAP for a patient with OSA or upper airway resistance) is usually the first step, followed by reevaluation for PLMS if needed.

Summary of common sleep disorders in women with epilepsy and recommended treatments

Insomnia	Behavioral interventions such as CBT, relaxation, and meditation
	Sleep hygiene counseling
	Pharmacotherapy: sedating ASM, antidepressants, and hypnotics such as melatonin
	Perimenopausal: non-hormone replacement therapy
	Menopausal: hormone replacement therapy (with caution)
OSA	CPAP
	Weight loss, positional therapy, dental appliance, and upper airway surgery
RLS/PLMS	Iron supplementation
	Limit caffeine intake
	Pharmacotherapy: gabapentin, pregabalin, benzodiazepines, and dopamine agonists

ASM: Antiseizure medication; CBT: Cognitive behavioral therapy; CPAP: Continuous positive airway pressure; OSA: Obstructive sleep apnea; PLMS: Periodic limb movement in sleep; RLS: Restless legs syndrome

Pregnancy and Sleep

Pregnancy results in multisystemic changes that can affect sleep and sleep disorders. Sleep disruption can be caused by nocturia, gastroesophageal reflux disease (GERD), rhinitis and nasal congestion, musculoskeletal discomfort, fetal movement, and psychosocial stressors.

Women in the first trimester report increased fatigue and daytime sleepiness, and often, total sleep time increases, although some report the onset of insomnia. These symptoms are usually due to hormonal effects on sleep, but unmasking of a preexisting sleep disorder should also be considered. In the second trimester, nocturnal awakenings increase, probably due to the emergence of nocturia and GERD as well as aggravation of SDB. Nearly one-third of women sleep less than 7 hours per night in the second trimester of pregnancy. During the third trimester, nocturnal awakenings, uterine contractions, fatigue, leg cramps, and shortness of breath all increase and are associated with a reduction in total sleep time. Women often try to compensate by napping or going to bed earlier. Changes in sleep architecture mainly affect the third trimester of gestation, with a reduction in total sleep duration, increased number of awakenings, and more superficial sleep with increase amounts of stage N1 sleep and reduction of N3 and REM sleep [41]. Pregnancy-related sleep disorders have been linked to adverse perinatal outcomes, including higher risk of gestational diabetes, cesarean delivery, and longer duration of labor [42].

The postpartum period has significant challenges to sleep as well, particularly with nighttime infant care. Postpartum women are more likely to report poor sleep quality, but this effect is reduced in women with a healthy lifestyle (not smoking, limited alcohol consumption, and regular physical activity). The amount of sleep disruption a woman experiences can depend on method of feeding, the infant's sleep pattern, support from a spouse or others, parity, anxiety and depression levels, and co-sleeping. Polysomnography studies have shown increased nocturnal awakenings, increased wakefulness after sleep onset, lower sleep efficiency, and shortened REM latency [42]. Hormonal changes probably also play a role in sleep deprivation postpartum. For example, even in the absence of infant care postpartum, sleep does not return to prepregnancy baseline. Others have reported that a number of the nocturnal awakenings are not related to care of the infant.

Many sleep medications are to be avoided in the context of pregnancy, and details are beyond the scope of this chapter. Assessment of objective sleep alterations during pregnancy is relevant in guiding appropriate therapeutic strategies for women reporting poor-quality sleep and daytime sleepiness. Treatment of the underlying sleep disorder may improve cognitive function and quality of life. Prior to administering treatment for sleep disorders in women with epilepsy, physicians must take into consideration (i) the risk for adverse pregnancy outcomes for women of childbearing age, (ii) the risk associated with adverse effects of drugs on nursing infants, and (iii) gender-specific changes in metabolism (women tend to clear some drugs, i.e., zolpidem, less effectively than men). If pharmacological treatment for sleep disorders is absolutely needed, patients are recommended to avoid breastfeeding near peak blood levels.

Sleep-Disordered Breathing in Pregnancy

Pregnant women are at increased risk of developing SDB, especially in the third trimester, and even though in most women the symptoms were absent before pregnancy, almost half report snoring and choking. Increased levels of estrogen and progesterone cause airway edema and nasal congestion, which probably accounts for the progressively increasing risk of snoring over the course of pregnancy. Weight gain and reduced diaphragmatic excursion may also contribute.

Women who are hypertensive at the time of birth are more likely to be snorers. Snoring causes sleep fragmentation and may contribute to symptoms of daytime sleepiness. The mechanism for elevated blood pressure may be due to autonomic activation associated with the arousals from sleep-related respiratory events, preventing the normal circadian decrease in blood pressure overnight. Treatment of upper airway resistance syndrome and snoring with CPAP in women with preeclampsia can significantly reduce blood pressure.

Obstructive sleep apnea is estimated to affect about 15% of pregnant women, and it has been associated with increased risk of gestational diabetes, hypertensive disorders, preeclampsia, preterm birth, and cesarean delivery [42]. Positive airway pressure (or CPAP) is the appropriate treatment for OSA and is considered safe in pregnancy.

Restless Legs Syndrome and Periodic Limb Movement in Sleep in Pregnancy

Restless legs syndrome is observed in 20–25% of otherwise healthy pregnant women, and usually occurs in the third trimester. Iron deficiency can cause or aggravate RLS. Young women are often iron deficient and, in pregnancy, volume expansion and hematopoiesis increase iron requirements. Multivitamins that are routinely recommended in pregnancy often contain inadequate amounts of replacement iron, and additional supplementation is appropriate for symptomatic women or women who have had RLS in previous pregnancies. Ferritin levels and other iron indices are usually measured. Iron is the rate-limiting step in the synthesis of dopamine in the brain, and in nonpregnant populations, dopamine agonists can effectively treat RLS. Dopamine circuits in the brain have also been implicated in mood disorders, suggesting a relationship between iron loss, RLS, and peripartum mood disorders [40].

Periodic limb movement in sleep is often associated with RLS, although the available studies do not show an increase in PLMS frequency in pregnant women compared to nonpregnant controls. Both RLS and PLMS can cause sleep disruption, with RLS usually resulting in sleep-onset insomnia. Nocturnal leg cramps should raise suspicion for PLMS because these may represent the culmination of a series of occult periodic limb movements [40].

Conservative measures for the treatment of RLS and PLMS include reducing caffeine and sleep loss and are often used preferentially in pregnancy. Reducing aggravating agents such as antidepressants may be considered. Iron management may be particularly important. Intravenous iron infusions may be an option for particularly symptomatic individuals. Dopamine agonists are the mainstay of treatment in nonpregnant populations. Opioids should be used with caution and are usually reserved for disabling refractory cases.

Menopause and Sleep

Sleep complaints in the perimenopausal period are common and are present in up to half of women. Perceived sleep changes mainly relate to difficulties falling asleep, having more fragmented sleep, nocturnal awakenings, and inability to resume sleep. Menopausal symptoms, particularly psychological changes and comorbid conditions such as depression, as well as vasomotor symptoms like hot flashes and night sweats contribute to subjective sleep difficulties.

Sleep patterns are known to change with normal aging, and older people tend to have reduced sleep efficiency, lighter sleep, and increased wakefulness after sleep onset. Independent of this, it has been suggested that menopause is associated with decreases in nocturnal melatonin secretion, resulting in circadian phase advance and early morning awakenings. Exogenous melatonin may help improve physical symptoms, mood, and subjective sleep quality in postmenopausal women. Many medical conditions and their treatments can have adverse effects on sleep and these become more common with age. Certain sleep disorders like OSA and RLS increase with age.

Sleep-Disordered Breathing

The risk of SDB increases about fourfold at the time of menopause, independent of age and body mass index, for hormonal reasons related to progesterone and testosterone that have already been described [23]. It is important to note that OSA in older age is associated with increased risk of cognitive impairment. Cognitive dysfunction due to OSA can sometimes be reversed with CPAP therapy. The OSA-associated risk of hypertension and stroke may further complicate comorbidities in older patients. The treatment for OSA in menopausal women is the same as elsewhere, except there might be an expanded role for hormonal therapy in selected circumstances.

Insomnia

The prevalence of insomnia increases in the premenopausal (~30%) to the postmenopausal period (~50–60%), which may be associated with the presence of vasomotor symptoms, age-related changes in sleep, and comorbid conditions [43]. In premenopausal women, night sweats may precipitate insomnia symptoms, but over time, other perpetuating factors and poor sleep hygiene may result in chronic insomnia. Non-HRT prescription medications such as fluoxetine, paroxetine, venlafaxine, and gabapentin have been reported to alleviate perimenopausal symptoms. Cognitive behavioral therapy may be effective in treating perimenopausal insomnia and should be considered as the first-line treatment of insomnia. Prolonged-released melatonin has good tolerability, safety, and efficacy on sleep and daytime function and should be considered as a first-line drug in women aged over 55 years [43]. Obstructive sleep apnea must be considered in the differential diagnosis of a perimenopausal woman complaining of insomnia because of increased prevalence and atypical presentation with insomnia in this population.

Hormone Replacement Therapy

Most studies have shown that both estrogen therapy alone and a combination of estrogen/progestogen HRT have some efficacy in improving subjective sleep quality and daytime sleepiness. Hormone replacement therapy also seems to have a modest effect in the treatment of OSA: a Sleep Heart Health study showed that the prevalence of OSA and SDB in women receiving HRT was found to be half that of women not taking HRT [44]. The possible mechanism is progesterone-related respiratory stimulation and upper airway dilatation.

Importantly, however, a Women's Health Initiative trial showed harm with HRT. This randomized, placebo-controlled trial found an increased risk of vascular disease and cancer in woman taking conjugated equine estrogens with medroxyprogesterone [45, 46]. The study has been criticized for not including women with severe menopausal symptoms, who would have been expected to derive the most benefit.

Currently, most physicians look for alternatives to HRT for the treatment of menopausal insomnia. Hormone replacement therapy may still have a role in the short-term treatment of women with severe menopausal symptoms, and in these circumstances, benefit to short-term quality of life must be weighed against the risk of long-term harm. For some women, the improvement in quality of life with HRT is dramatic. Estrogen is thought to mediate the harmful effects, and therefore the lowest effective dose of estrogen should be used, and HRT should be frequently reassessed to facilitate discontinuation when appropriate.

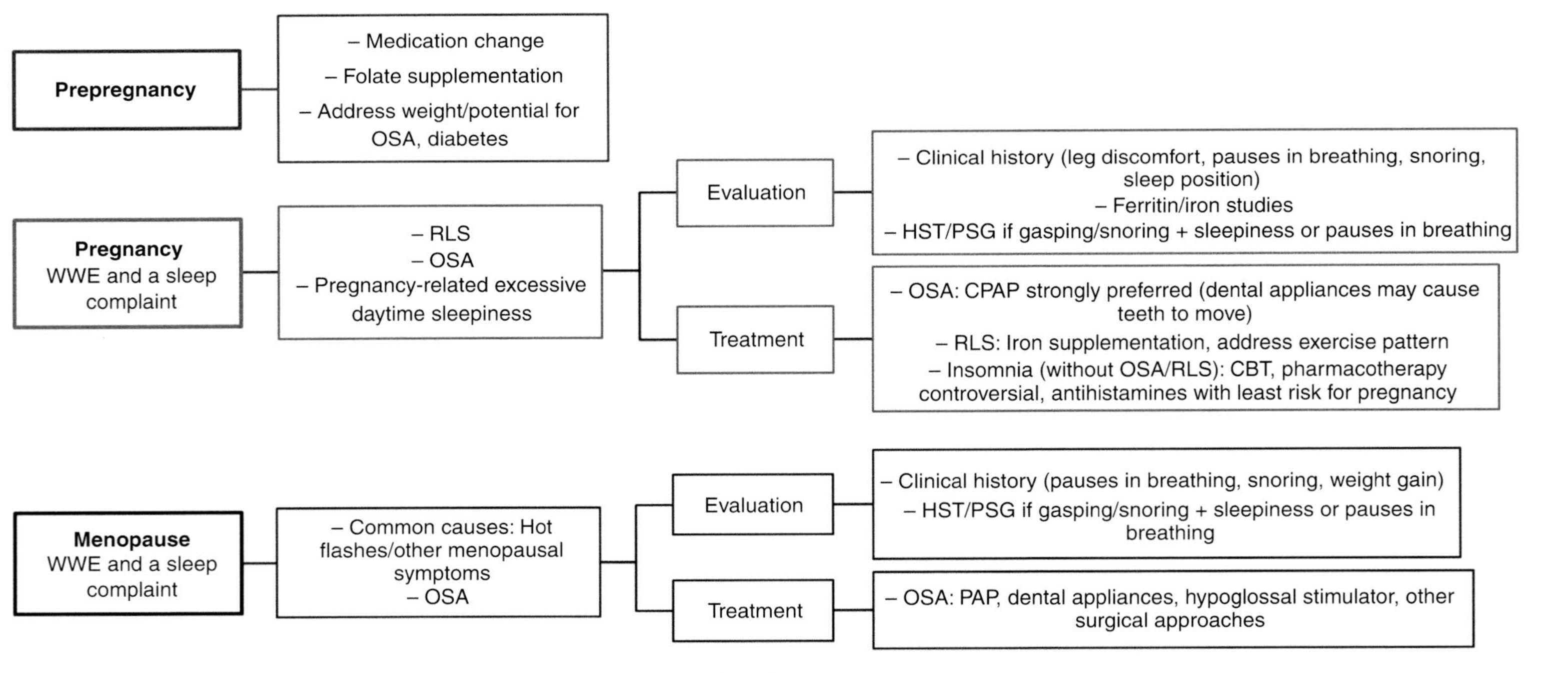

Figure 3.1 Evaluation and treatment of major sleep problems in women with epilepsy from prepregnancy to menopause
CBT: Cognitive behavioral therapy; CPAP: Continuous positive airway pressure; HST: Home sleep testing; OSA: Obstructive sleep apnea; PSG: Polysomnography; RLS: Restless legs syndrome; WWE: Women with epilepsy

Indications for Sleep Medicine Consultation and Polysomnography

It is important to note that sleep disruption can lead to cognitive impairments, and drowsiness is of major concern in patients who need to maintain alertness for safety reasons such as driving. Referral to a sleep specialist and/or sleep testing may be considered in the following circumstances:

- When a primary sleep disorder is suspected, especially SDB – for example, a history of snoring and sleepiness or witnessed apneas and so forth.
- When the patient exhibits sleepiness despite adequate sleep opportunity and narcolepsy or another central hypersomnia is suspected – the testing may include not only a polysomnogram, but also a daytime test called the Multiple Sleep Latency Test or other confirmatory tests.
- Where the diagnosis of nocturnal events is in question: distinguishing seizures from parasomnias particularly with complex profiles – the testing may include combining a standard polysomnogram and a standard 10–20 EEG recording.
- When comorbidities are multiple and lead to complex treatment decisions.
- When seizures or sleep symptoms are refractory to treatment, as this may be due to a primary sleep disorder.
- When safety concerns are present regarding nocturnal behaviors or alertness for driving.

Conclusion

Though minimal research has focused on sleep disorders in women with epilepsy, clinicians can extrapolate from what is currently known about sleep disorders in patients with epilepsy and sleep disorders in women. Sleep disorders in epilepsy are common, and the incidence and presentation of sleep disorders in women differs from that in men. Sleep disorders and epilepsy can exacerbate each other; therefore, optimal treatment of both aspects can be expected to produce the best outcome. Pregnancy is a particularly high-risk time for women with epilepsy, and correction of sleep disorders with a few simple interventions can improve the health of mother and baby. Menopause also has significant implications for sleep. Simple interventions often make dramatic differences to patients and their families – it may be as simple as changing the timing of ASM dosing or sleeping in the lateral decubitus position. Sleep disorders in women can be associated with significant morbidity and deterioration in quality of life and therefore warrant attention.

References

1. Bubrick EJ, Yazdani S, Pavlova MK. Beyond standard polysomnography: Advantages and indications for use of extended 10–20 EEG montage during laboratory sleep study evaluations. *Seizure*. 2014 Oct;**23**(9):699–702.
2. Vaughn BV, D'Cruz OF. Sleep and epilepsy. In *Clinical sleep disorders*. Carney PR, Berry RB, Geyer JD, eds. Philadelphia, PA: Ovid Technologies Inc., Lippincott Williams & Wilkins; 2005, pp. 403–19.
3. Pavlova MK, Lee JW, Yilmaz F, Dworetzky BA. Diurnal pattern of seizures outside the hospital: Is there a time of circadian vulnerability? *Neurology*. 2012 May 8;**78**(19):1488–92.

4. Khan S, Nobili L, Khatami R, et al. Circadian rhythm and epilepsy. *Lancet Neurol.* 2018 Dec 1;**17**(12):1098–108.
5. Anderson CT, Tcheng TK, Sun FT, Morrell MJ. Day-night patterns of epileptiform activity in 65 patients with long-term ambulatory electrocorticography. *J Clin Neurophysiol Off Publ Am Electroencephalogr Soc.* 2015 Oct;**32**(5):406–12.
6. Spencer DC, Sun FT, Brown SN, et al. Circadian and ultradian patterns of epileptiform discharges differ by seizure-onset location during long-term ambulatory intracranial monitoring. *Epilepsia.* 2016 Sep;**57**(9):1495–502.
7. Passarelli V, Castro LHM. Gender and age influence in daytime and nighttime seizure occurrence in epilepsy associated with mesial temporal sclerosis. *Epilepsy Behav EB.* 2015 Sep;**50**:14–17.
8. Baud MO, Kleen JK, Mirro EA, et al. Multi-day rhythms modulate seizure risk in epilepsy. *Nat Commun.* 2018 Jan 8;**9**(88):1–10.
9. Pavlova MK, Shea SA, Scheer FAJL, Bromfield EB. Is there a circadian variation of epileptiform abnormalities in idiopathic generalized epilepsy? *Epilepsy Behav EB.* 2009 Nov;**16**(3):461–7.
10. Sandhu MRS, Dhaher R, Gruenbaum SE, et al. Circadian-like rhythmicity of extracellular brain glutamate in epilepsy. *Front Neurol.* 2020;**11**(398):1–6.
11. Devinsky O, Hesdorffer DC, Thurman DJ, Lhatoo S, Richerson G. Sudden unexpected death in epilepsy: Epidemiology, mechanisms, and prevention. *Lancet Neurol.* 2016 Sep 1;**15**(10):1075–88.
12. Pavlova M. Sudden unexpected death in epilepsy: Assessing the risk factors. *Neurology.* 2020 Jan 28;**94**(4):e436–8.
13. Peter-Derex L, Klimes P, Latreille V, et al. Sleep disruption in epilepsy: Ictal and interictal epileptic activity matter. *Ann Neurol.* 2020 Nov;**88**(5):907–20.
14. Latreille V, Abdennadher M, Dworetzky BA, et al. Nocturnal seizures are associated with more severe hypoxemia and increased risk of postictal generalized EEG suppression. *Epilepsia.* 2017;**58**(9): e127–31.
15. Salvadé A, Ryvlin P, Rossetti AO. Impact of vagus nerve stimulation on sleep-related breathing disorders in adults with epilepsy. *Epilepsy Behav EB.* 2018 Feb;**79**:126–9.
16. Ng M, Pavlova M. Why are seizures rare in rapid eye movement sleep? Review of the frequency of seizures in different sleep stages. *Epilepsy Res Treat.* 2013;**2013**:932790.
17. Glick TH. The sleep-deprived electroencephalogram: Evidence and practice. *Arch Neurol.* 2002 Aug;**59**(8):1235–9.
18. Sinha SR. Basic mechanisms of sleep and epilepsy. *J Clin Neurophysiol Off Publ Am Electroencephalogr Soc.* 2011 Apr;**28**(2):103–10.
19. Chokroverty S, Montagna P. Sleep and epilepsy. In *Sleep disorders medicine: Basic science, technical considerations, and clinical aspects.* 3rd ed. Chokroverty S, ed. Philadelphia, PA: Saunders Elsevier; 2009. pp. 499–529.
20. Frauscher B, Gotman J. Sleep, oscillations, interictal discharges, and seizures in human focal epilepsy. *Neurobiol Dis.* 2019 Jul 1;**127**:545–53.
21. Scalise A, Desiato MT, Gigli GL, et al. Increasing cortical excitability: A possible explanation for the proconvulsant role of sleep deprivation. *Sleep.* 2006 Dec 1;**29**(12):1595–8.
22. Yeh WC, Lu SR, Wu MN, et al. The impact of antiseizure medications on polysomnographic parameters: A systematic review and meta-analysis. *Sleep Med.* 2021 May;**81**:319–26.
23. Andersen ML, Alvarenga TF, Mazaro-Costa R, Hachul HC, Tufik S. The association of testosterone, sleep, and sexual function in men and women. *Brain Res.* 2011 Oct 6;**1416**:80–104.
24. Herzog AG. Neuroactive properties of reproductive steroids. *Headache J Head Face Pain.* 2007;**47**(s2):S68–78.

25. Mong JA, Baker FC, Mahoney MM, et al. Sleep, rhythms, and the endocrine brain: Influence of sex and gonadal hormones. *J Neurosci Off J Soc Neurosci*. 2011 Nov 9;**31**(45):16107–16.
26. Driver HS, Mclean H, Kumar DV, et al. The influence of the menstrual cycle on upper airway resistance and breathing during sleep. *Sleep*. 2005 Apr 1;**28**(4):449–56.
27. Driver HS, Sloan EP. Women's sleep. In *Sleep disorders medicine: Basic science, technical considerations, and clinical aspects*. 3rd ed. Chokroverty S., ed. Philadelphia, PA: Saunders Elsevier; 2009. pp. 644–53.
28. American Academy of Sleep Medicine. *International classification of sleep disorders*. 3rd ed. Darien, IL: American Academy of Sleep Medicine; 2014.
29. van Golde EGA, Gutter T, de Weerd AW. Sleep disturbances in people with epilepsy: Prevalence, impact and treatment. *Sleep Med Rev*. 2011 Dec;**15**(6):357–68.
30. Latreille V, St Louis EK, Pavlova M. Co-morbid sleep disorders and epilepsy: A narrative review and case examples. *Epilepsy Res*. 2018 Sep;**145**:185–97.
31. Grigg-Damberger M, Andrews N, Wang L, Bena J, Foldvary-Schaefer N. Subjective and objective hypersomnia highly prevalent in adults with epilepsy. *Epilepsy Behav EB*. 2020 May;**106**:107023.
32. Bergmann M, Tschiderer L, Stefani A, et al. Sleep quality and daytime sleepiness in epilepsy: Systematic review and meta-analysis of 25 studies including 8,196 individuals. *Sleep Med Rev*. 2021 Jun;**57**:101466.
33. Arnedt JT, Owens J, Crouch M, Stahl J, Carskadon MA. Neurobehavioral performance of residents after heavy night call vs. after alcohol ingestion. *JAMA*. 2005 Sep 7;**294**(9):1025–33.
34. Macêdo PJOM, de Oliveira PS, Foldvary-Schaefer N, da Gomes M. Insomnia in people with epilepsy: A review of insomnia prevalence, risk factors and associations with epilepsy-related factors. *Epilepsy Res*. 2017 Sep;**135**:158–67.
35. Quigg M, Gharai S, Ruland J, et al. Insomnia in epilepsy is associated with continuing seizures and worse quality of life. *Epilepsy Res*. 2016 May;**122**:91–6.
36. Ahorsu DK, Lin CY, Imani V, et al. Testing an app-based intervention to improve insomnia in patients with epilepsy: A randomized controlled trial. *Epilepsy Behav EB*. 2020 Nov 1;**112**:107371.
37. Pavlova M, Sheikh LS. Sleep in women. *Semin Neurol*. 2011 Sep;**31**(4):397–403.
38. Lin Z, Si Q, Xiaoyi Z. Obstructive sleep apnoea in patients with epilepsy: A meta-analysis. *Sleep Breath Schlaf Atm*. 2017 May;**21**(2):263–70.
39. Latreille V, Willment KC, Sarkis RA, Pavlova M. Neuropsychological correlates of obstructive sleep apnea severity in patients with epilepsy. *Epileptic Disord Int Epilepsy J Videotape*. 2019 Feb 1;**21**(1):78–86.
40. Kohn M, Murray BJ. Sleep and quality of life in pregnancy. In *Sleep and quality of life in medical illnesses*. Verster JC, Pandi-Perumal SR, Streiner D, eds. Totowa, NJ: Humana Press; 2008. pp. 497–504.
41. Garbazza C, Hackethal S, Riccardi S, et al. Polysomnographic features of pregnancy: A systematic review. *Sleep Med Rev*. 2020 Apr;**50**:101249.
42. Pengo MF, Won CH, Bourjeily G. Sleep in women across the life span. *Chest*. 2018 Jul;**154**(1):196–206.
43. Proserpio P, Marra S, Campana C, et al. Insomnia and menopause: A narrative review on mechanisms and treatments. *Climacteric J Int Menopause Soc*. 2020 Dec;**23**(6):539–49.
44. Shahar E, Redline S, Young T, et al. Hormone replacement therapy and sleep-disordered breathing. *Am J Respir Crit Care Med*. 2003 May 1;**167**(9):1186–92.
45. Manson JE, Hsia J, Johnson KC, et al. Estrogen plus progestin and the risk of coronary heart disease. *N Engl J Med*. 2003 Aug 7;**349**(6):523–34.
46. Chlebowski RT, Kuller LH, Prentice RL, et al. Breast cancer after use of estrogen plus progestin in postmenopausal women. *N Engl J Med*. 2009 Feb 5;**360**(6):573–87.

Chapter 4

Hormonal Influences in Women with Epilepsy

Suchitra Joshi and Jaideep Kapur

Key Points

- Progesterone and estrogen are the primary female reproductive hormones.
- These hormones regulate neuronal activity indirectly via metabolites and directly via the classical steroid hormone receptors, progesterone and estrogen.
- The hormonal regulation of neuronal activity could manifest as catamenial epilepsy in women of reproductive age with epilepsy, which results from cyclic changes in seizure frequency coincident with menstrual cycle–linked hormonal fluctuations.
- Estrogen primarily exerts excitatory, proconvulsant effects through potentiation of glutamatergic transmission.
- Progesterone can suppress seizures through the metabolite allopregnanolone, a potent modulator of GABA-A receptors. In contrast, progesterone receptor activation has a seizure-promoting effect.

Introduction

Progesterone and estrogen are the principal female reproductive hormones; estradiol is the principal and most potent estrogen. The gonadotropin-releasing hormone secreted by the hypothalamus triggers the secretion of follicular-stimulating hormone (FSH). Follicular-stimulating hormone induces the maturation of ovarian follicles, which secrete estradiol, the principal estrogen in women. The corpus luteum formed following ovulation secretes progesterone. In the absence of pregnancy, the corpus luteum regresses and levels of estrogens and progesterone decrease. Additionally, adrenal glands synthesize these hormones in minor amounts. During pregnancy, the placenta is the primary source of these hormones.

Cholesterol converts to these hormones through enzymatic conversion, and steroidogenic organs express multiple enzymes regulating this conversion. The brain also expresses them; neurons and glia express the enzymes involved in steroid biosynthesis [1–3]. Thus, the brain can synthesize these steroid hormones and their neuroactive metabolites to maintain their levels independent of peripheral circulation [4].

The neuronal effects of these female reproductive hormones came to light when Hans Selye demonstrated the sedative and anesthetic effects of progesterone [5]. Since then, studies have revealed that progesterone and estrogen impact brain function under pathophysiological conditions. These hormones regulate neurotransmission and neuronal excitability in the neuroendocrine and limbic systems. Although seizures are primarily unpredictable, internal and external factors affect their occurrence. The female reproductive hormones are perhaps the most predominant and intensely studied internal factors regulating neuronal excitability and consequent seizure precipitation.

Cyclic changes take place in progesterone and estrogen levels during the reproductive years. Significant hormonal changes also occur at puberty, around menopause, and during pregnancy. Epilepsy onset may occur around puberty, or seizures may worsen [6, 7]. The perimenopausal hormone levels are erratic, and they decline after menopause. These changes could also affect seizure frequency. Seizure frequency eases after menopause, particularly in women with catamenial epilepsy [8]. Interestingly, hormone replacement therapy after menopause could increase seizure frequency [8, 9].

Catamenial Epilepsy

Hormonal regulation of seizures manifests in menstrual cycle–linked seizure exacerbation in women with epilepsy of childbearing age. This seizure exacerbation is called catamenial epilepsy when the seizure frequency is at least double at key days within the ovarian-menstrual cycle as opposed to the rest. The link between female reproductive hormones and seizures has been known for decades [10–12]; however, even today, no drug approved by the Food and Drug Administration (FDA) indicated explicitly for catamenial epilepsy is available. As many as 70% of women with epilepsy of childbearing age may experience menstrual cycle–linked seizure exacerbation, and the changes in seizure frequency in as many as 30% of the women fulfill the criteria for catamenial epilepsy, which remains the prevalent form of drug-refractory epilepsy in women. Since catamenial epilepsy is discussed in detail elsewhere in this book (Chapter 8), we will briefly discuss the link between hormonal fluctuations during the menstrual cycle and their influence on seizure frequency.

Using seizure diaries to identify seizure peaks and troughs, Herzog and colleagues identified three patterns – C1, C2, and C3 – of catamenial seizures based on the cycle phase linked to seizure precipitation [12]. The perimenstrual seizure exacerbation (C1) occurs around menses, whereas in the C2, more seizures occur at the time of ovulation. The third type, C3, occurs due to the inadequate luteal phase. Reproductive endocrine disorders are common in women with epilepsy [13–15], and mid-luteal progesterone rise may be abnormally low, which could lead to seizure exacerbation during the ovulatory, luteal, and perimenstrual phases. Even without a priori hormonal considerations, seizures follow a circa-lunar (the pattern repeating approximately every 29 days, similar to the length of a typical menstrual cycle) and ultra-lunar (periodicity occurring at < 29 days) periodicity; in a retrospective study, the best fit of more than 3,000 seizures from 100 patients revealed a rhythmic seizure exacerbation that occurred every 28 days, the duration of a menstrual cycle [16]. Patients with temporal lobe epilepsy, particularly with left-sided foci, are more prone to perimenstrual seizure exacerbation, with seizures peaking at the onset of menstruation [17]. On the other hand, seizures in patients with extra-temporal lobe foci or multiple foci are distributed randomly during the menstrual cycle.

The estrogen levels rise during the ovulatory phase of the menstrual cycle, followed by a rise in progesterone levels during the luteal phase. A high estrogen-to-progesterone ratio is proposed to cause periovulatory seizure precipitation. On the other hand, progesterone withdrawal causes perimenstrual seizure exacerbation. The seizures in the C3 type also occur because progesterone levels do not rise sufficiently during the luteal phase. Low progesterone levels are a common factor underlying the three patterns of catamenial seizures. This suggests that maintaining progesterone levels through exogenous administration could prevent catamenial worsening.

In a large clinical trial, women with and without catamenial epilepsy took natural progesterone (200 mg) or placebo three times daily on days 14–28 of menstrual cycles. Surprisingly, natural progesterone and placebo treatments were indistinguishable; the proportion of responders, women experiencing a 50% decline in seizure frequency, was similar between the progesterone and placebo-treated groups [18]. A predetermined post hoc logistical regression analysis revealed that women with C1 and C2 types of catamenial epilepsy were more likely to respond to the treatment. The anticipated primary outcome of the study was a reduction in seizure frequency in 30% of progesterone-treated women and 15% of placebo-treated patients. This outcome was achieved for women who experienced a threefold or more increase in seizures perimenstrually. Thus, although the treatment was not beneficial for all catamenial epilepsy patients, a subset of patients with a severe C1 type seizure exacerbation seemed to benefit from it. A study focused only on these patients is needed to test the therapeutic efficacy of progesterone for this type of seizure exacerbation. Importantly, this study highlights the complexity of the hormonal regulation of seizures and raises a need for animal studies to evaluate whether the activation of various cellular progesterone-signaling molecules uniformly dampens neuronal activity.

Animal Models of Catamenial Epilepsy

The reproductive cycles in mice and rats, called estrous cycles, are 4 or 5 days long and are accompanied by a cyclic rise and fall of progesterone and estrogen. Estrous cycle–linked hormonal fluctuations affect susceptibility to evoked seizures [19–21]. These changes also regulate susceptibility to prolonged seizures of status epilepticus [22]. The epileptic animal brain is distinct from that of non-epileptic animals because of neurodegeneration, altered network connections, and plasticity of neurotransmitter receptors. Hence, using epileptic animals will be ideal to understand the pathogenesis of catamenial epilepsy. The seizure burden also appears to fluctuate during the estrous cycle in epileptic animals [23]. However, many epileptic animals become acyclic or have irregular cycles [24, 25]. Thus, evaluating changes in seizures due to endogenous hormone cycling is difficult in experimental animals.

We used the pseudopregnancy model of Reddy and colleagues [26] to determine the mechanisms underlying perimenstrual seizure exacerbation. The female epileptic animals were treated with serum gonadotropins [25, 27]. These treatments cause a chronic elevation of the circulating progesterone levels. Ten days after initiating the hormone treatment, finasteride, an inhibitor of enzyme 5α-reductase, was administered to inhibit neurosteroid synthesis, preventing the conversion of progesterone to allopregnanolone, and it caused seizure exacerbation [25, 27]. Allopregnanolone administered to the finasteride-treated animals suppressed the seizure exacerbation, indicating that the reduced levels of allopregnanolone were a major contributing factor. Although this model mimics the perimenstrual decline in allopregnanolone levels, finasteride treatment causes the accumulation of progesterone. Thus, although this model is helpful to evaluate the role of endogenous and exogenous progesterone in controlling seizures, it does not fully replicate the perimenstrual hormonal milieu. Furthermore, other progesterone effector molecules, including progesterone receptors, membrane progesterone receptors (mPRs), and progesterone receptor membrane component 1 (PGRMC1), are also expressed in the brain. The chronically

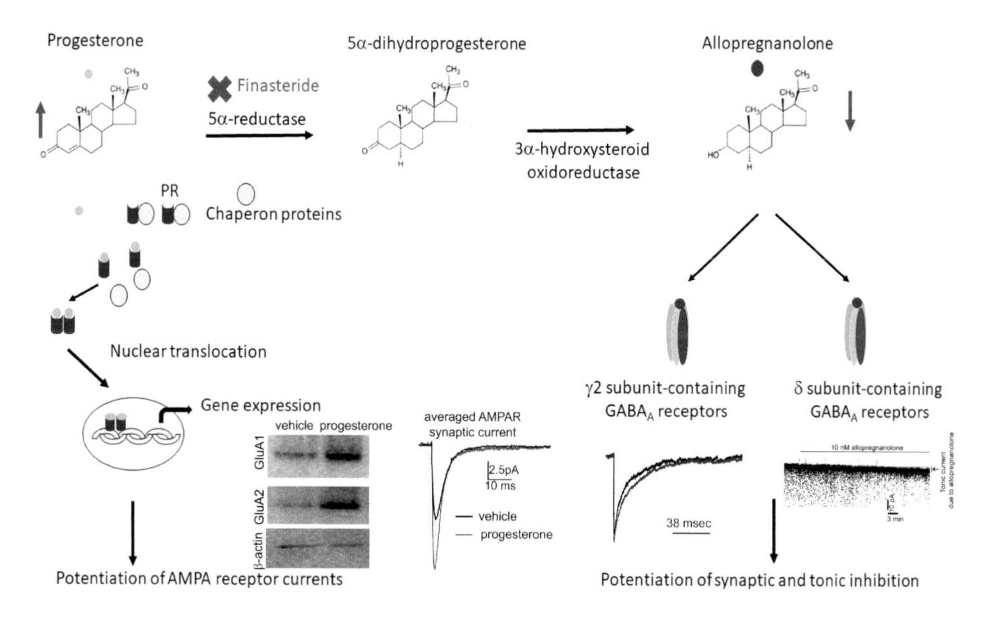

Figure 4.1 A schematic showing opposing actions of progesterone exerted through PRs and allopregnanolone. Progesterone is metabolized to allopregnanolone through enzymatic conversion. Finasteride blocks the activity of 5α-reductase, the enzyme regulating the rate-limiting step in the progesterone metabolism, leading to a decline in allopregnanolone levels and a concomitant increase in progesterone levels. Progesterone also binds to PRs. The PRs are kept sequestered in the cytoplasm through interaction with chaperon proteins; binding of progesterone to PRs leads to their dissociation from chaperon proteins, dimerization of the receptors, and translocation to the nucleus. Within the nucleus, PRs bind to the hormone response elements either alone or through interaction with other transcriptional regulators, and trigger gene expression. We have found that PR activation increases hippocampal AMPA receptor expression and potentiates AMPA receptor-mediated synaptic transmission of CA1 pyramidal neurons and entorhinal cortical neurons. This AMPA receptor plasticity could increase excitability of these neurons and exert a seizure-promoting effect. The progesterone metabolite allopregnanolone is a positive allosteric modulator of the synaptic and extrasynaptic GABA$_A$ receptors and potentiates the synaptic and tonic GABAergic inhibition. The potentiation of tonic current can be recorded as a change in the background current (holding current). The representative voltage-clamp recordings shown here are from hippocampal DGCs, which have a high expression of δ subunit-containing GABA$_A$ receptors. In the DGCs, the δ subunit-containing GABA$_A$ receptors, which have incomplete and slow desensitization, mediate most of the tonic current. In the tonic current recording trace shown here, application of allopregnanolone (10 nM) caused a shift in the baseline holding current, the extent of which corresponded to the potentiation of tonic current by allopregnanolone. The neurosteroids also potentiate the synaptic current and prolongation of the decay is seen following application of low nanomolar concentration of allopregnanolone. The representative trace shown here elucidates the decay before (black) and after (red) application of 10 nM allopregnanolone. These actions underlie the anticonvulsant effects of progesterone.

elevated progesterone levels in the hormone-treated animals, as well as an additional acute rise in progesterone levels due to blockade of its metabolism to allopregnanolone following finasteride treatment, could activate these effector molecules (Figure 4.1). As discussed later in this chapter, the role of other progesterone effector molecules like progesterone receptors in seizure regulation is starting to emerge (Table 4.1).

We developed another perimenstrual-like seizure exacerbation model devoid of the nonspecific effects of pregnant Meyer's serum gonadotropin (PMSG), human chorionic gonadotropin β subunit (β-HCG), and finasteride. We administered progesterone to the animals every day for a week to elevate its levels and then stopped the administration to induce progesterone withdrawal like that which happens during the perimenstrual period.

Table 4.1 Studies demonstrating anticonvulsant and seizure-promoting effects of progesterone

Study	Model	Results	Mechanism
[26]	Pseudopregnancy model in female rats: Day −2: Administration of pregnant mares' serum gonadotropin (20 IU/rat, s.c.) Day 0: Administration of human chorionic gonadotropin (β-HCG, 10 IU/rat, s.c.) Day 11: Administration of finasteride (100 mg/kg, i.p.) or vehicle (control) Day 12: Administration of pentylenetetrazol (PTZ, 30–100 mg/kg, s.c.)	Finasteride-treated animals were more sensitive to PTZ-induced seizures.	Anti-seizure effects of neurosteroids
[117]	Pseudopregnancy model in female rats 3 week progesterone capsule implantation followed by the capsule removal to cause progesterone withdrawal	Progesterone withdrawal increased the severity of seizures triggered by n-methyl-b-carboline–3-carboxamide or picrotoxin	Antiseizure effects of neurosteroids
[27]	Pseudopregnancy model in female epileptic rats	The frequency of recurrent spontaneous seizures was ~26 times that at the baseline during the 24 hours following finasteride administration. The seizure frequency was 11 times that at baseline following finasteride administration in animals without hormone treatment.	Antiseizure effects of neurosteroids
[118]	Case study in a woman with epilepsy Cyclic progesterone treatment for seizures 2 years followed by addition of finasteride for male pattern baldness	Seizures were controlled with cyclic progesterone treatment, but their frequency increased after the patient started to also take finasteride. The seizures were again controlled when the use of finasteride was stopped.	Antiseizure effects of neurosteroids

[25]	Pseudopregnancy model in female epileptic rats Administration of Ru–486 (10 mg/kg/day, i. p.) or vehicle (control) for the duration of hormone treatment Finasteride (100 mg/kg, i.p.) 10 days after β-HCG	Only a sixfold increase in seizures during the 24-hour period following finasteride administration in the Ru–486-treated animals compared to ~22-fold increase in seizure frequency in animals treated with the vehicle along with the hormones.	Antiseizure effects of neurosteroids and pro-seizure effects of progesterone receptor activation
[28]	(A) Progesterone treatment (50 mg/kg/day, i. p.) of female epileptic rats for a week followed by a week of progesterone withdrawal. Treatment of animals with Ru-486 (10 mg/kg/day, i.p.) or the vehicle during the duration of progesterone treatment (B) Treatment of female epileptic animals with PR agonist nestorone (3 mg/kg/day, s.c.) or vehicle for a week	(A) Seizure frequency increased during the week of progesterone withdrawal in vehicle-treated animals but not in the Ru-486–treated animals. (B) The animals experienced more seizures during the week of Nestorone treatment compared to the baseline seizure frequency.	Pro-seizure effects of progesterone receptor activation
[29]	Nestorone treatment (3 mg/kg/day, s. c.) for a week in female epileptic rats with PRs or with a global deletion of progesterone receptors	Nestorone did not increase the frequency of recurrent spontaneous seizures in rats lacking progesterone receptors.	Pro-seizure effects of progesterone receptor activation
[30]	Kindling of progesterone receptor mice	Mice with a global deletion of progesterone receptors kindled slower than the wild-type mice	Pro-seizure effects of progesterone receptor activation

As expected, progesterone withdrawal increased seizure frequency [28]. A doubling of seizures during one phase of the menstrual cycle compared to the other phases was set as a threshold for exacerbation in patients. We found that progesterone withdrawal alone, without finasteride, also caused seizure exacerbation in experimental animals [28]. Thus, progesterone withdrawal caused a seizure exacerbation similar to that observed in women. This was in contrast to a dramatic 15–20-fold increase in seizure frequency induced by finasteride. A near-complete depletion of all neurosteroids, including those derived from glucocorticoids, could account for the substantial rise in seizure frequency seen in finasteride-treated animals. Additionally, an acute increase in progesterone levels in finasteride-treated animals may activate other progesterone signaling molecules, increasing excitability.

Using both the neurosteroid-withdrawal model and the progesterone-withdrawal model of perimenstrual seizure exacerbation, we uncovered a role of progesterone receptors in regulating seizures. Treatment of animals with progesterone receptor antagonist Ru-486 with the hormone treatment attenuated the seizure precipitation triggered by neurosteroid withdrawal or progesterone withdrawal [25, 28]. Furthermore, the progesterone receptor activation with a specific agonist, nestorone, increased the frequency of spontaneous seizures [28]. These complementary approaches demonstrate a seizure-promoting role of progesterone receptor activation, which could counteract the anticonvulsant effects mediated through allopregnanolone. Pharmacological agents could have limitations such as limited bioavailability and potential off-target effects; however, studies using progesterone receptor knockout animals also support the seizure-promoting role of progesterone receptor signaling. Epileptic rats lacking progesterone receptors do not experience seizure exacerbation triggered by nestorone treatment [29]. Mice lacking progesterone receptor expression are also slower to kindle [30]. Progesterone is not always anticonvulsant; increased seizures were also found in women epilepsy patients taking hormonal contraceptives containing only progesterone [31, 32]. This increase in seizure burden could be due to the proconvulsant effects of progesterone receptor activation [Table 4.1].

It is also noteworthy that elevated progesterone levels in the hormone-treated animals did not reduce seizure frequency, which is similar to the findings of progesterone clinical trials [18, 33]. This lack of effect is perhaps due to opposing actions of allopregnanolone and progesterone receptor activation (Figure 4.1). Additionally, GABA-A receptors, which are targets of allopregnanolone, are also altered in epilepsy. The progesterone's anticonvulsant effect is observed commonly after acute administration and rapid depletion of neurosteroids; these studies miss the chronic action through progesterone receptor [34–38]. Progesterone receptors are nuclear hormone receptors and exert cellular effects through altered gene expression. This effect occurs over hours to days compared to the rapid impact of allopregnanolone exerted over minutes. Thus, a single dose of progesterone, studied acutely, has an anticonvulsant effect, but it disappears when repeated doses are given over a long time in chronically epileptic animals. As discussed earlier in this chapter, the human clinical trial also reveals a complex picture.

Allopregnanolone Mediates Progesterone's Anticonvulsant Effects

Progesterone exerts anticonvulsant effects through allopregnanolone. Finasteride blocks the activity of enzyme 5α-reductase, which regulates a rate-limiting step in the biosynthesis of allopregnanolone and other neurosteroids. Finasteride administration or 5α-reductase deletion prevents progesterone's anticonvulsant effects, whereas administration of allopregnanolone suppresses seizures [27, 36, 39, 40, 41]. Neurosteroids dampen neuronal excitability by potentiating GABAergic inhibition [42–45]. The rank order potency of allopregnanolone's anticonvulsant actions is similar to its actions on GABA-A receptors [46]. Allopregnanolone potentiates GABAergic inhibition via allosteric mechanisms at low concentrations or agonist-like activity at higher concentrations. Neurosteroids inhibit neurons to a varying degree because different neurons express different types of GABA-A receptor subtypes. For example, the GABA-A receptors containing a δ subunit are more sensitive to the allopregnanolone modulation than others [47, 48]. Neurosteroid regulation of neuronal activity is prominent in the hippocampal dentate granule cells (DGCs), which have a high expression of these receptors. The δ subunit-containing receptors mediate a steady background inhibition called tonic inhibition [42, 47]. The neurosteroid potentiation of tonic inhibition is reduced in mice lacking the δ subunit, and they are less effective in controlling neuronal excitability [22, 42, 49].

Epilepsy-associated alterations in the GABA-A receptor expression reduce the effectiveness of neurosteroids. The δ-subunit expression is reduced in epileptic animals, and this diminishes neurosteroid enhancement of tonic inhibition of DGCs [43, 50]. Additionally, neurosteroid sensitivity of granule cells is altered due to reduced expression of $\alpha 1\beta x\gamma 2$ subunit-containing and increased expression of $\alpha 4\beta x\gamma 2$-containing GABA-A receptors in epileptic animals. Neurosteroids are less effective on whole-cell GABA-evoked, synaptic, and tonic currents in granule cells of epileptic animals [43, 45, 50–52].

We confirmed these findings in experimental animal models and in human patients. The expression of α4 subunits was increased in cortical specimens obtained from pediatric epilepsy patients encompassing multiple pathologies. The potentiation of GABA-evoked currents by the neurosteroid allopregnanolone was decreased in Xenopus oocytes expressing GABA-A receptors isolated from epilepsy patients [53]. These findings suggest that the alterations seen in experimental animals agree with the findings in patients. Furthermore, mutations in two enzymes involved in neurosteroid biosynthesis, which causes allopregnanolone deficiency, are also associated with a female-limited epileptic encephalopathy [54]. Thus, the expression of GABA-A receptors with diminished neurosteroid sensitivity in epilepsy combined with declining allopregnanolone levels could be a major factor contributing to the perimenstrual seizure exacerbation.

The expression of δ subunit-containing receptors decreases soon after status epilepticus, an epileptogenic stimulus in experimental animals, whereas spontaneous seizures trigger the upregulation of $\alpha 4\beta x\gamma 2$ subunit-containing receptors [43, 52, 55]. The rapid diminution in neurosteroid potentiation of tonic current following status epilepticus could contribute to the impairment of dentate gating function [56, 57]. Thus, progesterone or allopregnanolone's control of neuronal excitability could also regulate epileptogenesis.

Progesterone's Proconvulsant Effects Exerted through Progesterone Receptor Activation

Progesterone receptors are also critical cellular progesterone-signaling molecules. The two main isoforms of progesterone receptors, PR-A and PR-B, mediate progesterone's genomic effects [58, 59]. The isoforms are encoded from a single locus, but their expression and function could differ in a region- and tissue-specific manner [60, 61]. Distinctions in their interaction with other transcription factors and co-activators also add to their regulatory effects' complexity. PR-B appears to be a better transcriptional activator than PR-A. Ligand-binding triggers dimerization and nuclear translocation of PRs and induction of gene expression.

Progesterone receptors are expressed widely in the brain, including limbic circuits comprised of the hippocampus, entorhinal cortex, and amygdala, associated with seizures in temporal lobe epilepsy [29, 62–64]. We have found that progesterone receptor activation potentiates AMPA receptor-mediated neurotransmission of CA1 and entorhinal cortical neurons and increases excitability [25, 29]. Nestorone is a specific progesterone receptor agonist that is free of actions at GABA-A and glucocorticoid receptors [65, 66]. Nestorone treatment increases AMPA receptor expression, similar to that triggered by progesterone [25]. The changes in AMPA receptor expression are accompanied by increased amplitude of the excitatory postsynaptic currents (EPSC) of CA1 neurons and increased frequency of EPSCs of entorhinal cortical neurons [25, 29]. Thus, potentiation of AMPA receptor-mediated glutamatergic transmission could contribute to the excitatory, proconvulsant effects of progesterone. Ru-486 treatment or knockdown of progesterone receptor expression blocks the AMPA receptor upregulation [25].

The progesterone receptor-regulated enhancement of glutamatergic transmission also occurs during the estrous cycle following the endogenous rise in progesterone [25]. The AMPA receptor-mediated synaptic transmission of CA1 neurons is stronger in rats in the estrus stage of the cycle than in the animals in the diestrus stage [25]. These fluctuations in glutamatergic transmission could contribute to estrous cycle–linked differences in excitability of CA1 and CA3 neurons and seizure susceptibility [22, 67, 68]. Indeed, the rats in the estrus stage of the cycle have a lower threshold for electroconvulsive and bicuculline-induced seizures than rats in the diestrus stage [19–21].

In addition to the potentiation of glutamatergic transmission, chronic progesterone treatment appears to suppress the expression of α2 subunits of GABA-A receptors since the termination of the treatment causes a significant upregulation of the subunit mRNA within 24 hours [69]. This enhancement in the progesterone receptor knockout animals is more than twice that in wild-type animals. This raises a possibility that the progesterone-progesterone receptor signaling keeps the α2 subunit expression suppressed, which could affect the strength of inhibitory neurotransmission. Together these studies revealed that progesterone receptor activation potentiates glutamatergic transmission and suppresses GABAergic transmission mediated by a subtype of receptors, increasing seizure susceptibility.

Neuronal Effects of Estrogens

Estradiol, the principal estrogen in women, exerts excitatory effects. Intravenous infusion of estradiol increased spike frequency in most women with focal-onset epilepsy that comprised the study group and triggered tonic-clonic seizures in some of them [10]. Estrogen primarily exerts proconvulsant effects in experimental animals [70]. Estradiol treatment shortens latency to kainate-induced seizures [71, 72], dose-dependently reduces the threshold to electroshock seizures [19], and promotes kindling triggered by stimulation of amygdala or administration of pentylenetetrazole (PTZ) [73, 74]. However, the estrogen effects are not uniformly proconvulsant and vary by the seizure focus location [70]. In some instances, the neuroprotective effects of estradiol have also been found; it could reduce seizure-induced neuronal loss [75–77].

The neuromodulatory effects of estrogens are commonly studied in the hippocampus. The density of dendritic spines fluctuates with the endogenous hormonal changes in female rats; the spines that harbor excitatory synapses are denser when estrogen levels are high [78, 79]. Administration of estradiol to ovariectomized animals also triggers spine formation [79]. Additionally, estradiol also upregulates the expression of synaptic proteins, including PSD95, synaptophysin, and syntaxin; enhances AMPA receptor expression; increases the number of synaptic boutons; and induces spine maturation [80–82]. Estradiol also increases depolarization-induced presynaptic glutamate release in cultured hippocampal neurons [83]. Together these changes potentiate glutamatergic transmission and could increase neuronal excitability. These long-term effects are exerted primarily through NMDA receptor activation [84, 85].

Additionally, acute application of 17β-estradiol potentiates glutamatergic transmission of hippocampal CA1 neurons in brain slices [86, 87]. These rapid changes are unlikely to involve genomic effects, which operate on a longer timescale and indicate the involvement of other cellular effectors. Estrogens are known to trigger long-term potentiation, which involves rapid surface membrane insertion of AMPA receptors. A similar mechanism could underlie the enhancement of excitatory postsynaptic currents found after the acute application of estrogens to the brain slices. Indeed, estradiol-induced synaptic excitability is blocked by AMPA receptor antagonist, but not by NMDA receptor antagonist [88]. The excitatory actions of estrogens also involve the suppression of GABAergic inhibition. Potential mechanisms underlying this effect may involve reduced presynaptic GABA release due to estrogen's inhibitory action on glutamic acid decarboxylase enzyme involved in GABA synthesis and decreased GABA binding to the receptors [89, 90].

The estrogens also exert cellular effects through estrogen receptors (ERs), which belong to the steroid hormone receptor family. The two isoforms of ERs, ER-α and ER-β, are also widely expressed in the central nervous system, including cortico-limbic regions that are critically associated with seizures [91–96]. Some regions have a predominant expression of one isoform over the other [97, 98]. Many of the estrogen's effects potentiating glutamatergic transmission are dependent on the signaling regulated by estrogen receptors [82]. Potentiation of glutamatergic transmission (long-term potentiation) underlies memory formation; this is also impaired in mice lacking estrogen receptors [99].

However, not all estrogen actions are excitatory and proconvulsant [100]. For example, treatment with diarylpropionitrile, an ER-β agonist, increases latency to PTZ-induced seizures [101]. A similar effect is not seen in animals treated with ER-α-modulating agent. ER-β deletion also appears to increase susceptibility to kainate-induced seizures [102]. Estrogen metabolites, including allopregnanolone, may contribute to these neuroprotective effects. The latency to PTZ-induced seizures is shorter in estrogen-treated 5α-reductase knockout mice than in wild-type mice [103]. Estrogens also protect neuropeptide Y (NPY)-expressing GABAergic interneurons from damage due to status epilepticus [104]. Since impairment of GABAergic inhibition plays a critical role in the breakdown of the dentate gating function, this neuroprotective effect could also alter epileptogenesis.

Hormones and Status Epilepticus

Status epilepticus (SE) is a condition of prolonged seizures arising due to failure of seizure termination mechanisms and activation of systems that could sustain abnormal neuronal activity for extended periods. Status epilepticus patients often have a history of epilepsy, and withdrawal from antiepileptic drugs is a factor underlying SE in patients [105]. Although women do not appear to be particularly susceptible to SE, female reproductive hormones seem to regulate susceptibility to SE and seizure intensity. We have found that blocking progesterone receptor signaling attenuates SE; rats with a global deletion of progesterone receptors experience shorter SE and less intense seizures [29]. Several brain regions are active during SE [106], and it is unclear whether all of them express progesterone receptors. However, our finding of progesterone receptor-regulated, fluctuating strength of AMPA receptor-mediated glutamatergic transmission during the female reproductive cycle could explain the varying susceptibility of experimental animals to SE during the estrous cycle. The strength of inhibitory neurotransmission also varies during the estrous cycle, and allopregnanolone-controlled induction of δ subunit-containing GABA-A receptors could be another factor contributing to the distinctions in SE susceptibility [22, 107]. Estrogen signaling also appears to play an important role in regulating seizure intensity during SE. Hippocampal estradiol levels rise during SE in experimental animals, and acute inhibition of estrogen synthesis suppresses kainate-induced electrographic and behavioral seizures [108].

Benzodiazepines are the first-line therapy for SE, but their efficacy declines with seizure progression linked to internalization of γ2 subunit-containing GABA-A receptors [109–112]. Novel treatment strategies are required to treat these seizures. The expression of functional δ subunit-containing GABA-A receptors is unaffected during experimental SE [111]. Neurosteroids that target these receptors could be potential therapeutic agents [113]. Inhibition of aromatase enzymes associated with rising estradiol levels during SE could also provide a novel therapeutic avenue.

Clinical Trials of Neurosteroids as Anticonvulsant Agents

The synthetic neurosteroid ganaxolone, which is more stable than the natural neurosteroid allopregnanolone, is under evaluation for anticonvulsant efficacy in clinical trials (Table 4.2). Ganaxolone treatment either alone or as add-on therapy with other antiepileptic agents seems to be well tolerated in pediatric and adult patients with refractory seizures of varying etiologies. However, these studies have not found a clear advantage of ganaxolone treatment in reducing seizure frequency, although a trend toward reduction was observed. Ganaxolone's lack of efficacy could be in part due to alterations in the GABA-A receptors occurring in epilepsy. The studies in experimental animals have shown that receptors with diminished neurosteroid sensitivity are expressed in the hippocampi of animals with epilepsy [43, 45, 50–52]. Human cortical tissue isolated from epilepsy patients also expresses GABA-A receptors with reduced neurosteroid sensitivity [53].

Ganaxolone treatment also appears to protect from seizures in patients with CDKL5 deficiency disorder (CDD), a rare, X-linked, developmental, and epileptic encephalopathy characterized by developmental impairment and treatment-refractory seizures [114]. In another open-label flexible-dose exploratory trial study, ganaxolone reduced seizure frequency in patients with PCDH19 epilepsy, which is characterized by early-onset seizures [115]. Since these patients have lower circulating allopregnanolone levels, supplemental neurosteroids could potentiate GABAergic inhibition and control seizures.

The synthetic neurosteroid brexanolone was also tested for treatment of super-refractory SE. In this study, intravenous administration of brexanolone as an add-on to anesthetic third-line agents in pediatric and adult patients with super-refractory SE seemed

Table 4.2 Outcomes of the ganaxolone clinical trials

Study design	Treatment	Patients	Seizure type	Add on to AEDs	Treatment duration	outcomes	conclusions	Reference
Randomized and double-blind	(A) Ganaxolone (1,500 mg/d on day 1, 1,875 mg/d on days 2 to 8) (B) Placebo	18–69 years old, men and women	complex partial seizures with or without secondary generalization	No	8 days of treatment	(A) 50% of patients (12 of the 24) remained seizure-free (B) 25% (7 of the 28) patients remained seizure-free	A trend toward seizure control	[119]
Open-label	Ganaxolone up to 36 mg/kg/day	5–15 years old	partial or generalized seizures including myoclonic and epileptic spasms	Yes	Dose escalation for up to 16 days followed by maintenance phase up to 8 weeks	At week 8 of maintenance, 25% (n = 4 of the 15) of patients had ≥ 50% reduction in seizures, 13% (n = 2 of the 15) of patients had 25–49% reduction in seizures, 60% (n = 9 of the 15) nonresponders	A moderate to substantial reduction in seizures in 50% of patients	[120]
Double-blind, placebo-controlled	(A) Ganaxolone (B) Placebo	18–69 years old, men and women	Partial onset with or without secondarily generalization	Yes	Dose escalation for 6 days to 1,500 mg/kg/day, then maintenance for 8 weeks	(A) 17.6% reduction in seizure frequency compared to that at baseline (n = 98) during	Ganaxolone reduced the frequency of partial-onset seizures	[121]

Table 4.2 (cont.)

Study design	Treatment	Patients	Seizure type	Add on to AEDs	Treatment duration	outcomes	conclusions	Reference
						combined titration +maintenance phases (B) 2% increase in seizure frequency (n = 49)		
Open-label	Ganaxolone	2 month to 5 year old	Infantile spasms	Yes	Dose escalation by week 4 and subsequent maintenance for 2 months, followed by 2 weeks withdrawal	33% (n = 5 of the 15) substantial responders, >50% reduction in seizures 33% (n = 5 of the 15) moderate responders, 25–50% decrease in seizure frequency 33% (5 of the 15) non-responders, <25% decrease in seizures	Ganaxolone was well-tolerated and adverse effects were mild.	[122]

to improve the outcome of SE, including successful weaning of the anesthetic agent without seizure recurrence [116]. However, the findings of the subsequent placebo-controlled trial (NCT022477618) have been disappointing, as brexanolone and placebo did not differ with regard to efficacy in tapering of coma-inducing drugs without seizure recurrence.

Conclusions

The female reproductive hormones are potent neuromodulators, and they play an important role in regulating neuronal excitability and seizure susceptibility. Their cyclic fluctuations underlie the reproductive cycle–linked seizure exacerbation in women with epilepsy. Progesterone exerts acute anticonvulsant and neuroprotective effects but increases excitability and seizures when administered repeatedly or for a longer duration. These distinctions are due to the involvement of distinct cellular signaling molecules and opposing effects on inhibitory and excitatory neurotransmission. Estrogens primarily exert a proconvulsant effect. The dynamic changes in the levels of these hormones and activation of complex cellular signaling pathways underlie catamenial seizure exacerbation, and a thorough understanding of their acute and chronic effects on neuronal function is required before these hormones can be efficaciously used for therapeutic intervention.

References

1. Stoffel-Wagner B. Neurosteroid metabolism in the human brain. *European Journal of Endocrinology*. 2001;**145**(6):669–79.
2. Rupprecht R, Rammes G, Eser D, et al. Translocator protein (18 kD) as target for anxiolytics without benzodiazepine-like side effects. *Science*. 2009;**325**(5939):490–3.
3. Avallone R, Lucchi C, Puja G, et al. BV-2 microglial cells respond to rotenone toxic insult by modifying pregnenolone, 5α-dihydroprogesterone and pregnanolone levels. *Cells*. 2020;**9**(9):2091.
4. Bixo M, Bäckström T, Winblad B, Selstam G, Andersson A. Comparison between pre- and postovulatory distributions of oestradiol and progesterone in the brain of the PMSG-treated rat. *Acta Physiol Scand*. 1986;**128**(2):241–6.
5. Selye H. Anaesthetic effects of steroid hormones. *Proc. Soc. Exp. Biol. Med*. 1941;**46**:116–21.
6. Klein P, Van Passel-Clark LM, Pezzullo JC. Onset of epilepsy at the time of menarche. *Neurology*. 2003;**60**(3):495–7.
7. Herzog AG, Mandle HB, MacEachern DB. Does the age of seizure onset relate to menarche and does it matter? *Seizure*. 2019;**69**:1–6.
8. Harden CL, Pulver MC, Ravdin L, Jacobs AR. The effect of menopause and perimenopause on the course of epilepsy. *Epilepsia*. 1999;**40**(10):1402–7.
9. Harden CL, Herzog AG, Nikolov BG, et al. Hormone replacement therapy in women with epilepsy: A randomized, double-blind, placebo-controlled study. *Epilepsia*. 2006;**47**(9):1447–51.
10. Logothetis J, Harner R, Morrell F, Torres, F. The role of estrogens in catamenial exacerbation of epilepsy. *Neurology*. 1959;**9**(5):352–60.
11. Bäckström T. Epileptic seizures in women related to plasma estrogen and progesterone during the menstrual cycle. *Acta Neurologica Scandinavica*. 1976;**54**(4):321–47.
12. Herzog AG, Klein P, Ransil BJ. Three patterns of catamenial epilepsy. *Epilepsia*. 1997;**38**(10):1082–8.
13. Herzog AG, Seibel MM, Schomer DL, Vaitukaitis JL, Geschwind N. Reproductive endocrine disorders in women with partial

seizures of temporal lobe origin. *Arch Neurol.* 1986;**43**(4):341–6.

14. Bilo L, Meo R, Valentino R, et al. Characterization of reproductive endocrine disorders in women with epilepsy. *J Clin Endocrin Metab.* 2001;**86**(7):2950–6.
15. Bauer J, Isojärvi JIT, Herzog AG, et al. Reproductive dysfunction in women with epilepsy: Recommendations for evaluation and management. *J Neurol Neurosurg Psych.* 2002;**73**(2):121.
16. Quigg M, Fowler KM, Herzog AG, et al. Circalunar and ultralunar periodicities in women with partial seizures. *Epilepsia.* 2008;**49**(6):1081–5.
17. Quigg M, Smithson SD, Fowler KM, et al. Laterality and location influence catamenial seizure expression in women with partial epilepsy. *Neurology.* 2009;**73**(3):223–7.
18. Herzog AG, Fowler KM, Smithson SD, et al. Progesterone vs. placebo therapy for women with epilepsy: A randomized clinical trial. *Neurology.* 2012;**78**(24):1959–66.
19. Woolley DE, Timiras PS. The gonad–brain relationship: Effects of female sex hormones on electroshock convulsions in the rat. *Endocrinology.* 1962;**70**(2):196–209.
20. Finn DA, Gee KW. The estrus cycle, sensitivity to convulsants and the anticonvulsant effect of a neuroactive steroid. *J Pharmacol Exp Therap.* 1994;**271**(1):164–70.
21. Tan M, Tan U. Sex difference in susceptibility to epileptic seizures in rats: Importance of estrous cycle. *Int J Neurosci.* 2001;**108**(3–4):175–91.
22. Maguire JL, Stell BM, Rafizadeh M, Mody I. Ovarian cycle-linked changes in GABAA receptors mediating tonic inhibition alter seizure susceptibility and anxiety. *Nat Neurosci.* 2005;**8**(6):797–804.
23. Li J, Leverton LK, Naganatanahalli LM, Christian-Hinman CA. Seizure burden fluctuates with the female reproductive cycle in a mouse model of chronic temporal lobe epilepsy. *Exp Neurol.* 2020;**334**:113492.
24. Scharfman HE, Malthankar-Phatak GH, Friedman D, et al. A rat model of epilepsy in women: A tool to study physiological interactions between endocrine systems and seizures. *Endocrinology.* 2009;**150**(9):4437–42.
25. Joshi S, Sun H, Rajasekaran K, et al. A novel therapeutic approach for treatment of catamenial epilepsy. *Neurobiol Dis.* 2018;**111**:127–37.
26. Reddy DS, Kim HY, Rogawski MA. Neurosteroid withdrawal model of perimenstrual catamenial epilepsy. *Epilepsia.* 2001;**42**:328–36.
27. Lawrence C, Martin BS, Sun C, Williamson J, Kapur J. Endogenous neurosteroid synthesis modulates seizure frequency. *Ann. Neurol.* 2010;**67**(5):689–93.
28. Shiono S, Williamson J, Kapur J, Joshi S. Progesterone receptor activation regulates seizure susceptibility. *Ann Clin Trans Neurol.* 2019;**6**(7):1302–10.
29. Shiono S, Sun H, Batabyal T, et al. Limbic progesterone receptor activity enhances neuronal excitability and seizures. *Epilepsia.* 2021;**62**(8):1946–59.
30. Reddy DS, Mohan A. Development and persistence of limbic epileptogenesis are impaired in mice lacking progesterone receptors. *J Neurosci.* 2011;**31**(2):650–8.
31. Herzog AG, Mandle HB, Cahill KE, Fowler KM, Hauser WA. Differential impact of contraceptive methods on seizures varies by antiepileptic drug category: Findings of the Epilepsy Birth Control Registry. *Epilepsy Beh.* 2016;**60**:112–17.
32. Mandle HB, Cahill KE, Fowler KM, et al. Reasons for discontinuation of reversible contraceptive methods by women with epilepsy. *Epilepsia.* 2017;**58**(5):907–14.
33. Dana-Haeri J, Richens A. Effect of norethisterone on seizures associated with menstruation. *Epilepsia.* 1983;**24**(3):377–81.

34. Kokate TG, Cohen AL, Karp E, Rogawski MA. Neuroactive steroids protect against pilocarpine- and kainic acid-induced limbic seizures and status epilepticus in mice. *Neuropharmacology.* 1996;**35**(8):1049–56.
35. Frye CA, Scalise TJ, Bayon LE. Finasteride blocks the reduction in ictal activity produced by exogenous estrous cyclicity. *J Neuroendocrinol.* 1998;**10**(4):291–6.
36. Kokate TG, Banks MK, Magee T, Yamaguchi S, Rogawski MA. Finasteride, a 5α-reductase inhibitor, blocks the anticonvulsant activity of progesterone in mice. *J Pharmacol Exp Ther.* 1999;**288**(2):679–84.
37. Frye CA, Scalise TJ. Anti-seizure effects of progesterone and α,5α-THP in kainic acid and perforant pathway models of epilepsy. *Psychoneuroendocrinology.* 2000;**25**(4):407–20.
38. Reddy DS, Castaneda DC, O'Malley BW, Rogawski MA. Anticonvulsant activity of progesterone and neurosteroids in progesterone receptor knockout mice. *J Pharmacol Exp Therap.* 2004;**310**(1):230–9.
39. Frye CA, Manjarrez J, Camacho-Arroyo I. Infusion of 3α,5α-THP to the pontine reticular formation attenuates PTZ-induced seizures. *Brain Res.* 2000;**881**(1):98–102.
40. Frye C, Rhodes M, Walf A, Harney J. Progesterone reduces pentylenetetrazol-induced ictal activity of wild-type mice but not those deficient in type I 5α-reductase. *Epilepsia.* 2002;**43**:14–17.
41. Reddy DS, Ramanathan G. Finasteride inhibits the disease-modifying activity of progesterone in the hippocampus kindling model of epileptogenesis. *Epilepsy Behav.* 2012;**25**(1):92–7.
42. Stell BM, Brickley SG, Tang CY, Farrant M, Mody I. Neuroactive steroids reduce neuronal excitability by selectively enhancing tonic inhibition mediated by δ subunit-containing GABAA receptors. *Proc. Natl. Acad. Sci. U. S. A.* 2003;**100**(24):14439–44.
43. Peng Z, Huang CS, Stell BM, Mody I, Houser CR. Altered expression of the δ subunit of the GABAA receptor in a mouse model of temporal lobe epilepsy. *J Neurosci.* 2004;**24**(39):8629–39.
44. Sun C, Mtchedlishvilli Z, Erisir A, Kapur J. Diminished neurosteroid sensitivity of synaptic inhibition and altered location of the α4 subunit of GABAA receptors in an animal model of epilepsy. *J Neurosci.* 2007;**27**(46):12641–50.
45. Zhang N, Wei W, Mody I, Houser CR. Altered localization of GABAA receptor subunits on dentate granule cell dendrites influences tonic and phasic inhibition in a mouse model of epilepsy. *J Neurosci.* 2007;**27**(28):7520–31.
46. Kokate TG, Svensson BE, Rogawski MA. Anticonvulsant activity of neurosteroids: Correlation with gamma-aminobutyric acid-evoked chloride current potentiation. *J Pharmacol. Exp. Ther.* 1994;**270**(3):1223–9.
47. Saxena NC, MacDonald RL. Assembly of GABAA receptor subunits: Role of the delta subunit. *J Neurosci.* 1994;**14**(11 Pt 2):7077–86.
48. Bianchi MT, MacDonald RL. Neurosteroids shift partial agonist activation of GABA(A) receptor channels from low- to high-efficacy gating patterns. *J Neurosci.* 2003;**23**(34):10934–43.
49. Glykys J, Mann EO, Mody I. Which GABAA receptor subunits are necessary for tonic inhibition in the hippocampus? *J Neurosci.* 2008;**28**(6):1421–6.
50. Rajasekaran K, Joshi S, Sun C, Mtchedlishvilli Z, Kapur J. Receptors with low affinity for neurosteroids and GABA contribute to tonic inhibition of granule cells in epileptic animals. *Neurobiol Dis.* 2010;**40**(2):490–501.
51. Mtchedlishvili Z, Bertram EH, Kapur J. Diminished allopregnanolone enhancement of GABAA receptor currents in a rat model of chronic temporal lobe epilepsy. *J Physiol.* 2001;**537**(Pt 2):453–65.
52. Joshi S, Rajasekaran K, Williamson J, Kapur J. Neurosteroid-sensitive δ-GABAA

receptors: A role in epileptogenesis? *Epilepsia*. 2017;**58**(3):494–504.

53. Joshi S, Roden WH, Kapur J, Jansen LA. Reduced neurosteroid potentiation of GABAA receptors in epilepsy and depolarized hippocampal neurons. *Ann Clin Transl Neurol*. 2020;**7**(4):527–42.
54. Tan C, Shard C, Ranieri E, et al. Mutations of protocadherin 19 in female epilepsy (PCDH19-FE) lead to allopregnanolone deficiency. *Human Mol Gene*. 2015;**24**(18):5250–9.
55. Grabenstatter HL, Cogswell M, Cruz Del Angel Y, et al. Effect of spontaneous seizures on GABAA receptor α4 subunit expression in an animal model of temporal lobe epilepsy. *Epilepsia*. 2014;**55**(11):1826–33.
56. Lothman EW, Stringer JL, Bertram EH. The dentate gyrus as a control point for seizures in the hippocampus and beyond. *Epilepsy Res Suppl*. 1992;**7**:301–13.
57. Pathak HR, Weissinger F, Terunuma M, et al. Disrupted dentate granule cell chloride regulation enhances synaptic excitability during development of temporal lobe epilepsy. *J Neurosci*. 2007;**27**(51):14012–22.
58. Spelsberg TC, Steggles AW, O'Malley BW. Progesterone-binding components of chick oviduct. 3. Chromatin acceptor sites. *J Biol Chem*. 1971;**246**(13):4188–97.
59. Schrader WT, O'Malley BW. Progesterone-binding components of chick oviduct. IV. Characterization of purified subunits. *J Biol Chem*. 1972;**247**(1):51–9.
60. Brinton RD, Thompson RF, Foy MR, et al. Progesterone receptors: Form and function in brain. *Front Neuroendocrinol*. 2008;**29**(2):313–39.
61. Joshi S, Kapur J. Neurosteroid regulation of GABAA receptors: A role in catamenial epilepsy. *Brain Res*. 2018;**1703**:31–40.
62. Guerra-Araiza C, Villamar-Cruz O, González-Arenas A, Chavira R, Camacho-Arroyo I. Changes in progesterone receptor isoforms content in the rat brain during the oestrous cycle and after oestradiol and progesterone treatments. *J Neuroendocrinol*. 2003;**15**(10):984–90.
63. Waters EM, Torres-Reveron A, McEwen BS, Milner TA. Ultrastructural localization of extranuclear progestin receptors in the rat hippocampal formation. *J Comp Neurol*. 2008;**511**(1):34–46.
64. Mitterling KL, Spencer JL, Dziedzic N, et al. Cellular and subcellular localization of estrogen and progestin receptor immunoreactivities in the mouse hippocampus. *J Comp Neurol*. 2010;**518**(14):2729–43.
65. Kumar N, Koide SS, Tsong YY, Sundaram K. Nestorone-«: A progestin with a unique pharmacological profile. *Steroids*. 2000;**65**(10):629–36.
66. Kumar N, Fagart J, Liere P, et al. Nestorone-« as a novel progestin for nonoral contraception: Structure–activity relationships and brain metabolism studies. *Endocrinology*. 2017;**158**(1):170–82.
67. Scharfman HE, Mercurio TC, Goodman JH, Wilson MA, Maclusky NJ. Hippocampal excitability increases during the estrous cycle in the rat: A potential role for brain-derived neurotrophic factor. *J Neurosci*. 2003;**23**(37):11641–52.
68. Scharfman HE, Goodman JH, Rigoulot MA, et al. Seizure susceptibility in intact and ovariectomized female rats treated with the convulsant pilocarpine. *Exp Neurol*. 2005;**196**(1):73–86.
69. Reddy DS, Gangisetty O, Wu X. PR-independent neurosteroid regulation of α2-GABAA receptors in the hippocampus subfields. *Brain Res*. 2017;**1659**(S C):142–7.
70. Veliskova J. The role of estrogens in seizures and epilepsy: The bad guys or the good guys? *Neuroscience*. 2006;**138**(3):837–44.
71. Woolley CS. Estradiol facilitates kainic acid-induced, but not flurothyl-induced, behavioral seizure activity in adult female rats. *Epilepsia*. 2000;**41**(5):510–15.
72. Ledoux VA, Smejkalova T, May RM, Cooke BM, Woolley CS. Estradiol

facilitates the release of neuropeptide Y to suppress hippocampus-dependent seizures. *J Neurosci*. 2009;**29**(5):1457–68.

73. Horn AC, Buterbaugh GG. Estrogen alters the acquisition of seizures kindled by repeated amygdala stimulation or pentylenetetrazol administration in ovariectomized female rats. *Epilepsia*. 1986;**27**(2):103–8.
74. Edwards HE, Burnham WM, Mendonca A, Bowlby DA, MacLusky NJ. Steroid hormones affect limbic afterdischarge thresholds and kindling rates in adult female rats. *Brain Res*. 1999;**838**(1–2):136–50.
75. Velíšková J, Velíšek L, Galanopoulou AS, Sperber EF. Neuroprotective effects of estrogens on hippocampal cells in adult female rats after status epilepticus. *Epilepsia*. 2000;**41**(s6):S30–S35.
76. Galanopoulou AS, Alm EM, Velíšková J. Estradiol reduces seizure-induced hippocampal injury in ovariectomized female but not in male rats. *Neurosci Lett*. 2003;**342**(3):201–5.
77. Hoffman GE, Moore N, Fiskum G, Murphy AZ. Ovarian steroid modulation of seizure severity and hippocampal cell death after kainic acid treatment. *Exp Neurol*. 2003;**182**(1):124–34.
78. Woolley CS, Gould E, Frankfurt M, McEwen BS. Naturally occurring fluctuation in dendritic spine density on adult hippocampal pyramidal neurons. *J Neurosci*. 1990;**10**(12):4035–9.
79. Woolley CS, McEwen BS. Roles of estradiol and progesterone in regulation of hippocampal dendritic spine density during the estrous cycle in the rat. *J Comp Neurol*. 1993;**336**(2):293–306.
80. Woolley CS, McEwen BS. Estradiol mediates fluctuation in hippocampal synapse density during the estrous cycle in the adult rat. *J Neurosci*. 1992;**12**(7):2549–54.
81. Brake WG, Alves SE, Dunlop JC, et al. Novel target sites for estrogen action in the dorsal hippocampus: An examination of synaptic proteins. *Endocrinology*. 2001;**142**(3):1284–9.
82. Waters EM, Mitterling K, Spencer JL, et al. Estrogen receptor alpha and beta specific agonists regulate expression of synaptic proteins in rat hippocampus. *Brain Res*. 2009;**1290**:1–11.
83. Yokomaku D, Numakawa T, Numakawa Y, et al. Estrogen enhances depolarization-induced glutamate release through activation of phosphatidylinositol 3-kinase and mitogen-activated protein kinase in cultured hippocampal neurons. *Mol Endocrinol*. 2003;**17**(5):831–44.
84. Foy MR, Xu J, Xie X, et al. 17beta-estradiol enhances NMDA receptor-mediated EPSPs and long-term potentiation. *J Neurophysiol*. 1999;**81**(2):925–9.
85. Smith CC, McMahon LL. Estradiol-induced increase in the magnitude of long-term potentiation is prevented by blocking NR2B-containing receptors. *J Neurosci*. 2006;**26**(33):8517–22.
86. Teyler TJ, Vardaris RM, Lewis D, Rawitch AB. Gonadal steroids: Effects on excitability of hippocampal pyramidal cells. *Science*. 1980;**209**(4460):1017–18.
87. Oberlander JG, Woolley CS. 17β-Estradiol acutely potentiates glutamatergic synaptic transmission in the hippocampus through distinct mechanisms in males and females. *J Neurosci*. 2016;**36**(9):2677–90.
88. Wong M, Moss RL. Long-term and short-term electrophysiological effects of estrogen on the synaptic properties of hippocampal CA1 neurons. *J Neurosci*. 1992;**12**(8):3217–25.
89. Wallis CJ, Luttge WG. Influence of estrogen and progesterone on glutamic acid decarboxylase activity in discrete regions of rat brain. *J Neurochem*. 1980;**34**(3):609–13.
90. O'Connor LH, Nock B, McEwen BS. Regional specificity of GABAA receptor regulation by estradiol. *Neuroendocrinology*. 1988;**47**(6):473–81.
91. Weiland NG, Orikasa C, Hayashi S, McEwen BS. Distribution and hormone regulation of estrogen receptor immunoreactive cells in the hippocampus of male and female rats. *J Comp Neurol*. 1997;**388**(4):603–12.

92. Milner TA, McEwen BS, Hayashi S, et al. Ultrastructural evidence that hippocampal alpha estrogen receptors are located at extranuclear sites. *J Comp Neurol.* 2001;**429**(3):355–71.

93. Kalita K, Szymczak S, Kaczmarek L. Non-nuclear estrogen receptor β and α in the hippocampus of male and female rats. *Hippocampus.* 2005;**15**(3):404–12.

94. Milner TA, Ayoola K, Drake CT, et al. Ultrastructural localization of estrogen receptor β immunoreactivity in the rat hippocampal formation. *J Comp Neurol.* 2005;**491**(2):81–95.

95. Weiser MJ, Foradori CD, Handa RJ. Estrogen receptor beta in the brain: From form to function. *Brain Res Rev.* 2008;**57**(2):309–20.

96. Almey A, Milner TA, Brake WG. Estrogen receptors in the central nervous system and their implication for dopamine-dependent cognition in females. *Hormones Beh.* 2015;**74**:125–38.

97. Shughrue PJ, Lane MV, Merchenthaler I. Comparative distribution of estrogen receptor-α and -β mRNA in the rat central nervous system. *J Comp Neurol.* 1997;**388**(4):507–25.

98. Mitra SW, Hoskin E, Yudkovitz J, et al. Immunolocalization of estrogen receptor β in the mouse brain: Comparison with estrogen receptor α. *Endocrinology.* 2003;**144**(5):2055–67.

99. Day M, Sung A, Logue S, Bowlby M, Arias R. Beta estrogen receptor knockout (BERKO) mice present attenuated hippocampal CA1 long-term potentiation and related memory deficits in contextual fear conditioning. *Beh Brain Res.* 2005;**164**(1):128–31.

100. Velísková J, De Jesus G, Kaur R, Velísek L. Females, their estrogens, and seizures. *Epilepsia.* 2010;**51**(S3):141–4.

101. Frye CA, Ryan A, Rhodes M. Antiseizure effects of 3α-androstanediol and/or 17β-estradiol may involve actions at estrogen receptor β. *Epilepsy Beh.* 2009;**16**(3):418–22.

102. Wang Z, Xie R, Yang X, et al. Female mice lacking ERβ display excitatory/inhibitory synaptic imbalance to drive the pathogenesis of temporal lobe epilepsy. *Theranostics.* 2021;**11**(12):6074–89.

103. Osborne DM, Frye CA. Estrogen increases latencies to seizures and levels of 5α-pregnan-3α-ol-20-one in hippocampus of wild-type, but not 5α-reductase knockout, mice. *Epilepsy Beh.* 2009;**16**(3):411–14.

104. Velísková J, Velísek L. Beta-estradiol increases dentate gyrus inhibition in female rats via augmentation of hilar neuropeptide Y. *J Neurosci.* 2007;**27**(22):6054–63.

105. Leitinger M, Trinka E, Giovannini G, et al. Epidemiology of status epilepticus in adults: A population-based study on incidence, causes, and outcomes. *Epilepsia.* 2019;**60**(1):53–62.

106. Dabrowska N, Joshi S, Williamson J, et al. Parallel pathways of seizure generalization. *Brain.* 2019;**142**(8):2336–51.

107. Maguire J, Mody I. Neurosteroid synthesis-mediated regulation of GABAA receptors: Relevance to the ovarian cycle and stress. *J Neurosci.* 2007;**27**(9):2155–62.

108. Sato SM, Woolley CS. Acute inhibition of neurosteroid estrogen synthesis suppresses status epilepticus in an animal model. *Elife.* 2016;**5**:e12917.

109. Kapur J, MacDonald RL. Rapid seizure-induced reduction of benzodiazepine and Zn^{2+} sensitivity of hippocampal dentate granule cell GABAA receptors. *J Neurosci.* 1997;**17**(19):7532–40.

110. Naylor DE, Liu H, Wasterlain CG. Trafficking of GABAA receptors, loss of inhibition, and a mechanism for pharmacoresistance in status epilepticus. *J Neurosci.* 2005;**25**(34):7724–33.

111. Goodkin HP, Joshi S, Mtchedlishvili Z, Brar J, Kapur J. Subunit-specific trafficking of GABAA receptors during

status epilepticus. *J Neurosci.* 2008;**28**(10):2527–38.

112. Terunuma M, Xu J, Vithlani M, et al. Deficits in phosphorylation of GABAA receptors by intimately associated protein kinase C activity underlie compromised synaptic inhibition during status epilepticus. *J Neurosci.* 2008;**28**(2):376–84.
113. Rogawski MA, Loya CM, Reddy K, Zolkowska D, Lossin C. Neuroactive steroids for the treatment of status epilepticus. *Epilepsia.* 2013;**54**(6):93–8.
114. Knight EMP, Amin S, Bahi-Buisson N, et al. Safety and efficacy of ganaxolone in patients with CDKL5 deficiency disorder: Results from the double-blind phase of a randomised, placebo-controlled, phase 3 trial. *Lancet Neurol.* 2022;**21**:417–27.
115. Lappalainen J, Chez M, Sullivan J, et al. A multicenter, open-label trial of ganaxolone in children with PCDH19 epilepsy (P5.236). *Neurology.* 2017;**88**.
116. Rosenthal ES, Claassen J, Wainwright MS, et al. Brexanolone as adjunctive therapy in super-refractory status epilepticus. *Ann Neurol.* 2017;**82**:342–52.
117. Moran MH, Smith SS. Progesterone withdrawal I: Pro-convulsant effects. *Brain Res.* 1998;**807**:84–90.
118. Herzog AG, Frye CA. Seizure exacerbation associated with inhibition of progesterone metabolism. *Ann Neurol.* 2003;**53**:390–1.
119. Laxer K, Blum D, Abou-Khalil BW, et al. Assessment of ganaxolone's anticonvulsant activity using a randomized, double-blind, presurgical trial design. Ganaxolone Presurgical Study Group. *Epilepsia.* 2000;**41**:1187–94.
120. Pieribone VA, Tsai J, Soufflet C, et al. Clinical evaluation of ganaxolone in pediatric and adolescent patients with refractory epilepsy. *Epilepsia.* 2007;**48**:1870–4.
121. Sperling MR, Klein P, Tsai J. Randomized, double-blind, placebo-controlled phase 2 study of ganaxolone as add-on therapy in adults with uncontrolled partial-onset seizures. *Epilepsia.* 2017;**58**:558–64.
122. Kerrigan JF, Shields WD, Nelson TY, et al. Ganaxolone for treating intractable infantile spasms: A multicenter, open-label, add-on trial. *Epilepsy Res.* 2000;**42**:133–9.

Antiseizure Medications and Hormones

Mona Sazgar

Key Points

- Drug-specific endocrine side effects of antiseizure medications (ASMs) are seen in both men and women with epilepsy.
- Hepatic enzyme-inducing ASMs may increase the breakdown of testosterone and decrease the bioavailability of estradiol, resulting in menstrual disorders, anovulatory cycles, and polycystic ovarian syndrome (PCOS).
- Carbamazepine (CBZ), phenytoin (PHT), and valproic acid (VPA) can inhibit sperm motility according to both in vivo and in vitro studies.
- Valproic acid is associated with increased risk of developing PCOS, hyperandrogenism, anovulatory cycles, and menstrual irregularities.
- Polycystic ovarian syndrome occurs in 4–7% of women of reproductive age in the general population but in 10–25% of women with epilepsy.
- Lamotrigine (LTG) and levetiracetam (LEV) are not associated with drug-specific endocrine or sexual side effects.
- In people with epilepsy, the risk of bone fracture is two to six times higher than the risk in the general population.
- Risk factors for bone loss include duration and severity of epilepsy, ASMs, female sex, menopause, sedentary lifestyle, smoking, excessive alcoholic beverage intake, inadequate sun exposure, and certain endocrine conditions.
- Most ASMs, irrespective of whether they are hepatic enzyme-inducing or non-enzyme-inducing, may result in low bone mineral density (BMD), hypocalcemia, and vitamin D deficiency, which may occur early during treatment.
- Providers caring for patients with epilepsy should consider monitoring of calcium and vitamin D levels and periodic BMD examinations in their patients for early detection of upcoming bone loss.
- In patients on long-term ASM therapy, only high doses of vitamin D at 4,000 IU/d for adults and 2,000 IU/d for children substantially increased BMD.
- Among ASMs, VPA, gabapentin (GBP), vigabatrin (VGB), pregabalin (PGB), CBZ, and primidone (PRM) are associated with weight gain. On the other hand, topiramate (TPM), zonisamide (ZNS), and felbamate (FBM) are associated with weight loss.
- Nearly one-third of patients on ASMs develop thyroid hormonal abnormalities.
- Thyroid hormonal abnormalities including subclinical hypothyroidism are reported with epilepsy patients taking hepatic enzyme-inducing ASMs such as phenobarbital (PB), PHT, CBZ, and oxcarbazepine (OXC), as well as VPA, but not with LTG, LEV, TPM, tiagabine (TGB), and VGB.

- Hyponatremia is commonly associated with CBZ, OXC, and eslicarbazepine (ESL), and is likely due to syndrome of inappropriate antidiuretic hormone (SIADH) secretion. There are several case reports of hyponatremia induced by VPA, LTG, and LEV.

Introduction

Antiseizure medications (ASMs) can result in endocrine-related side effects, including polycystic ovaries, decreased libido, erectile dysfunction, change in glucose metabolism and weight, bone loss, and abnormal thyroid function. Microsomal hepatic enzyme-inducing ASMs may impact sex hormones and result in lower levels of bioavailable testosterone and estradiol and subsequently contribute to sexual dysfunction, menstrual irregularities, and problems with fertility. Some non-enzyme-inducing ASMs such as valproic acid (VPA) also are associated with endocrine disturbances such as polycystic ovary and weight gain. This chapter will explore the endocrine side effects and hormonal changes caused by ASMs.

Reproductive and Endocrine Effects of Antiseizure Medications

A prospective study of pregnancy in women with epilepsy seeking conception (the WEPOD study) found that women with epilepsy without a history of infertility or related disorders seeking pregnancy had similar likelihood of achieving pregnancy compared with their peers [1]. However, most women with epilepsy in this study were taking lamotrigine (LTG) and levetiracetam (LEV) monotherapy (73.5%). Drug-specific endocrine effects of seizure medications are found in both women and men with epilepsy. Certain ASMs may contribute to sexual dysfunction by a variety of mechanisms. Antiseizure medications influence the metabolism of the central and peripheral endocrine hormones and their binding proteins [2]. Some hepatic cytochrome P450 enzyme-inducing ASMs increase the breakdown of biologically active testosterone, resulting in hyposexuality in men and women with epilepsy. They also decrease the bioavailability of estradiol, resulting in menstrual disorders, anovulatory cycles, and polycystic ovaries [2]. Most of the non-enzyme-inducing ASMs such as gabapentin (GBP), pregabalin (PGB), benzodiazepines, and VPA enhance GABAergic transmission, which in turn has specific effects on sexual function [2]. To discuss the effects of ASMs on sexual function, this chapter will divide the effects of ASMs into two separate categories based on hepatic enzyme-inducing activity versus non-enzyme-inducing ASMs.

Hepatic Enzyme-Inducing Antiseizure Medications

Carbamazepine (CBZ), phenobarbital (PB), and phenytoin (PHT) are all hepatic microsomal enzyme-inducing ASMs (EIASMs). Long-term treatment with these medications results in low levels of free testosterone and estradiol and therefore high levels of sex-hormone-binding globulin (SHBG) concentrations in people with epilepsy [3–6]. This in turn may lead to menstrual irregularities, sexual dysfunction, and reduced fertility. Carbamazepine and PHT use was associated with inhibition of sperm motility in both in vitro and in vivo studies. Long-term CBZ use is also linked to morphologically abnormal sperms [7, 8]. In a study by Svalheim and colleagues, 63 men and 30 women treated with CBZ monotherapy found that satisfaction with their sexual lives was lower in women on CBZ compared with the control group and with women on LTG and LEV [9]. Despite all of the hormonal endocrine changes associated with the use of ASMs, a population-based study in Finland did not find a statistically significant reduction in birth rate in people with epilepsy taking CBZ compared with a cohort without epilepsy [10].

Phenytoin is also associated with increased risk for sexual dysfunction. Mattson and colleagues reported that 11% of 110 patients treated with PHT for 1 year experienced impotence [11]. Another cross-sectional study of 25 men taking PHT for at least 3 months also found worse sexual function compared with the control group [12].

Oxcarbazepine (OXC) follows a different metabolic pathway than CBZ. It is metabolized by reduction rather than oxidation and converts to its monohydroxy derivative (MHD) active metabolite. Oxcarbazepine is a weak inducer of CYP3A4, but in high doses, it can affect serum testosterone levels and induce changes in sperm morphology [13]. Oxcarbazepine has been reported to decrease endogenous estrogen by 50% and progesterone by 58%, and it reduces testosterone levels by 25%. Oxcarbazepine results in DHEA and androstenedione levels going up by 30% and 20% [13]. Despite such reports, other studies suggest improvement in sexual function after switching from CBZ to OXC [14].

Topiramate (TPM) is associated with sexual dysfunction in both men and women with epilepsy. A recent systematic review of 17 publications by Chen and colleagues found that self-reported incidence of TPM-associated sexual dysfunction and disorder of libido is about 9%, and orgasmic disorders are reported by 2.6% of patients [16]. Sexual dysfunction reported by a European database of 11,972 patients with suspected adverse drug reaction was at a rate of 0.6% [15]. Men mainly reported erectile dysfunction as opposed to women reporting anorgasmia [16]. The effect of TPM on sexual function can be either central and related to interference at the limbic and cortico-striatal loop or through affecting peripheral spinal and autonomic neurons. Substitution or reduction in dose resulted in recovery from symptoms [16].

Non-Enzyme-Inducing Antiseizure Medications

Valproate (VPA) may affect serum androgen concentration and reduce follicle-stimulating hormone (FSH) levels in men. A recent meta-analysis and systematic review of the literature to evaluate the effect of VPA in reproductive endocrine function in men with epilepsy found that long-term VPA treatment leads to significant decrease in FSH and testosterone and alters DHEA, luteinizing hormone (LH), insulin, C-peptide, and carnitine ratios [17]. There is evidence that VPA can contribute to dysregulation of sex hormones, reduced sperm motility, altered sperm morphology, and small testicular size in men with epilepsy [18–20]. These alterations may result in sexual and reproductive dysfunction in men with epilepsy [21–24].

In women with epilepsy, VPA is associated with increased risk of developing polycystic ovary syndrome (PCOS), hyperandrogenism, anovulatory cycles, and menstrual irregularities [25–29]. Polycystic ovary syndrome is characterized by enlarged ovaries with multiple small cysts and a hyper-vascularized, androgen-secreting stroma, leading to the associated signs of androgen excess (hirsutism, alopecia, acne), obesity, and menstrual cycle disturbance (oligomenorrhea or amenorrhea) [30]. It occurs in 4–7% of women of reproductive age in the general population but in 10–25% of women with epilepsy [31, 32].

Since the 1990s, several studies have been published on the reproductive and endocrine effects of VPA. A cross-sectional study in 1993 of 238 women with epilepsy showed that menstrual disorders were common in women taking VPA monotherapy (45%). Polycystic ovary syndrome and hyperandrogenism were seen in 90% of women on VPA monotherapy, especially if VPA was started before age 20 [33]. A subsequent prospective, randomized, open-label, multicenter, 12-month study evaluated the occurrence of PCOS in women taking VPA versus LTG monotherapy. At baseline the prevalence of PCOS was 45%. More women on VPA monotherapy developed PCOS (54% on VPA vs. 38% on LTG).

A recent study of VPA and LTG monotherapy in Indian women with epilepsy found significantly elevated testosterone levels at 6 months and 12 months of VPA monotherapy, a higher rate of hirsutism, menstrual disturbance, weight gain, and PCOS. Substitution of VPA with LTG resulted in significant reduction in mean testosterone levels and mean body weight, suggesting that the endocrine side effects of VPA are at least partly reversible.

Lamotrigine does not have hepatic enzyme-inducing properties, and LTG monotherapy is reported to cause minimal sexual effects in men and even improvement in sexual function in women [6, 34]. Gil-Nagel and colleagues reported that of 141 patients treated with LTG for a period of 8 months, 79 initiated the treatment and 62 were switched to LTG for better seizure control [34]. Women who started the LTG treatment reported significant improvement in Changes in Sexual Functioning Questionnaire (CSFQ) scores in all dimensions of sexual desire, frequency, interest, pleasure, arousal, excitement, and interest. Women who had substitution of previous ASMs with LTG reported improvement in sexual desire and frequency. Men reported improvement only in one dimension (pleasure and orgasm) [34]. Another study, by Svalheim and colleagues, found a greater degree of satisfaction with sexual function in 40 women on LTG monotherapy compared with 30 women using CBZ monotherapy [9]. Despite these larger-scale studies suggesting lack of sexual dysfunction in patients treated with LTG, there is a case report of a 56-year-old man with intermittent nonadherence to LTG secondary to sexual dysfunction, including reversible lack of libido and trouble with orgasm and ejaculation that every time resolved with withholding LTG for 72 hours [35].

Levetiracetam was studied as a monotherapy and was not associated with drug-specific endocrine or sexual side effects in men and women. Per this study by Svalheim and colleagues, women treated with LTG and LEV were more satisfied with their sexual function than patients treated with CBZ and healthy controls [9]. This finding is in contrast with animal studies that showed LEV affecting reproductive endocrine function [36, 37]. Another study examined the semen quality, sexual function, and sex hormone levels in men with epilepsy treated with LEV, OXC, and LTG. They found no changes in sexual function and sex hormone levels. Semen quality was decreased even before treatment in all these patients. There are case reports of LEV-associated hypersexuality [38], as well as loss of libido and anhedonia [39]. The effect is postulated to be due to changing in the balance of dopamine/serotonin ratio.

Gabapentin and PGB (GABA analog ASMs) have frequently been reported in case series regarding their contribution to sexual dysfunction. Gabapentin was reported to be associated with loss of libido, erectile dysfunction, ejaculatory dysfunction, and anorgasmia [40–44]. Erectile dysfunction, anorgasmia, and loss of libido were also reported in a case series of patients treated with PGB [45]. The mechanism suggested is increased GABA levels in the central nervous system; these medications may impede vasoactive intestinal peptide and nitric oxide, which are essential for sexual arousal [45]. On the contrary, GBP was used in a randomized, placebo-controlled trial on 89 women with vulvodynia and resulted in improved sexual function and increase in sexual arousal [46].

Table 5.1 Antiseizure medications and sexual function

Antiseizure medications	Effect on sexual function
PHT, CBZ, PRM, PB	Menstrual irregularities, sexual dysfunction, reduced fertility Decreased libido, impotence, hyposexuality, changes in semen quality
VPA	PCOS, menstrual irregularity, anovulatory cycles Decreased libido, impotence Retrograde ejaculation
OXC	Few reports of decreased sexual function, ejaculation disorder Reports of improved sexual function when switched from CBZ
LTG	Improvement in pleasure and orgasm in men and desire/ frequency in women
LEV	Enhanced sexual function in women Erectile dysfunction, decreased libido
TPM	Erectile dysfunction, premature ejaculation
GBP, PGB	Erectile dysfunction, anorgasmia, decreased libido, impotence, abnormal ejaculation
ZNS	Erectile dysfunction, decreased libido
LCM	Erectile dysfunction, decreased libido

PHT: phenytoin, CBZ: carbamazepine, PRM: primidone, PB: phenobarbital, VPA: valproic acid, OXC: oxcarbazepine, LTG: lamotrigine, LEV: levetiracetam, TPM: topiramate, GBP: gabapentin, PGB: pregabalin, ZNS: zonisamide, LCM: lacosamide

Lacosamide (LCM) was reported to be associated with severe loss of libido and erectile dysfunction in a 27-year-old man with posttraumatic focal epilepsy. The side effect resolved after withdrawing the medication and replacing it with another ASM [47].

Zonisamide (ZNS) reportedly contributed to erectile dysfunction in a 33-year-old man. The symptoms resolved after discontinuation of the medication [48]. There is lack of large population-based studies to provide conclusive guidance regarding the potential adverse sexual effects of LCM, ZNS, and other newer ASMs. Table 5.1 summarizes what is reported in the literature regarding the effects of ASMs on sexual function.

Multiple factors contribute to ASM-induced sexual dysfunction. Changes in the levels of biologically active sex hormones and disturbance of neurotransmission may contribute to disorders of reproductive and endocrine function. In addition, psychological factors related to ASMs such as depression and anxiety may lead to decreased libido, anorgasmia, and erectile dysfunction. Sexual dysfunction is often underreported and has negative impact on quality of life of persons with epilepsy. It is important to actively question patients regarding satisfaction with their sexual life and to identify potential ASM-related sexual endocrine side effects. One may consider replacing the seizure medication and treating the anxiety and depression to address the problem and the potential negative impact on the lives of people with epilepsy.

Antiseizure Medications and Bone Health

Certain ASMs are independent risk factors for bone loss and result in predisposition to fractures. Bone diseases were reported in about 50% of patients on ASMs. The cumulative drug load and duration and severity of epilepsy can contribute to progressive reduction in bone mineral density (BMD). In people with epilepsy, the risk of bone fracture is two to six times higher than the risk in general population [49–51]. This is likely due to altered bone metabolism, decreased bone density, seizure-related falls and trauma, and ASM-induced loss of balance [52]. Risk factors for bone loss include duration and severity of epilepsy, ASMs, female sex, menopause, sedentary lifestyle, smoking, excessive alcoholic beverage intake, inadequate sun exposure, and certain endocrine conditions.

Hepatic CYP450 enzyme-inducing ASMs such as CBZ, PHT, PB, and primidone (PRM) and benzodiazepines (BZDs) have long been associated with decreased BMD and abnormal bone metabolism. Several mechanisms have been suggested for ASM-induced bone disease. Enzyme-inducing ASMs and VPA may affect specific isoenzymes involved in vitamin D metabolism and result in accelerated vitamin D metabolism, therefore lowering vitamin D levels and interfering with normal absorption of calcium. Secondary hyperparathyroidism has been reported in patients taking ASMs [53]. Antiseizure medications may also affect the proliferation of chondrocytes in the growth plate, resulting in bone loss [54]. Enzyme-inducing ASMs can reduce the capacity of thyroid chief cells to secrete calcitonin. Some ASMs can increase serum homocysteine by lowering the folate levels. Folate is thought to have a role in preserving nitric oxide synthase activity in bone cells, stimulating osteoblasts and inhibiting bone catabolism and loss. It has been found that (independent to age and sex) for each standard deviation increase in the homocysteine level the risk of fracture increased by 30% [55].

Several studies have reported decreased BMD, osteopenia, and osteoporosis of hip and lumbar spine with CBZ [2, 56–58], PHT [59–61], VPA [2, 59, 60, 62], TPM [63, 64], and OXC [58, 65]. Sato and colleagues reported a BMD reduction of 14% with VPA therapy and 13% with PHT [59]. A recent study of adult patients newly diagnosed with epilepsy treated with VPA, LTG, and LEV monotherapy found that VPA altered bone turnover while LTG and LEV did not exert harmful effects on bone health [66]. The same author(s) investigated the long-term effects of LTG and VPA and found that particularly when combined, they can cause short stature, low BMD, and reduced bone formation [67]. In a study of bone metabolism and bone density in premenopausal women with epilepsy receiving ASM monotherapy (PHT, CBZ, VPA, and LTG), PHT altered bone metabolism and increased bone turnover while CBZ and VPA were associated with low calcium levels. Lamotrigine did not result in low calcium levels or increased bone turnover markers [68].

Another prospective longitudinal study also found that BMD and vitamin D were not affected by 6 months of LTG therapy [69]. Koo and colleagues did not find any harmful effect of LEV on bone density [70]. However, at least one study has reported reduced BMD in adults treated with LEV [71]. Koo also studied the effects of ZNS after 13 months of monotherapy in epilepsy patients and concluded that long-term ZNS monotherapy does not negatively affect bone health in drug-naive patients with epilepsy [72]. Takahashi and colleagues found that chronic ZNS administration to rats can cause reduced BMD [73]. Long-term GBP use in several studies was associated with fractures [74] and bone loss in the hip and spine [75–77]. Table 5.2 summarizes the current known effects of ASMs on bone metabolism.

Table 5.2 Effects of antiseizure medications on bone metabolism

Antiseizure medications	Bone effect
PHT	↓BMD/ ↓Vitamin D/ ↓ Calcium/ Rickets or Osteomalacia
CBZ	↓BMD/ ↓Vitamin D/ ↓ Calcium/ Rickets or Osteomalacia
PRM	↓BMD/ ↓Vitamin D
PB	↓BMD/ ↓Vitamin D, ↓ Calcium
VPA	↓BMD/ ↓Vitamin D/ osteopenia, osteoporosis/ shorter stature
OXC	↓BMD/↓Vitamin D/ ↓ Calcium
LTG	No significant clinical effect
LEV	No significant clinical effect
TPM	↓BMD/ osteopenia, osteoporosis/ mild ↓ Calcium
GBP	↓BMD
ZNS	No significant clinical effect/ ↓BMD in rats

PHT: phenytoin, CBZ: carbamazepine, PRM: primidone, PB: phenobarbital, VPA: valproic acid, OXC: oxcarbazepine, LTG: lamotrigine, LEV: levetiracetam, TPM: topiramate, GBP: gabapentin, ZNS: zonisamide

In summary, epilepsy patients treated with ASMs are at risk for bone loss and fractures. Most ASMs, irrespective of whether they are hepatic enzyme-inducing or non-enzyme-inducing, may result in low BMD, hypocalcemia, and vitamin D deficiency, which may occur early during treatment and initially remain asymptomatic. Neurologists caring for patients with epilepsy should consider monitoring calcium and vitamin D levels and periodic BMD examinations in their patients for early detection of upcoming bone loss. The Society for Endocrinology guidelines recommend 25-hydroxyvitamin D concentrations should be maintained at greater than 30 ng/mL, which may require at least 1,500 IU/d to 2,000 IU/d of vitamin supplementation. Mikati and colleagues in two parallel, randomized, controlled trials showed that in patients on long-term ASM therapy, only high doses of vitamin D at 4,000 IU/d for adults and 2,000 IU/d for children substantially increased BDM [78]. Dual-energy X-ray absorptiometry (DEXA) scans should be performed periodically to monitor BMD. In case osteopenia or osteoporosis are detected, consideration should be given to increasing calcium and vitamin D supplementation, replacing enzyme-inducing ASMs, using bisphosphonates or other therapeutic agents, and referring the patient to an endocrinologist. Other treatment modalities for bone loss may include estrogens and hormonal therapy, parathyroid hormone (teriparatide), and estrogen agonist/antagonist (raloxifene). Table 5.3 summarizes the current considerations for bone health in patients taking ASMs.

Antiseizure Medications and Hormonal Control of Glucose Metabolism and Weight

Antiseizure medications may alter weight, causing either weight gain or weight loss. Among ASMs, VPA, GBP, vigabatrin (VGB), PGB, CBZ, and perampanel (PRM) are associated with

Table 5.3 Recommendations for bone health in patients with epilepsy

No osteopenia or osteoporosis	Detected osteopenia or osteoporosis
Monitor calcium and vitamin D twice a year	Increase vitamin D supplementation to 4,000 IU or above to achieve a level >30 ng/mL
DEXA scan every 2 years	Lifestyle modifications to avoid falls
Calcium (1,200 mg) and vitamin D supplement (600 IU) to aim for a vitamin D level above 30 ng/mL	Consider switch to NEIASMs if safe
Smoking cessation	Consider bisphosphonates
Limit excessive alcohol and caffeine consumption	Consider estrogen and hormonal therapy, and estrogen agonist/ antagonist
Weight-bearing exercises	Consider parathyroid hormone

DEXA: dual energy x-ray absorptiometry, NEIASM: non-enzyme-inducing antiseizure medication

weight gain. On the other hand, TPM, ZNS, and felbamate (FBM) are associated with weight loss. Weight gain induced by ASMs has several health and psychological consequences, including self-confidence and body image issues, hypertension, type II diabetes, dyslipidemia, and accelerated atherosclerosis. Lack of adherence to ASM due to weight gain may affect compliance with medication.

The mechanism by which this occurs may involve ASMs' effects on lipid and glucose metabolism and have an underlying genetic cause. Insulin and leptin are the key neuropeptides recognized by the brain for regulation of food intake and energy expenditure [79, 80]. The action of leptin in the hypothalamus for regulation of food intake and body weight is known to be mediated by orexigenic signals such as neuropeptide Y and galanin. Ghrelin, a peptide hormone secreted by the stomach and the proximal small intestine, is known to stimulate appetite and food intake [81]. Some studies correlate ASM-induced weight gain with alteration of these hormonal peptides.

Valproate has been associated with an average of 10% weight gain in up to 71% of patients. The weight gain is more prominent in postpubertal girls compared with boys and prepubertal children [82, 83]. Valproic acid can cause weight gain by several mechanisms. It interferes with hepatic insulin metabolism, leading to hyperinsulinemia [79, 80]. In a normal state, insulin is a peptide hormone involved in energy metabolism. Following a meal, increase in the levels of blood glucose stimulates insulin secretion (SIADH) and subsequent promotion of glycogen storage in the liver and muscle to convert excess glucose to fatty acid and triglycerides in fatty tissue. Valproic acid inhibits GLUT-1 activity, resulting in reduced glucose transport. It can also increase serum leptin levels, which is strongly associated with increased body mass index (BMI) [84, 85]. In a study by Gungor and colleagues, VPA increased ghrelin levels after 6 months in prepubertal children taking VPA compared with control, likely leading to stimulation of appetite and increased food intake [86]. Finally, several neurohormonal factors are suggested to be involved in VPA-induced weight gain, including increased glucagon-like peptide [87], neuropeptide Y [81, 88, 89], galanin [81], and GABA [90, 91].

Pregabalin may contribute to weight gain via enhancement of GABA transmission. A meta-analysis of 43, 525 patients treated with PGB showed weight gain of greater than 7% for 16% of patients irrespective of their gender, baseline BMI and age. Patients treated with a dose of 600 mg of PGB gained 12–14% weight compared to 6% of the placebo [92, 93].

Topiramate and ZNS are associated with weight loss in adults and children. Weight loss is reported in 6–15% of adults treated with TPM [94] and 35% of those treated with ZNS [95]. The mechanism proposed for TPM is reduction in serum galanin [96] and stimulation of lipoprotein lipase [97, 98]. Zonisamide is associated with low serum leptin and inhibition of lipogenesis [99]. Topiramate and ZNS both work through inhibition of mitochondrial carbonic anhydrase isoforms. In fact, both TPM and ZNS are approved as anti-obesity drugs in certain regions [100].

Felbamate is a GABA receptor modulator and NMDA receptor blocker. It can cause weight loss in 75% of children and adolescents [101]. The mechanism of weight loss for FBM and its possible effects on glucose and energy homeostasis is not well known. It can have an anorexic effect.

Commonly used ASMs can cause weight gain or loss, and the mechanism of weight change with ASMs is not well understood. The treating neurologist should consider the potential for endocrine disturbance and contribution to comorbidities in patients with epilepsy before prescribing ASMs. In patients with morbid obesity, VPA is better avoided, and in patients with anorexia and low body mass, TPM or ZNS should not be considered as first-line treatment.

Thyroid Hormones and Antiseizure Medications

The prevalence of thyroid dysfunction in adults in the general population ranges from 1% to 10% [102, 103]. Nearly one-third of patients on ASMs develop thyroid hormonal abnormalities. Thyroid hormonal abnormalities, including subclinical hypothyroidism, are reported with epilepsy patients taking hepatic EIASMs such as PB, PHT, CBZ, VPA, and OXC [104–107], but not with LTG, LEV, TPM, tiagabine (TGB), and VGB [106, 108]. These hormonal changes are reversible by discontinuing the offending ASM or supplementing L-thyroxine.

Risk factors for subclinical hypothyroidism include young age, polytherapy with more than one ASM, and long duration of therapy greater than 6 months. Goiter is reported with CBZ, VPA, and their combination [109]. Thyroid enlargement (goiter) is seen in 18.2% of children and 26% of adults on long-term ASMs, specifically if treated with CBZ and VPA [110, 111]. Hyperthyroidism has not been associated with ASMs. The main mechanism for reduced concentrations of free and bound thyroid hormone in patients on EIASMs such as PB, CBZ, PHT, and OXC is accelerated hormonal metabolism and increased turnover of thyroid hormones. Antiseizure medications also can alter protein binding and interfere with the function of the hypothalamic-pituitary-thyroid axis. Valproic acid is metabolized in the liver by glucuronide conjugation and oxidation. Both T4 and T3 are metabolized to a small extent by glucuronide conjugation and oxidation. Induction of uridine diphosphate glucuronosyltransferases may be involved as a possible additional mechanism for thyroid hormone changes with ASMs [112].

In clinical practice, there is no recommendation for routine testing of thyroid function tests in patients on ASMs. Since the use of older ASMs such as PB, PHT, CBZ, and VPA is associated with adverse metabolic comorbid conditions, it is reasonable to monitor patients at higher risk for thyroid disease such as patients on polytherapy with multiple EIASMs, pregnant patients, and patients with an adverse metabolic profile.

Antiseizure Medications and Antidiuretic Hormone-Related Hyponatremia

Sodium has an important function, and its normal concentration is 135–145 mmol/L. Acute hyponatremia may have serious consequences, including headache, nausea, vomiting, fatigue, irritability, and confusion. Severe hyponatremia can result in increased intracranial pressure, cerebral herniation, convulsions, coma, and death [113]. Treatment with some of the ASMs is associated with hyponatremia. Hyponatremia is commonly associated with CBZ, OXC, and eslicarbazepine (ESL) acetate [114–116]. There are several case reports of hyponatremia induced by VPA [117], LTG [118], and LEV [119].

Carbamazepine-induced hyponatremia and its antidiuretic effects have been known since 1966 [120]. The largest study included 573 patients treated with CBZ and reported 28 (4.8%) with sodium below 135 mmol/L [121]. A smaller study of 16 patients on CBZ found 5 with CBZ-induced hyponatremia (31.3%) [122]. The first 3 months of initiation of therapy is the high-risk period for developing CBZ-induced hyponatremia [123]. The risk is dose dependent and the higher the dose of CBZ, the more significant the risk of hyponatremia. When the level of CBZ reaches greater than 6 mcg/mL, the risk of hyponatremia is increased 3.5-fold [124].

Oxcarbazepine in a multicenter, retrospective study was found to be associated with lower-than-normal sodium levels in 23% of the patients [125]. Dong and colleagues reported the rate of hyponatremia in 97 patients treated with OXC and found that 29.9% had sodium below 134 and 12.4% below 129 mmol/ L [114]. Like with CBZ, serum sodium levels are negatively correlated with the dose of OXC.

Eslicarbazepine acetate, a third-generation ASM, was associated with 0.6–1.5% hyponatremia in ESL-treated patients participating in clinical trials [126]. Post-marketing experience revealed that 5.1% of patients treated with ESL developed serum sodium levels of 125–134 mmol/L and 1.5% developed serum sodium levels below 125 mmol/L [127]. The decrease in sodium levels is more likely to happen in the first two months of treatment. Like with CBZ and OXC, ESL-induced hyponatremia is dose dependent [127].

There are case reports of hyponatremia induced by VPA [128–131], LTG [118], LEV [132], and GBP [133]. Hyponatremia induced by VPA may be more likely in older patients and in patients with low baseline serum sodium levels treated with high dosages of VPA.

The most likely mechanism for ASM-induced hyponatremia is a syndrome of inappropriate antidiuretic hormone (SIADH) secretion [128–130, 134]. High antidiuretic hormone levels, low plasma osmolality, high urinary sodium, and high urine osmolality are observed in patients with SIADH. The antidiuretic properties of CBZ and OXC may be explained by activating the vasopressin 2 receptor (V2 R)/aquaporin 2 (AQP2) pathway. Carbamazepine and OXC can induce renal water absorption by directly activating the V2 R-protein G complex and upregulating AQP2 expression [135]; SIADH is likely involved in VPA-induced hyponatremia as well [128]. Lamotrigine affects voltage sensitive sodium channels, reducing calcium conductance, inducing SIADH and hyponatremia [118]. Aldosterone may also play a role in OXC-induced hyponatremia. Increased aldosterone in the serum of OXC-treated patients may be a compensatory response to prevent additional decrease in sodium levels [136].

It is recommended to obtain a baseline sodium level prior to starting OXC, ESL, and CBZ in epilepsy patients. Serum sodium should be retested at least a week after the start of these medications. If there is a drop of sodium below 130 mmol/L, more frequent monitoring is recommended at the discretion of the treating physician. Lowering the dose of OXC, ESL, and CBZ and fluid restriction can help normalize the sodium levels. However, if serum sodium levels continue to decline below 125 mmol/L, drug withdrawal should be considered.

Hyponatremia is common in patients treated with OXC, CBZ, and ESL, likely due to SIADH. Hyponatremia is rarely reported with VPA, LTG, LEV, and LTG. The symptoms may be subtle and missed. Elderly patients, high doses of ASMs, low baseline sodium levels, polytherapy, and female gender are risk factors for developing ASM-induced hyponatremia. Neurologists treating patients with OXC, CBZ, and ESL should monitor sodium levels at least in the first 3 months after initiation of treatment and be aware of the signs and symptoms associated with this potentially deadly ASM-induced side effect.

References

1. Pennell PB, French JA, Harden CL, et al. Fertility and birth outcomes in women with epilepsy seeking pregnancy. *JAMA Neurol.* 2018;**75**(8):962–9.
2. Hamed SA. The effect of epilepsy and antiepileptic drugs on sexual, reproductive and gonadal health of adults with epilepsy. *Expert Rev Clin Pharmacol.* 2016;**9**(6):807–19.
3. Macphee GJ, Larkin JG, Butler E, Beastall GH, Brodie MJ. Circulating hormones and pituitary responsiveness in young epileptic men receiving long-term antiepileptic medication. *Epilepsia.* 1988;**29**(4):468–75.
4. Isojarvi JI. Serum steroid hormones and pituitary function in female epileptic patients during carbamazepine therapy. *Epilepsia.* 1990;**31**(4):438–45.
5. Murialdo G, Galimberti CA, Gianelli MV, et al. Effects of valproate, phenobarbital, and carbamazepine on sex steroid setup in women with epilepsy. *Clin Neuropharmacol.* 1998;**21**(1):52–8.
6. Herzog AG. Differential impact of antiepileptic drugs on the effects of contraceptive methods on seizures: Interim findings of the Epilepsy Birth Control Registry. *Seizure.* 2015;**28**:71–5.
7. Chen SS, Shen MR, Chen TJ, Lai SL. Effects of antiepileptic drugs on sperm motility of normal controls and epileptic patients with long-term therapy. *Epilepsia.* 1992;**33**(1):149–53.
8. Roste LS, Tauboll E, Haugen TB, et al. Alterations in semen parameters in men with epilepsy treated with valproate or carbamazepine monotherapy. *Eur J Neurol.* 2003;**10**(5):501–6.
9. Svalheim S, Tauboll E, Luef G, et al. Differential effects of levetiracetam, carbamazepine, and lamotrigine on reproductive endocrine function in adults. *Epilepsy Behav.* 2009;**16**(2):281–7.
10. Artama M, Isojarvi JI, Auvinen A. Antiepileptic drug use and birth rate in patients with epilepsy: A population-based cohort study in Finland. *Hum Reprod.* 2006;**21**(9):2290–5.
11. Mattson RH, Cramer JA, Collins JF, et al. Comparison of carbamazepine, phenobarbital, phenytoin, and primidone in partial and secondarily generalized tonic-clonic seizures. *N Engl J Med.* 1985;**313**(3):145–51.
12. Herzog AG, Drislane FW, Schomer DL, et al. Differential effects of antiepileptic drugs on sexual function and hormones in

men with epilepsy. *Neurology*. 2005;**65**(7):1016–20.

13. Lofgren E, Tapanainen JS, Koivunen R, Pakarinen A, Isojarvi JI. Effects of carbamazepine and oxcarbazepine on the reproductive endocrine function in women with epilepsy. *Epilepsia*. 2006;**47**(9):1441–6.
14. Luef G, Kramer G, Stefan H. Oxcarbazepine treatment in male epilepsy patients improves pre-existing sexual dysfunction. *Acta Neurol Scand*. 2009;**119**(2):94–9.
15. European Database of Suspected Adverse Drug Reaction Reports: Topiramate. Accessed on December 18, 2016.
16. Chen LW, Chen MY, Chen KY, et al. Topiramate-associated sexual dysfunction: A systematic review. *Epilepsy Behav*. 2017;**73**:10–17.
17. Zhao S, Wang X, Wang Y, et al. Effects of valproate on reproductive endocrine function in male patients with epilepsy: A systematic review and meta-analysis. *Epilepsy Behav*. 2018;**85**:120–8.
18. Hamed SA, Moussa EM, Tohamy AM, et al. Seminal fluid analysis and testicular volume in adults with epilepsy receiving valproate. *J Clin Neurosci*. 2015;**22**(3):508–12.
19. Xiaotian X, Hengzhong Z, Yao X, et al. Effects of antiepileptic drugs on reproductive endocrine function, sexual function and sperm parameters in Chinese Han men with epilepsy. *J Clin Neurosci*. 2013;**20**(11):1492–7.
20. Ocek L, Tarhan H, Uludag FI, et al. Evaluation of sex hormones and sperm parameters in male epileptic patients. *Acta Neurol Scand*. 2018;**137**(4):409–16.
21. Isojarvi JI, Lofgren E, Juntunen KS, et al. Effect of epilepsy and antiepileptic drugs on male reproductive health. *Neurology*. 2004;**62**(2):247–53.
22. Hamed SA. Neuroendocrine hormonal conditions in epilepsy: Relationship to reproductive and sexual functions. *Neurologist*. 2008;**14**(3):157–69.
23. Kose-Ozlece H, Ilik F, Cecen K, Huseyinoglu N, Serim A. Alterations in semen parameters in men with epilepsy treated with valproate. *Iran J Neurol*. 2015;**14**(3):164–7.
24. Verrotti A, Loiacono G, Laus M, et al. Hormonal and reproductive disturbances in epileptic male patients: Emerging issues. *Reprod Toxicol*. 2011;**31**(4):519–27.
25. Verrotti A, Mencaroni E, Cofini M, et al. Valproic acid metabolism and its consequences on sexual functions. *Curr Drug Metab*. 2016;**17**(6):573–81.
26. Prabhakar S, Sahota P, Kharbanda PS, et al. Sodium valproate, hyperandrogenism and altered ovarian function in Indian women with epilepsy: A prospective study. *Epilepsia*. 2007;**48**(7):1371–7.
27. Meador K, Reynolds MW, Crean S, Fahrbach K, Probst C. Pregnancy outcomes in women with epilepsy: A systematic review and meta-analysis of published pregnancy registries and cohorts. *Epilepsy Res*. 2008;**81**(1):1–13.
28. Sahota P, Prabhakar S, Kharbanda PS, et al. Seizure type, antiepileptic drugs, and reproductive endocrine dysfunction in Indian women with epilepsy: A cross-sectional study. *Epilepsia*. 2008;**49**(12):2069–77.
29. Pack AM. Implications of hormonal and neuroendocrine changes associated with seizures and antiepileptic drugs: A clinical perspective. *Epilepsia*. 2010;**51** Suppl 3:150–3.
30. Balen A. Pathogenesis of polycystic ovary syndrome: The enigma unravels? *Lancet*. 1999;**354**(9183):966–7.
31. Bauer J, Cooper-Mahkorn D. Reproductive dysfunction in women with epilepsy: Menstrual cycle abnormalities, fertility, and polycystic ovary syndrome. *Int Rev Neurobiol*. 2008;**83**:135–55.
32. Knochenhauer ES, Key TJ, Kahsar-Miller M, et al. Prevalence of the polycystic ovary syndrome in unselected black and white women of the southeastern United States: A prospective study. *J Clin Endocrinol Metab*. 1998;**83**(9):3078–82.
33. Isojarvi JI, Laatikainen TJ, Pakarinen AJ, Juntunen KT, Myllyla VV. Polycystic

ovaries and hyperandrogenism in women taking valproate for epilepsy. *N Engl J Med.* 1993;**329**(19):1383–8.

34. Gil-Nagel A, Lopez-Munoz F, Serratosa JM, et al. Effect of lamotrigine on sexual function in patients with epilepsy. *Seizure.* 2006;**15**(3):142–9.

35. Kaufman KR, Coluccio M, Sivaraaman K, Campeas M. Lamotrigine-induced sexual dysfunction and non-adherence: Case analysis with literature review. *BJPsych Open.* 2017;**3**(5):249–53.

36. Svalheim S, Tauboll E, Surdova K, et al. Long-term levetiracetam treatment affects reproductive endocrine function in female Wistar rats. *Seizure.* 2008;**17**(2):203–9.

37. Tauboll E, Gregoraszczuk EL, Tworzydo A, Wojtowicz AK, Ropstad E. Comparison of reproductive effects of levetiracetam and valproate studied in prepubertal porcine ovarian follicular cells. *Epilepsia.* 2006;**47**(9):1580–3.

38. Metin SZ, Ozmen M, Ozkara C, Ozmen E. Hypersexuality in a patient with epilepsy during treatment of levetiracetam. *Seizure.* 2013;**22**(2):151–2.

39. Calabro RS, Italiano D, Militi D, Bramanti P. Levetiracetam-associated loss of libido and anhedonia. *Epilepsy Behav.* 2012;**24**(2):283–4.

40. Kaufman KR, Struck PJ. Gabapentin-induced sexual dysfunction. *Epilepsy Behav.* 2011;**21**(3):324–6.

41. Brannon GE, Rolland PD. Anorgasmia in a patient with bipolar disorder type 1 treated with gabapentin. *J Clin Psychopharmacol.* 2000;**20**(3):379–81.

42. Dalal A, Zhou L. Gabapentin and sexual dysfunction: Report of two cases. *Neurologist.* 2008;**14**(1):50–1.

43. Labbate LA, Rubey RN. Gabapentin-induced ejaculatory failure and anorgasmia. *Am J Psychiatry.* 1999;**156**(6):972.

44. Clark JD, Elliott J. Gabapentin-induced anorgasmia. *Neurology.* 1999;**53**(9):2209.

45. Hamed SA. Sexual dysfunctions induced by pregabalin. *Clinical Neuropharmacology.* 2018;**41**(4):116–22.

46. Bachmann GA, Brown CS, Phillips NA, et al. Effect of gabapentin on sexual function in vulvodynia: A randomized, placebo-controlled trial. *Am J Obstet Gynecol.* 2019;**220**(1):89e1–e8.

47. Calabro RS, Magaudda A, Nibali VC, Bramanti P. Sexual dysfunction induced by lacosamide: An underreported side effect? *Epilepsy Behav.* 2015;**46**:252–3.

48. Maschio M, Saveriano F, Dinapoli L, Jandolo B. Reversible erectile dysfunction in a patient with brain tumor-related epilepsy in therapy with zonisamide in add-on. *J Sex Med.* 2011;**8**(12):3515–17.

49. Nicholas JM, Ridsdale L, Richardson MP, Grieve AP, Gulliford MC. Fracture risk with use of liver enzyme inducing antiepileptic drugs in people with active epilepsy: Cohort study using the general practice research database. *Seizure.* 2013;**22**(1):37–42.

50. Sheik Ahmad B, Hill KD, O'Brien TJ, et al. Falls and fractures in patients chronically treated with antiepileptic drugs. *Neurology.* 2012;**79**(2):145–51.

51. Souverein PC, Webb DJ, Petri H, et al. Incidence of fractures among epilepsy patients: A population-based retrospective cohort study in the General Practice Research Database. *Epilepsia.* 2005;**46**(2):304–10.

52. Pack AM. Treatment of epilepsy to optimize bone health. *Curr Treat Options Neurol.* 2011;**13**(4):346–54.

53. Telci A, Cakatay U, Kurt BB, et al. Changes in bone turnover and deoxypyridinoline levels in epileptic patients. *Clin Chem Lab Med.* 2000;**38**(1):47–50.

54. Lee HS, Wang SY, Salter DM, et al. The impact of the use of antiepileptic drugs on the growth of children. *BMC Pediatr.* 2013;**13**:211.

55. Golbahar J, Hamidi A, Aminzadeh MA, Omrani GR. Association of plasma folate, plasma total homocysteine, but not methylenetetrahydrofolate reductase C667 T polymorphism, with bone mineral density in postmenopausal Iranian women: A cross-sectional study. *Bone.* 2004;**35**(3):760–5.

56. Nilsson OS, Lindholm TS, Elmstedt E, Lindback A, Lindholm TC. Fracture incidence and bone disease in epileptics receiving long-term anticonvulsant drug treatment. *Arch Orthop Trauma Surg.* 1986;**105**(3):146–9.
57. Linde J, Molholm Hansen J, Siersbaek-Nielsen K, Fuglsang-Fredriksen V. Bone density in patients receiving long-term anticonvulsant therapy. *Acta Neurol Scand.* 1971;**47**(5):650–1.
58. Mintzer S, Boppana P, Toguri J, DeSantis A. Vitamin D levels and bone turnover in epilepsy patients taking carbamazepine or oxcarbazepine. *Epilepsia.* 2006;**47**(3):510–15.
59. Sato Y, Kondo I, Ishida S, et al. Decreased bone mass and increased bone turnover with valproate therapy in adults with epilepsy. *Neurology.* 2001;**57**(3):445–9.
60. Nissen-Meyer LS, Svalheim S, Tauboll E, et al. Levetiracetam, phenytoin, and valproate act differently on rat bone mass, structure, and metabolism. *Epilepsia.* 2007;**48**(10):1850–60.
61. Moro-Alvarez MJ, Diaz Curiel M, de la Piedra C, Marinoso ML, Carrascal MT. Bone disease induced by phenytoin therapy: Clinical and experimental study. *Eur Neurol.* 2009;**62**(4):219–30.
62. Boluk A, Guzelipek M, Savli H, et al. The effect of valproate on bone mineral density in adult epileptic patients. *Pharmacol Res.* 2004;**50**(1):93–7.
63. Heo K, Rhee Y, Lee HW, et al. The effect of topiramate monotherapy on bone mineral density and markers of bone and mineral metabolism in premenopausal women with epilepsy. *Epilepsia.* 2011;**52**(10):1884–9.
64. Zhang J, Wang KX, Wei Y, et al. [Effect of topiramate and carbamazepine on bone metabolism in children with epilepsy]. *Zhongguo Dang Dai Er Ke Za Zhi.* 2010;**12**(2):96–8.
65. Cansu A, Yesilkaya E, Serdaroglu A, et al. Evaluation of bone turnover in epileptic children using oxcarbazepine. *Pediatr Neurol.* 2008;**39**(4):266–71.
66. Guo Y, Lin Z, Huang Y, Yu L. Effects of valproate, lamotrigine, and levetiracetam monotherapy on bone health in newly diagnosed adult patients with epilepsy. *Epilepsy Behav.* 2020;**113**:107489.
67. Guo CY, Ronen GM, Atkinson SA. Long-term valproate and lamotrigine treatment may be a marker for reduced growth and bone mass in children with epilepsy. *Epilepsia.* 2001;**42**(9):1141–7.
68. Pack AM, Morrell MJ, Marcus R, et al. Bone mass and turnover in women with epilepsy on antiepileptic drug monotherapy. *Ann Neurol.* 2005;**57**(2):252–7.
69. Kim SH, Lee JW, Choi KG, Chung HW, Lee HW. A 6-month longitudinal study of bone mineral density with antiepileptic drug monotherapy. *Epilepsy Behav.* 2007;**10**(2):291–5.
70. Koo DL, Joo EY, Kim D, Hong SB. Effects of levetiracetam as a monotherapy on bone mineral density and biochemical markers of bone metabolism in patients with epilepsy. *Epilepsy Res.* 2013;**104**(1–2):134–9.
71. Beniczky SA, Viken J, Jensen LT, Andersen NB. Bone mineral density in adult patients treated with various antiepileptic drugs. *Seizure.* 2012;**21**(6):471–2.
72. Koo DL, Nam H. Effects of zonisamide monotherapy on bone health in drug-naive epileptic patients. *Epilepsia.* 2020;**61**(10):2142–9.
73. Takahashi A, Onodera K, Kamei J, et al. Effects of chronic administration of zonisamide, an antiepileptic drug, on bone mineral density and their prevention with alfacalcidol in growing rats. *J Pharmacol Sci.* 2003;**91**(4):313–18.
74. Jette N, Lix LM, Metge CJ, et al. Association of antiepileptic drugs with nontraumatic fractures: A population-based analysis. *Arch Neurol.* 2011;**68**(1):107–12.
75. Ensrud KE, Walczak TS, Blackwell TL, et al. Antiepileptic drug use and rates of hip bone loss in older men: A prospective study. *Neurology.* 2008;**71**(10):723–30.

76. Vestergaard P. Effects of antiepileptic drugs on bone health and growth potential in children with epilepsy. *Paediatr Drugs.* 2015;**17**(2):141–50.

77. Andress DL, Ozuna J, Tirschwell D, et al. Antiepileptic drug-induced bone loss in young male patients who have seizures. *Arch Neurol.* 2002;**59**(5):781–6.

78. Mikati MA, Dib L, Yamout B, et al. Two randomized vitamin D trials in ambulatory patients on anticonvulsants: Impact on bone. *Neurology.* 2006;**67**(11):2005–14.

79. Pylvanen V, Knip M, Pakarinen A, et al. Serum insulin and leptin levels in valproate-associated obesity. *Epilepsia.* 2002;**43**(5):514–17.

80. Luef G, Abraham I, Trinka E, et al. Hyperandrogenism, postprandial hyperinsulinism and the risk of PCOS in a cross sectional study of women with epilepsy treated with valproate. *Epilepsy Res.* 2002;**48**(1–2):91–102.

81. Cansu A, Serdaroglu A, Camurdan O, Hirfanoglu T, Cinaz P. Serum insulin, cortisol, leptin, neuropeptide Y, galanin and ghrelin levels in epileptic children receiving valproate. *Horm Res Paediatr.* 2011;**76**(1):65–71.

82. Egger J, Brett EM. Effects of sodium valproate in 100 children with special reference to weight. *Br Med J (Clin Res Ed).* 1981;**283**(6291):577–81.

83. Verrotti A, la Torre R, Trotta D, Mohn A, Chiarelli F. Valproate-induced insulin resistance and obesity in children. *Horm Res.* 2009;**71**(3):125–31.

84. Vorbrodt AW, Dobrogowska DH, Kozlowski PB, et al. Immunogold study of effects of prenatal exposure to lipopolysaccharide and/or valproic acid on the rat blood-brain barrier vessels. *J Neurocytol.* 2005;**34**(6):435–46.

85. Hamed SA, Fida NM, Hamed EA. States of serum leptin and insulin in children with epilepsy: Risk predictors of weight gain. *Eur J Paediatr Neurol.* 2009;**13**(3):261–8.

86. Gungor S, Yucel G, Akinci A, et al. The role of ghrelin in weight gain and growth in epileptic children using valproate. *J Child Neurol.* 2007;**22**(12):1384–8.

87. Martin CK, Han H, Anton SD, Greenway FL, Smith SR. Effect of valproic acid on body weight, food intake, physical activity and hormones: Results of a randomized controlled trial. *J Psychopharmacol.* 2009;**23**(7):814–25.

88. Aydin K, Serdaroglu A, Okuyaz C, Bideci A, Gucuyener K. Serum insulin, leptin, and neuropeptide y levels in epileptic children treated with valproate. *J Child Neurol.* 2005;**20**(10):848–51.

89. Brill J, Lee M, Zhao S, Fernald RD, Huguenard JR. Chronic valproic acid treatment triggers increased neuropeptide y expression and signaling in rat nucleus reticularis thalami. *J Neurosci.* 2006;**26**(25):6813–22.

90. Tokgoz H, Aydin K, Oran B, Kiyici A. Plasma leptin, neuropeptide Y, ghrelin, and adiponectin levels and carotid artery intima media thickness in epileptic children treated with valproate. *Childs Nerv Syst.* 2012;**28**(7):1049–53.

91. Biton V, Mirza W, Montouris G, et al. Weight change associated with valproate and lamotrigine monotherapy in patients with epilepsy. *Neurology.* 2001;**56**(2):172–7.

92. Beydoun A, Uthman BM, Kugler AR, et al. Safety and efficacy of two pregabalin regimens for add-on treatment of partial epilepsy. *Neurology.* 2005;**64**(3):475–80.

93. Ben-Menachem E. Weight issues for people with epilepsy: A review. *Epilepsia.* 2007;**48** Suppl 9:42–5.

94. Gilliam FG, Veloso F, Bomhof MA, et al. A dose-comparison trial of topiramate as monotherapy in recently diagnosed partial epilepsy. *Neurology.* 2003;**60**(2):196–202.

95. Yang J, Lee MS, Joe SH, Jung IK, Kim SH. Zonisamide-induced weight loss in schizophrenia: Case series. *Clin Neuropharmacol.* 2010;**33**(2):104–6.

96. Shi RF, Wang KL, Li QH, et al. [Changes of body weight and galanin in epileptic children treated with topiramate].

Zhonghua Er Ke Za Zhi. 2007;**45**(3):199–202.

97. Richard D, Picard F, Lemieux C, et al. The effects of topiramate and sex hormones on energy balance of male and female rats. *Int J Obes Relat Metab Disord.* 2002;**26**(3):344–53.
98. Picard F, Deshaies Y, Lalonde J, Samson P, Richard D. Topiramate reduces energy and fat gains in lean (Fa/?) and obese (fa/fa) Zucker rats. *Obes Res.* 2000;**8**(9):656–63.
99. Kim DW, Yoo MW, Park KS. Low serum leptin level is associated with zonisamide-induced weight loss in overweight female epilepsy patients. *Epilepsy Behav.* 2012;**23**(4):497–9.
100. Gadde KM, Allison DB, Ryan DH, et al. Effects of low-dose, controlled-release, phentermine plus topiramate combination on weight and associated comorbidities in overweight and obese adults (CONQUER): A randomised, placebo-controlled, phase 3 trial. *Lancet.* 2011;**377**(9774):1341–52.
101. Bergen DC, Ristanovic RK, Waicosky K, Kanner A, Hoeppner TJ. Weight loss in patients taking felbamate. *Clin Neuropharmacol.* 1995;**18**(1):23–7.
102. Tunbridge WM, Vanderpump MP. Population screening for autoimmune thyroid disease. *Endocrinol Metab Clin North Am.* 2000;**29**(2):239–53.
103. Samuels MH. Subclinical thyroid disease in the elderly. *Thyroid.* 1998;**8**(9):803–13.
104. Hamed SA, Hamed EA, Kandil MR, et al. Serum thyroid hormone balance and lipid profile in patients with epilepsy. *Epilepsy Res.* 2005;**66**(1–3):173–83.
105. Isojarvi JI, Pakarinen AJ, Myllyla VV. Thyroid function with antiepileptic drugs. *Epilepsia.* 1992;**33**(1):142–8.
106. Yilmaz U, Yilmaz TS, Akinci G, Korkmaz HA, Tekgul H. The effect of antiepileptic drugs on thyroid function in children. *Seizure.* 2014;**23**(1):29–35.
107. Tanaka K, Kodama S, Yokoyama S, et al. Thyroid function in children with long-term anticonvulsant treatment. *Pediatr Neurosci.* 1987;**13**(2):90–4.
108. Aygun F, Ekici B, Aydinli N, et al. Thyroid hormones in children on antiepileptic therapy. *Int J Neurosci.* 2012;**122**(2):69–73.
109. Mikati MA, Tarabay H, Khalil A, et al. Risk factors for development of subclinical hypothyroidism during valproic acid therapy. *J Pediatr.* 2007;**151**(2):178–81.
110. Hegedus L, Hansen JM, Luhdorf K, et al. Increased frequency of goiter in epileptic patients on long-term phenytoin or carbamazepine treatment. *Clin Endocrinol (Oxf).* 1985;**23**(4):423–9.
111. Chakova L, Karakhanian E, Dimitrov H, Lutakova E. Effect of antiepileptic drugs on the thyroid gland in children with epilepsy (preliminary report). *Folia Med (Plovdiv).* 1998;**40**(1):80–3.
112. Benedetti MS, Whomsley R, Baltes E, Tonner F. Alteration of thyroid hormone homeostasis by antiepileptic drugs in humans: Involvement of glucuronosyltransferase induction. *Eur J Clin Pharmacol.* 2005;**61**(12):863–72.
113. Lu X, Wang X. Hyponatremia induced by antiepileptic drugs in patients with epilepsy. *Expert Opin Drug Saf.* 2017;**16**(1):77–87.
114. Dong X, Leppik IE, White J, Rarick J. Hyponatremia from oxcarbazepine and carbamazepine. *Neurology.* 2005;**65**(12):1976–8.
115. Kellinghaus C, Berning S, Stogbauer F. Use of oxcarbazepine for treatment of refractory status epilepticus. *Seizure.* 2014;**23**(2):151–4.
116. Kim YS, Kim DW, Jung KH, et al. Frequency of and risk factors for oxcarbazepine-induced severe and symptomatic hyponatremia. *Seizure.* 2014;**23**(3):208–12.
117. Gupta E, Kunjal R, Cury JD. Severe hyponatremia due to valproic acid toxicity. *J Clin Med Res.* 2015;7(9):717–19.
118. Mewasingh L, Aylett S, Kirkham F, Stanhope R. Hyponatraemia associated with lamotrigine in cranial diabetes insipidus. *Lancet.* 2000;**356**(9230):656.

119. Belcastro V, Costa C, Striano P. Levetiracetam-associated hyponatremia. *Seizure*. 2008;**17**(4):389–90.
120. Braunhofer J, Zicha L. [Does tegretal offer new possibilities of therapy in several neurologic and endocrine diseases? A clinical electroencephalographic and thin-layer chromatographic study]. *Med Welt*. 1966;**36**:1875–80.
121. Kalff R, Houtkooper MA, Meyer JW, et al. Carbamazepine and serum sodium levels. *Epilepsia*. 1984;**25**(3):390–7.
122. Henry DA, Lawson DH, Reavey P, Renfrew S. Hyponatraemia during carbamazepine treatment. *Br Med J*. 1977;**1**(6053):83–4.
123. Kuz GM, Manssourian A. Carbamazepine-induced hyponatremia: Assessment of risk factors. *Ann Pharmacother*. 2005;**39**(11):1943–6.
124. Lahr MB. Hyponatremia during carbamazepine therapy. *Clin Pharmacol Ther*. 1985;**37**(6):693–6.
125. Friis ML, Kristensen O, Boas J, et al. Therapeutic experiences with 947 epileptic out-patients in oxcarbazepine treatment. *Acta Neurol Scand*. 1993;**87**(3):224–7.
126. Tambucci R, Basti C, Maresca M, Coppola G, Verrotti A. Update on the role of eslicarbazepine acetate in the treatment of partial-onset epilepsy. *Neuropsychiatr Dis Treat*. 2016;**12**:1251–60.
127. Sperling MR, Abou-Khalil B, Harvey J, et al. Eslicarbazepine acetate as adjunctive therapy in patients with uncontrolled partial-onset seizures: Results of a phase III, double-blind, randomized, placebo-controlled trial. *Epilepsia*. 2015;**56**(2):244–53.
128. Beers E, Van Puijenbroek EP, Bartelink IH, Van der Linden CM, Jansen PA. Syndrome of inappropriate antidiuretic hormone secretion (SIADH) or hyponatraemia associated with valproic acid: Four case reports from the Netherlands and a case/non-case analysis of VigiBase. *Drug Saf*. 2010;**33**(1):47–55.
129. Ikeda K, Moriyasu H, Yasaka M, Oita J, Yamaguchi T. [Valproate-related syndrome of inappropriate secretion of antidiuretic hormone (SIADH): A case report]. *Rinsho Shinkeigaku*. 1994;**34**(9):911–13.
130. Miyaoka T, Seno H, Itoga M, et al. Contribution of sodium valproate to the syndrome of inappropriate secretion of antidiuretic hormone. *Int Clin Psychopharmacol*. 2001;**16**(1):59–61.
131. Branten AJ, Wetzels JF, Weber AM, Koene RA. Hyponatremia due to sodium valproate. *Ann Neurol*. 1998;**43**(2):265–7.
132. Nasrallah K, Silver B. Hyponatremia associated with repeated use of levetiracetam. *Epilepsia*. 2005;**46**(6):972–3.
133. Wilton LV, Shakir S. A postmarketing surveillance study of gabapentin as add-on therapy for 3,100 patients in England. *Epilepsia*. 2002;**43**(9):983–92.
134. Inamura T, Kuba H, Morioka T, et al. [Carbamazepine-induced hyponatremia]. *No Shinkei Geka*. 1999;**27**(1):85–7.
135. Berghuis B, De Haan GJ, Van den Broek MP, et al. Epidemiology, pathophysiology and putative genetic basis of carbamazepine- and oxcarbazepine-induced hyponatremia. *Eur J Neurol*. 2016;**23**(9):1393–9.
136. Isojarvi JI, Huuskonen UE, Pakarinen AJ, Vuolteenaho O, Myllyla VV. The regulation of serum sodium after replacing carbamazepine with oxcarbazepine. *Epilepsia*. 2001;**42**(6):741–5.

Genetic Epilepsies in Females

Paula Teixeira Marques and Danielle M. Andrade

Key Points

- Different genetic epilepsy syndromes may be differently expressed in men and women.
- Epilepsy syndromes with pathogenic genetic variants involving the X chromosome have distinct sex-dependent phenotypes (Rett syndrome, *CDKL5* deficiency disorder, subcortical band heterotopia, periventricular heterotopia, *PCDH19* epilepsy, and Aicardi syndrome).
- Genetic generalized epilepsy has a slightly higher incidence in females.
- Juvenile myoclonic epilepsy has a female preference with some familial forms having a predominantly maternal transmission.

Introduction

The incidence of epilepsy and unprovoked seizures is slightly higher in males compared to females. This difference is mainly due to men's greater exposure to risk factors leading to lesional epilepsy and acute symptomatic seizures such as traumatic brain injury. Conversely, the most common form of epilepsy, idiopathic (or genetic) generalized epilepsy (GGE), which is genetically determined, has a slightly higher incidence in women and is more frequently transmitted to offspring by the women affected with epilepsy than by men [1, 2]. The reason for this sex difference in GGEs is not well understood but might be associated with sex hormones [2]. This theory likely explains why after menopause the risk difference between men and women tends to equilibrate [2]. The epilepsy syndromes limited to females are frequently associated with pathogenic variants in genes located on the X chromosome. Here we describe the clinical and genetic factors associated with them and a summary of clinical, electrographic, and genetic characteristics (see also Table 6.1).

Why Is It Important to Recognize These Syndromes and How to Diagnose Them?

Recognizing these epilepsy syndromes not only helps in understanding the prognosis of patients with these conditions, but it also might aid the clinician in selecting appropriate treatment. In addition, the presence of some of these genetic variants in carrier women may explain spontaneous miscarriages. Counseling of patients and family members is important when there is risk of the pathogenic variant being passed on to offspring. In cases where the mother carries a X-linked variant, risk of transmission is 50% for girls and 50% for boys.

Table 6.1 Epilepsy syndromes limited to females and their key features

Condition	Seizure onset	Seizure types	Comorbidities and other clinical features	EEG	Genetics	Treatment
Rett syndrome (RTT)	Typically stage 3 between 2 and 10 years, but as late as 20 years	Focal impaired awareness seizures, tonic-clonic, tonic, and myoclonic seizures	Hypotonia, abnormal gait, microcephaly, ASD, constipation, reflux, air swallowing, sleep cycle abnormalities, self-injuring, delayed reaction to pain, scoliosis, and extrapyramidal disturbances	Follows the four stages of the disease. Stage 1: EEG can be normal. Stage 2: focal spikes in the centrotemporal regions with involvement of the motor cortex that coincides with the motor symptoms. Stage 3: abnormal sleep, bilateral pseudo-periodic delta activity and generalized rhythmic spike discharges, Stage 4: mostly slowing of the background activity that can have a pattern of theta in central and frontal regions and	X-linked *MECP2* pathogenic variants found in 95% of typical and 73.2% of atypical cases.	Pharmacoresistant

				can be accompanied by multifocal epileptiform activity and generalized spike and wave.		
CDKL5 Deficiency disorder (CDD)	Infantile spasms, focal and generalized seizures from birth to 3 months of age	Epileptic spasms, evolving to generalized or mixed focal and generalized with spasms, tonic, and tonic-clonic seizures. Migrating focal seizures can also occur.	Limited ability to walk, inability to speak, limited hand skills and purposeless hand movements, lack of eye contact due to cortical visual impairment, constipation, circadian problems, breathing irregularities, and hypotonia	Hypsarrhythmia and evolution often includes focal or generalized slowing, focal and generalized epileptiform activity. Slowing of background activity	X-linked *CDKL5* pathogenic variants	Pharmacoresistant, depending on stage. CBD, fenfluramine in recent studies. There may be a role of sodium channel blocker in focal seizures.
Subcortical band heterotopia (SBH)	Varied seizure types such as GTCS, focal seizures with impaired awareness	Lennox–Gastaut syndrome, typically focal or generalized epilepsy, can have tonic-clonic,	Feeding and swallowing difficulties, decreasing head circumference, disturbed muscle	Background can show focal and generalized slowing. Interictal EEG can include focal and multifocal discharges as well	X-linked DCX pathogenic variants	Pharmacoresistant, role of surgery uncertain but probably related to poor outcomes

Table 6.1 (cont.)

Condition	Seizure onset	Seizure types	Comorbidities and other clinical features	EEG	Genetics	Treatment
	between 1 month and 16 years	myoclonic seizures, atypical absences and drop attacks.	tone, immobility, scoliosis	as generalized spike and waves, with less than a 3 Hz frequency.		
Periventricular nodular heterotopia (PNH)	Focal seizures in adolescence or adulthood, ranging from 7 to 40 years of age	Uncomplicated febrile convulsions to GTCS, focal seizures as the prominent epileptic symptom	Cognitive and developmental delay, cardiac valve disease, aortic dilation, chronic obstructive lung disease, skeletal abnormalities, chronic obstipation, Ehlers–Danlos-like phenotype affecting connective tissues and persistent ductus arteriosus in the newborn	Background usually normal but can show diffuse slowing in more severely affected patients. Interictal changes in the form of focal, multifocal spikes, focal slowing and is some cases generalized spike and wave discharges may occur, especially during sleep.	X-linked FLNA pathogenic variants, 50% inherited, 50% de novo	Resective or ablative surgery if single nodule identified.
PCDH19 Epilepsy	Febrile seizures and clusters between 3 and 36	Afebrile clusters, may evolve to non- convulsive or convulsive status	Mild-to-profound ID and ASD; aggression, hyperactivity, suicidal ideation,	Interictal EEG can show focal and generalized discharges. The background can	X-linked *PCDH19* pathogenic variants	Pharmacoresistant, LEV, CLB, Bromide, Ganaloxone.

	months of age, as late as 20 years of age	epilepticus. Focal seizures with hypomotor manifestations, hemiclonic, focal unaware that evolve to bilateral tonic-clonic, atonic, myoclonic and absence seizures.	obsessive behaviors, schizophrenia. Earlier onset of seizures (<12 months) is associated with more severe ID	exhibit focal and generalized slowing. May show photoparoxysmal responses. Focal seizures more common, especially with onset in frontotemporal regions.		
Aicardi syndrome	Asymmetric or unilateral focal seizures between 3 and 4 months of age.	Infantile spasms, myoclonic, tonic, atonic, generalized tonic-clonic, atypical absence, focal seizures, and reflex audiogenic seizures	Hypotonia (early sign), microcephaly (not all patients), visual disability, scoliosis, spasticity, reflux constipation, feeding problems	Background can show burst suppression pattern with hemispheric asymmetry. Interictal EEG multifocal spikes, bilateral independent bursts of high voltage irregular slow waves and fast waves, diffuse asynchronous slow spike and wave complexes, asynchronous hypsarrhythmia	Causative gene not yet discovered. Some cases are associated with chromosomal translocations with breakpoints in the Xp22 region	Pharmacoresistant, CBD [16], callostomy if partial agenesis of corpus callosum

Table 6.1 (cont.)

Condition	Seizure onset	Seizure types	Comorbidities and other clinical features	EEG	Genetics	Treatment
Juvenile myoclonic epilepsy (JME)	Myoclonic jerks, usually in the morning period, and generalized tonic-clonic seizures	Seizures triggered by photosensitivity, sleep deprivation, alcohol intake, menses, and cognitive tasks	Psychiatric comorbidities appear in 21% of patients; 74% of patients with JME for 20 years or more develop at least one unfavorable social outcome	Usually normal background, interictal finding is of bursts of generalized and irregular spike and waves and polyspikes and waves in a frequency of 3–5 Hz and with a frontocentral predominance.	One of the most heritable forms of epilepsy. Female preference, some familial forms of JME have a maternal transmission	First line: VPA (avoid in women at childbearing age), Second line: LTG, LEV, TPM

Note: *all patients with epilepsies considered pharmacoresistant in these cases may try palliative treatments such as a vagus nerve stimulator, deep brain stimulator and ketogenic or other low-glycemic diets and callostomy if drop seizures. Abbreviations: ASD = autism spectrum disorder, CBD = cannabidiol, CDD = *CDKL5* deficiency disorder, CLB = clobazam, EEG = electroencephalogram, GTCS = generalized tonic-clonic seizure, JME = juvenile myoclonic epilepsy, LEV = levetiracetam, LTG = lamotrigine, MRI = magnetic resonance imaging, PNH = periventricular nodular heterotopia, RTT = Rett syndrome, SBH = subcortical band heterotopia, TPM = topiramate, VPA = valproic acid

Since boys have only one X chromosome, they may receive only the abnormal copy of the gene. If this happens in genes associated with periventricular nodular heterotopia, subcortical band heterotopia, *CDKL5* deficiency disorder (CDD), or *MECP2* deficiency, the pathology caused by having only the abnormal variant can be much more severe than that seen in women (who have one normal and one abnormal copy of the same gene on their two X chromosomes). Such severe pathology may not be compatible with life, leading to miscarriage or early mortality. Finally, the severity of symptoms may be associated to the random X-chromosome inactivation, which can lead to a higher or lower number of neurons expressing the abnormal gene.

In GGE and juvenile myoclonic epilepsy (JME), most cases have a complex inheritance pattern – that is, the phenotype is caused by several hundreds (or thousands) of variants of small effect in different regions of the genome, possible in concert with environmental factors. As such, the risk of transmission to offspring is usually lower than that of an X-linked gene, and it varies across studies. One study, from Pal and colleagues showed that the overall risk of epilepsy in first-degree relatives of patients with GGE (including JME and non-JME) was 8%. That risk could increase to 15.8% in the presence of absence seizures [3]. In the rare cases where GGE has a Mendelian inheritance, transmission will be up to 50% of offspring if autosomal dominant and 25% of offspring if autosomal recessive, as expected in Mendelian cases.

When suspecting a genetic etiology for epilepsy, several genetic tests can be requested. One recent meta-analysis showed that whole-exome sequencing had the highest cost-effectiveness in diagnosing epilepsies, with 45% yield, followed by an epilepsy panel (23%) and a chromosomal microarray (8%) [4]. Ordering genetic testing might also be influenced by the availability of these tests and, in some centers, familiarity of the clinician with genetic testing and/or availability of genetic counselors.

Rett Syndrome

Rett syndrome (RTT) can affect up to 1 in 10,000 girls; it is considered one of the most common genetic causes of developmental and intellectual impairment in females [6].

Clinical manifestations: Typical RTT can be divided into four clinical stages: early onset, rapid destructive, plateau and late motor deterioration. Patients with classic (typical) RTT have early normal development (until 6–12 months) before the clinical symptoms appear. This is followed by a period of stagnation or regression in cognitive and social skills, loss of language, and loss of purposeful hand movements, causing lifelong dependence. Hypotonia can be one of the earlier symptoms. Abnormal gait and growth failure also become evident in the following months and years. Microcephaly is an important, but not universal manifestation. Head circumference is normal until 3 months but falls to the second percentile by 2 years. Length is also normal at birth but falls to the fifth percentile by 7 years [6]. Other manifestations of RTT include periods of inconsolable crying during early infancy [7]. Later, stereotypic (midline) hand movements, autism, constipation, gastroesophageal reflux, air swallowing, sleep cycle abnormalities, breathing problems (apnea and/or hyperventilation), inappropriate laughing/ screaming, episodes self-injurious behavior, peripheral vasomotor disturbances, small and cold hands and feet, diminished response to pain, and scoliosis can be a part of the syndrome [7, 8]. Extrapyramidal disturbances are common and include oculogyric crisis, dystonia, chorea, tremor, bruxism, truncal ataxia, proximal myoclonus, rigidity, spasticity, bradykinesia, and hypomimia [8]. An evolution from a hyperkinetic to a hypokinetic state can also occur [8].

Epilepsy is frequently associated with RTT and negatively impacts the quality of life of patients and caregivers, being an important contributor to the severity of RTT. In typical RTT, seizures can start between the ages of 3 and 20 years.

Seizure characteristics: Frequency can vary from one or two seizures per year, monthly seizures, weekly seizures, and daily seizures. Those with more frequent seizures are overall more severely affected [9]. Seizures presenting in the first year of life are usually more difficult to control than seizures appearing later [10]. Seizure types include focal with impaired awareness with focal or multifocal onset, febrile seizures, generalized tonic-clonic seizures, atypical absences, myoclonic seizures, and focal-to-bilateral tonic-clonic seizures [11]. The most common seizure types are focal with impaired awareness and generalized tonic-clonic seizures [10]. Individuals who have no genetic variants identified are less commonly affected by epilepsy and usually have a later onset of seizures [10]. Electrical status epilepticus during sleep (ESES) can be seen in up to 10% of patients [12]. Other risk factors for severe forms of epilepsy include microcephaly, developmental delay in the first 10 months of life, absence of walking, and certain pathogenic variants in the *MECP2* gene [9, 11]. Some paroxysmal events called seizures by parents can be non-epileptic events. Examples of such behaviors include apnea, hyperventilation, behavioral arrest or "freezing" episodes, inappropriate screaming or laughter, dystonia, tremulousness, and limpness. Glaze and colleagues reported that only one-third of such parent-reported seizure behaviors were associated with ictal EEG findings [13].

Treatment: Currently, there are no specific treatments for RTT, but recent studies have identified rational molecular targets for drug therapies in mouse models. Some of these targets are being tested on clinical trials, specifically in patients with the *MECP2* pathogenic variant [14]. Previous studies have reported efficacy to different antiseizure medications (ASMs), but large studies comparing them are not yet available. A study from Glaze and colleagues described carbamazepine (CBZ), lamotrigine (LMT), and levetiracetam (LEV) as frequently used ASMs while valproic acid (VPA) was only rarely prescribed [9, 15].

Life expectancy: Patients with RTT tend to stabilize clinically into adulthood. Most patients with typical RTT live at least until 45 years of age. Patients with atypical forms may live longer [16]. Therefore, adult neurologists should become familiar with the condition and with the need for a multidisciplinary approach. Cardiac abnormalities and frequent, pharmacoresistant seizures may increase the chances of sudden death. Other causes of hospitalization include pneumonia, respiratory distress, rectal bleeding, decline in ambulation, and inability to eat or drink [7].

Radiology/pathology: The brains of most RTT patients are small and do not grow after 4 years of age. There is no evidence of brain degeneration or of macroscopic malformation of cortical development. However, there is a striking decrease in the dendritic trees of selected cortical areas, chiefly projection neurons of the motor, association, and limbic cortices. This may result from abnormalities of trophic factors [17].

Electroencephalography: In classical RTT, the EEG follows the four stages of the disease. In stage 1, seizures are not prominent and EEG can be normal. In stage 2, there are focal spikes in the centrotemporal regions with involvement of the motor cortex that coincides with the motor symptoms. Seizures are frequent in Stage 3, and in this phase, abnormal sleep patterns can be observed along with bilateral synchronous pseudo-periodic delta activity and generalized rhythmic spike discharges. In stage 4, seizures are no longer prominent, and the EEG shows mostly slowing of the background activity in central and frontal regions and can be accompanied by multifocal epileptiform activity and generalized spike and wave. These findings are not pathognomonic for RTT and although some features such as slow spike and wave might resemble Lennox–Gastaut syndrome, there is absence of paroxysmal fast activity.

Genetics: The *MECP2* (methyl-CpG-binding protein 2) gene causes 95% of typical RTT cases, and up to 73.2% of atypical RTT cases. *MECP2* maps to chromosome Xq28 and silences the gene by binding to methylated CpG islands in other genes' promoters and repressing their transcription. However, so far it is not clear which genes are affected by *MECP2*. *MECP2* associates with histone deacetylase (HDAC) in order to silence other genes. Since valproic acid is an HDAC inhibitor, some experts suggest that its use in patients with RTT may worsen phenotype (although the dose needed to inhibit HDAC may be supra-therapeutic). Genotype–phenotype correlation is not precise, but some genetic variants are associated with more severe phenotypes such as early truncating variants, large deletions, and specific point mutations [11].

Why does RTT affect predominantly females? Given the random brain inactivation of one of the X chromosomes, it is likely that some *MECP2* expression allows women to survive but is not enough to prevent the symptoms. Given that all *MECP2* expressed in male embryos derives from the only X chromosome carrying this gene with the pathogenic variant, these embryos cannot survive or rarely do, but are more severely affected. Possible exceptions are cases of Klinefelter syndrome, where a male has two X chromosomes, or mosaics [11, 15]. *MECP2* duplication is a different syndrome that manifests in men. Women who have this duplication do not have symptoms but are at risk of having boys with the syndrome. An *MECP2* duplication in males causes a neurodevelopmental disorder characterized by mild dysmorphic features (brachycephaly, mid-face hypoplasia, depressed nasal bridge), infantile hypotonia, developmental delay to profound intellectual disability, absent or minimal speech, seizures (focal and/or generalized), autism, progressive spasticity, and severe respiratory infections [11, 19].

CDKL5 Deficiency Disorder

For several years, CDD was considered an atypical Rett syndrome, known as Hanefeld variant. It can affect up to 1 in 40,000 to 1 in 60,000 people.

Clinical manifestations: CDD patients may manifest seizures from birth but more commonly at the third month of life. Infantile spasms are seen in up to 50% of cases, but multiple types of focal and generalized seizures are often combined in this condition. In addition, CDD patients often have limited ability to walk, inability to speak, limited hand skills and purposeless hand movements, lack of eye contact due to cortical visual impairment, constipation, circadian rhythm problems, breathing irregularities, and hypotonia [9, 10, 20–22].

Seizure types: Patients with CDD may present with early-onset infantile spasms and migrating focal seizures from the first weeks of life [10]. Later, epilepsy tends to be generalized or mixed focal and generalized, including epileptic spasms, tonic, and tonic-clonic seizures [23]. Three phases can be distinguished in CDD: (1) early-onset, at times pharmacoresponsive seizures, (2) epileptic encephalopathy, and (3) refractory multifocal and myoclonic epilepsy.

Treatment: The epilepsy associated with CDD is refractory and difficult to treat in most cases. One study by Devinsky has shown the efficacy of cannabidiol (purified CBD oil) in reducing seizures in patients with CDD [24]. A more recent study has shown the efficacy of fenfluramine in the treatment of patients with CDD [25]. Sodium channel blockers such as CBZ, oxcarbazepine, and lacosamide have been shown to be effective in younger patients with focal features and no history of West syndrome [26].

Life expectancy: Life expectancy is not well known for this condition, although non-medical references describe patients who are 40 years old.

Radiology/pathology: Neuroimaging is usually normal but may show cortical atrophy or white matter hyperintensities [23]. Literature reports of pathology are scarce, but one case report describes the brain as the only organ with abnormalities in a postmortem examination. The findings included brain and cerebellar atrophy and ventricular enlargement, gliosis in the cerebral cortex with preservation of the hexalaminar layers, neuronal heterotopias in the white matter of the cerebellar vermis, and gliosis of the cerebellar cortex with loss of Purkinje cells and axonal torpedoes [23].

Electroencephalography: In CDD, the EEG at onset can vary from hypsarrhythmia to mild abnormalities [23]. Infantile spasms can occur in the absence of hypsarrhythmia [23]. Other abnormalities may include focal, multifocal, and generalized epileptiform abnormalities and slowing of the background activity [23].

Genetics: The *CDKL5* (cyclin-dependent kinase-like 5) gene is located on chromosome Xp22.13. *CDKL5* possesses kinase activity and can auto-phosphorylate as well as mediate *MECP2* phosphorylation, suggesting that these two genes belong to the same molecular pathway. Indeed, the *CDKL5* and *MECP2* genes' expressions overlap during neural maturation and synaptogenesis, and these two genes interact in vitro and in vivo [27].

Why does CDD affect predominantly females? Similar to RTT, in CDD, there is random inactivation of X chromosomes, allowing women to survive, while in male embryos the condition is usually lethal. Rare males with RTT-like symptoms with encephalopathy and early seizures have been shown to have *CDKL5* pathogenic variants.

Subcortical Band Heterotopia

Subcortical band heterotopia (SBH) is also known as double cortex syndrome. This is a malformation of cortical development of the neuronal migration type.

Clinical manifestations: Patients with SBH may have mild to severe cognitive delay and almost all patients have epilepsy, which is drug-resistant in 65% of them. Seizure and cognitive dysfunction severity are thought to be related to the thickness of the subcortical band [28]. Other clinical manifestations include developmental delay, moderate-to-severe language impairment, and behavioral problems [29]. The overwhelming majority of affected patients are females, although males have been rarely described with SBH. As in most other X-linked epilepsies in males with *DCX* pathogenic variants, the phenotype is more severe with lissencephaly, mental retardation, and seizures that are usually much more difficult to control than in females [30].

Seizure characteristics: Seizure types are varied, as is age of onset. About 50% of these epilepsy patients have focal seizures, and the remaining 50% have generalized epilepsy, often within the spectrum of Lennox–Gastaut syndrome. About one-third can have tonic-clonic or myoclonic seizures, atypical absences, and drop attacks [31].

Treatment: Currently, no specific ASMs are recommended for SBH. Treatment with resective surgery demonstrated poor outcomes in one article that described six patients, suggesting these patients are not good candidates for surgery [32]. However, another article reported one patient with a good outcome after a left temporal lobectomy, despite the imaging showing bilateral band heterotopia.

Life expectancy: The long-term outcomes depend on severity of seizures and the life span might be shortened in patients with refractory seizures.

Radiology/pathology: Subcortical band heterotopia is characterized by bilateral bands of heterotopic gray matter located in the white matter between the cortex and ventricles. The bands usually extend from the frontal to the occipital regions, usually with a frontal predominance (anterior–posterior gradient; see Figure 6.1) [29]. Rarely the bands are only frontal or only occipitoparietal. The heterotopic gray matter consists of a superficial zone of disorganized neurons, an intermediate zone of neurons with rudimentary columnization, and a deeper zone where heterotopia may break into nodules. The overlying cortex is usually normal, although rarely SBH can merge frontally with the pachygyric cortex [29, 33].

Electroencephalography: The findings correlated with the multiple seizure types that can occur in these patients. Interictal EEG can include focal and multifocal discharges as well as generalized spike and waves, with a frequency of less than 3 Hz. The background can show focal or generalized slowing [31].

Genetics: The majority of patients with identified pathogenic genetic variants carry an abnormality on the X-linked *DCX* gene [34]. *DCX* pathogenic genetic variants are seen in 100% of familial cases and in 53–84% of sporadic, diffuse, or anteriorly predominant band heterotopia cases [35, 36].

Multiplex ligation-dependent probe amplification has increased the detection of large genomic deletions involving the *DCX* gene in patients with no identifiable pathogenic single nucleotide variants on gene sequencing [37]. Maternal germ-line or mosaic *DCX* pathogenic variants can occur in 10% of the cases of SBH [28]. *DCX* codes for doublecortin, a protein expressed during embryogenesis in migrating neurons and in the cortical plate [36]. Both

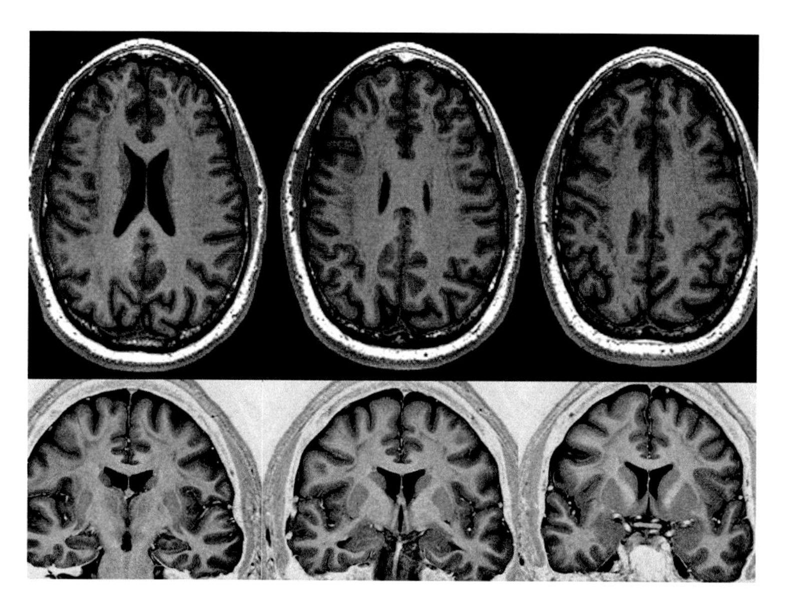

Figure 6.1 Subcortical band heterotopia. Bilateral areas of heterotopic gray matter are seen running along the anterior–posterior axis (arrowheads), forming long bands. Courtesy of Dr. Timo Krings

DCX and *LIS1* appear to interact and to enhance tubulin polymerization in order to maintain proper microtubule function [38]. Proper microtubule functioning is necessary for neuronal migration, and *DCX* appears to be regulated by phosphorylation through *CDK5* [29].

Why are most patients with SBH females? The proposed mechanism is that in females, the neurons with the mutant gene inactive (due to the random inactivation of X chromosomes) migrate normally to the cortex. Those neurons with the mutant gene active migrate abnormally and form the SBH. It is believed that surviving male embryos carrying a pathogenic variant of the *DCX* gene develop lissencephaly instead of SBH. Rare cases of SBH in males were seen in patients with somatic mosaicism, suggesting that somatic mosaicism in males is the equivalent of X inactivation in females [29, 30]. Some males may inherit a mutated *DCX* gene from their mothers. Interestingly, it was demonstrated that a few women with mild intellectual disability – with or without epilepsy, but with normal MRIs – had children affected with SBH and lissencephaly. Some of these women had children with a mild phenotype, suggesting the pathogenic variant was mild also in the female carriers. However, in another two families, the probands were severely affected, likely reflecting a severe variant in the carrier mothers. Skewed X inactivation was observed in these carriers' lymphocytes. Although this same mechanism cannot be proven to occur in the brain, it might explain the heterogeneity in the female carriers [39].

Periventricular Nodular Heterotopia

Periventricular nodular heterotopia (PNH) is also considered as a malformation of the cortical development of the neuronal migration type.

Clinical manifestations: About 90% of the patients have a refractory epilepsy that may start only during adolescence or adulthood. Most patients have normal intelligence, but cognitive and developmental delay can also be observed. Cognitive dysfunction might manifest only as difficulty in reading, processing speed and executive function. Associated clinical features in patients with *FLNA* pathogenic variants can include cardiac valve disease, aortic dilation, chronic obstructive lung disease, skeletal abnormalities, chronic obstipation, Ehlers–Danlos-like phenotype affecting connective tissues, and persistent ductus arteriosus in the newborn [40, 41].

Seizure characteristics: In the classical form of PNH, epilepsy begins in the second decade of life with focal seizures that have a low frequency at onset. Even though the frequency of seizures might increase, they typically disappear later or become very rare. Nonclassical forms, considered as PNH-plus, might involve focal epilepsy, which is more difficult to treat, and these patients can have associated intellectual disability and other neurological deficits. Drop attacks have also been described [42, 43].

Treatment: For patients presenting with refractory epilepsy, they might be eligible for a resective or ablative surgery, especially in cases where a single nodule is identified as the main epileptic generator and is located in a non-eloquent area [40].

Life expectancy: Considering classical forms have a "benign" course, life span should be normal in these patients. In the group with PNH plus, life span might be shortened by refractory seizures or associated comorbidities [43].

Radiology: Periventricular nodular heterotopia caused by *FLNA* is typically easy to identify on brain MRI as nodules localized across the lateral ventricles that predominate anteriorly or posteriorly. They can be unilateral, bilateral, single, or multiple. The anterior predominant PNH is more associated with *FLNA* variants. The posterior predominant can be associated with other genes [40].

Electroencephalography: Background is usually normal but can show diffuse slowing in more severely affected patients. Interictal changes usually occur in the form of focal, multifocal spikes, focal slowing, and in some cases, generalized spike and wave discharges may occur, especially during sleep. The focal changes can correlate with the anatomical localization of the periventricular nodules. The EEG may also be completely normal [40, 41].

Genetics: The most frequent cause of the classical X-linked form of PNH is single nucleotide pathogenic variants or deletions of the *FLNA* gene. This gene encodes filamin A, a protein that regulates reorganization of the actin cytoskeleton. Other genes have been associated with PNH, such as *ARFGEF2, INTS8, MCPH1, FAT4, DCHS1, NEDD4 L,* and *ERMARD.* Copy number variants have also been associated with PNH, including 22q11.2 deletion syndrome, whose sufferers also exhibit other clinical symptoms such as schizophrenia, hypocalcemia, dysmorphic features, and heart defects [45–47].

Why are most patients with PNH females? The classical form of PNH is associated with a pathogenic variant in the *FLNA* gene, which localizes to the X chromosome. Therefore, this condition is inherited in an X-linked manner. Male embryos carrying this mutated *FLNA* may not survive pregnancy or may die in the neonatal period. As such, this gene is associated with high miscarriage rates or high infantile mortality in boys [43]. About 50% of females inherit the pathogenic genetic variant from their mother and 50% will have a de novo pathogenic genetic variant [48].

PCDH19 Epilepsy

Different from the previous X-linked epilepsies, *PCDH19* epilepsy is an X-linked disease that may be recognized by the analysis of large pedigrees with multiple affected females linked through unaffected male relatives [49]. The pattern of transmission is more difficult to recognize in small pedigrees with only one affected female.

Clinical manifestations: Initially this syndrome was described as a *SCN1A*-negative Dravet syndrome but the phenotype can be quite distinctive, especially as patients get older [50]. Sixty-seven percent of patients with *PCDH19* epilepsy have borderline intellect or intellectual disability varying from mild to profound. Obsessive features are seen in more than 30%, aggressive behavior in 25%, and autism spectrum disorders in 22% [51]. The early psychomotor development can vary from normal to severely abnormal. Onset of psychosis during adulthood is common, and these patients should be carefully monitored for psychiatric disorders, which can include schizophrenia [52]. Interestingly, in one family, five male carriers had obsessive traits and controlling, rigid, and inflexible personalities [53].

Seizure characteristics: Seizures in *PCDH19* epilepsy usually start between 3 and 36 months of age. Initially, febrile seizures are seen in 63% of patients. However, subsequent seizures are mainly afebrile. Seizure clusters are a common feature, being reported in almost all patients. These clusters may evolve to nonconvulsive or convulsive status epilepticus and can be refractory to conventional therapy [54]. Seizure types vary from hemiclonic, focal unaware that evolve to bilateral tonic-clonic, atonic, myoclonic, and absence. Focal seizures, especially with hypomotor manifestations, and behavior arrest are the most common type at onset and throughout life. Affective symptoms such as fearful screaming seem to be a common feature. In contrast with Dravet syndrome, late onset of myoclonic, absence, and tonic seizures is rare and photosensitivity is rarely described [50]. In some families, patients stop having seizures after the age of 12 years. The clinical severity also varies. Some patients may have seizures controlled after a certain age, while others may have intractable seizures and several episodes of status epilepticus can occur in one-third of the patients [51, 53].

Treatment: No clinical trials have evaluated the efficacy of ASMs in patients with *PCDH19* epilepsy. A small case series suggested intravenous corticoid therapy was effective for seizure clusters [55]. The role of steroids is recently being explored in clinical trials through the use of ganaxolone as an ASM, showing some promising results [56]. Another study, which included 58 patients, demonstrated good results with clobazam and bromide [50]. Despite the known psychiatric side effects of levetiracetam, a study from Sadleir and colleagues showed this drug was effective in two cohorts of females with *PCDH19* epilepsy where 42% and 76% of females became seizure free for longer than 12 months, respectively, suggesting this medication should be trialed early on [57].

Life expectancy: No studies report the long-term outcomes of these patients. Considering their seizures stabilize over time, they might have a normal life expectancy.

Radiology: Most patients with *PCDH19* epilepsy exhibit normal brain MRI. However, patients with hippocampal sclerosis, focal cortical dysplasia, and periventricular nodular heterotopia have been reported [50].

Electroencephalography: Interictal EEG can show focal and generalized discharges. The background can also exhibit focal and generalized slowing. The majority of seizures have a focal onset, even though generalized onset has also been reported. The most frequent ones have onset on the frontotemporal regions, but posterior onset can also happen [50].

Genetics: *PCDH19* epilepsy is caused by pathogenic variants involving the protocadherin 19 (*PCDH19*) gene, which also localizes to the X chromosome. The protein encoded by this gene is a member of the delta-2 protocadherin subclass of the cadherin superfamily. The encoded protein is thought to be a calcium-dependent, cell-adhesion protein primarily expressed in the brain. Three transcript variants encoding different isoforms have been found for this gene [58].

Why does *PCDH19* epilepsy affect mainly females? This condition is different from those described earlier in this chapter, where affected males die in utero or have a more severe phenotype. Here, the males with pathogenic *PCDH19* variants are usually normal and can reproduce. Dibbens and colleagues proposed the following mechanism:

> Since the *PCDH19* gene is subject to X inactivation, hemizygous transmitting males likely have a homogenous population of *PCDH19*-mutated cells, while affected females behave like mosaics comprising *PCDH19*-mutated cells and *PCDH19*-wildtype cells. This tissue mosaicism may scramble cell-cell communication which manifests clinically as *PCDH19* epilepsy. The absence of *PCDH19* function in males may be compensated by the related but non-paralogous procadherin gene *PCDH11Y*, a Y chromosome gene expressed in human brain. *PCDH11Y* has an X chromosome paralogue, *PCDH11X*, that has strong sequence similarity. [58]

Aicardi Syndrome

Aicardi syndrome is also a neurodevelopmental disorder affecting mainly girls.

Clinical manifestations: Aicardi syndrome (AS) is characterized by a triad of corpus callosum (partial or total) agenesis, infantile spasms, and chorioretinal lacunae. Most patients have severe intellectual disability, optic disc or nerve coloboma or hypoplasia, malformation of cortical development, and vertebral and rib deformities [59]. Dysmorphic features are common and include prominent premaxilla, upturned nasal tip, decreased angle of the nasal bridge, and sparse lateral eyebrows. Externally apparent microphthalmia is present in up to 25% of cases. Vascular malformations or vascular malignancy can also occur [59].

Seizure characteristics: Epilepsy in AS can range from mild (rarely) to very severe [63], with several forms of pharmacoresistant seizures. Seizures types include infantile spasms, myoclonic, tonic, atonic, generalized tonic-clonic, atypical absence, focal seizures, and reflex audiogenic seizures [61]. Seizures usually appear early, at 3–4 months of age, and are often asymmetric or unilateral [59, 61].

Treatment: Patients with AS should be treated with a multidisciplinary approach because of their many comorbidities. Seizures are very frequently resistant to treatment in these patients. A study by Devinsky and colleagues has shown a 50% decrease from the median baseline number of seizures with purified CBD oil [24]. In cases where there is partial agenesis of the corpus callosum, a corpus callosotomy may be considered [62].

Life expectancy: There is little information on the life expectancy of girls with AS. One report on 69 patients demonstrated a median age of survival of 18.5 (+/−4 years) [63]. But the authors have patients as old as 37 years old in their adult genetic epilepsy clinic (personal experience).

Radiology: The largest study of girls with AS showed that in addition to the known total or partial agenesis of corpus callosum, all patients had polymicrogyria that was predominantly frontal and perisylvian, and often associated with under-opercularization. Periventricular nodular heterotopia was also present in all patients. Cerebellar abnormalities were seen in 95% of cases. Tectal enlargement was seen in 10 out of 23 cases studied. Single or multiple cysts were observed in 21 out of 23 cases [64]. Other abnormalities previously described include pachygyria, papilloma of the choroid plexus, and basal ganglia dysmorphisms [59, 64].

Electroencephalography: The classical features of AS are a burst suppression pattern with hemispheric asymmetry (split EEG) due to the absence of the corpus callosum. Interictal EEG can show multifocal spikes, bilateral and independent bursts of high-voltage irregular slow and fast waves, and diffuse asynchronous slow spike and wave complexes. A pattern of asynchronous hypsarrhythmia can also be observed [65].

Genetics: Aicardi syndrome is a sporadic disease. Given that almost all cases are seen in females, this condition is thought to be an X-linked disorder with lethality in the hemizygous male embryo. Nevertheless, a causative gene is yet to be discovered. Some cases are associated with chromosomal translocations with breakpoints in the Xp22 region.

Juvenile Myoclonic Epilepsy

Juvenile myoclonic epilepsy (JME) affects 5–10% of all patients with epilepsy, making it one of the most common epilepsy subtypes [66]. Although it affects both men and women, there is a female preference. In addition, some familial forms of JME have a maternal transmission [1, 2].

Clinical manifestations: Patients with JME present with myoclonic jerks, usually in the morning period, and generalized tonic-clonic seizures. These patients classically have photosensitivity and their seizures are triggered by sleep deprivation, alcohol intake, menses, and cognitive tasks (praxis induction). Some atypical JME patients, especially those belonging to multiplex families, may have a history of absence or very rarely astatic (atonic) seizures in addition to myoclonus and generalized tonic-clonic seizures. Seizure onset in typical JME patients is between 8 and 20 years and seizures usually continue for life [67].

Treatment: Regardless of the commonality of JME, no double-blind randomized, placebo-controlled trials have been conducted comparing different drugs for treatment of this disease. Some experts advocate for valproate as the most effective drug in treating JME, although it should be avoided in women of childbearing age. Second-line therapies include lamotrigine, levetiracetam, and topiramate [66].

Life expectancy: Life expectancy for JME patients is normal. Unfortunately, 74% of patients with JME for 20 years or more develop at least one unfavorable social outcome such as unemployment or unplanned pregnancy [68]. Even though the rate of remission for seizures is high in these patients, only a minority of them remain seizure free without medication [66].

Radiology/pathology: No structural brain abnormalities are seen on routine MRI of patients with JME. However, studies with morphometric T1-weighted MRI have shown abnormalities in gray matter that can be increased [69] or decreased in the mesial frontal lobe of these patients [70].

Electroencephalography: Usually the EEG background on these patients is within normal limits. The classical interictal finding is bursts of generalized and irregular spike and waves and polyspikes and waves in a frequency of 3–5 Hz and with a frontocentral predominance. These bursts might also appear in the form of fragments, especially in the frontal regions. Focal interictal discharges can also be seen in some cases [71].

Genetics: Juvenile myoclonic epilepsy is one of the most heritable forms of epilepsy; however, the precise mechanism of transmission is not clear. Large efforts have been employed to identify the genetic basis of common epilepsies such as the GGE and specifically the JME subtypes. Juvenile myoclonic epilepsy is highly genetically determined, with concordance rates in monozygotic twins of up to 94% [73]. In extremely rare families (less than 1%), JME is inherited in Mendelian fashion, and in these families, diseased genes have been identified, including *EFHC1*, *CACNB4*, *CASR*, *GABRD*, *CLCN2*, and *GABRA1* [74, 75]. Other studies have demonstrated polymorphisms in *GRM4*, *CX36*, and *BRD2* to be significantly associated with JME. Not all multiplex families have "pure" JME. Multiplex families of JME probands are divided into: (1) families where all affected have classic JME (72%); (2) families where some or most individuals present with childhood absence epilepsy, which later evolves into JME as they grow older (18%); (3) families where JME patients also develop adolescence-onset absence seizures (7%); and (4) families with individuals who also develop astatic (atonic) seizures (3%) [78]. In groups (1) and (2), there is a higher maternal than paternal transmission. In groups (3) and (4), the maternal/paternal transmission rate is equal. No specific genes were associated with maternal/paternal transmission [67].

Other genetic abnormalities such as copy number variants have been described as a risk factor for JME [76]. Recently, it was demonstrated that sporadic cases of GGE have a 4.5 higher burden of variants (as calculated by polygenic risk score) compared to controls. So far, this has been seen in the non-Finnish European population. A JME-specific increased polygenic risk score has not yet been demonstrated [77].

Conclusion

So far, genetic forms of epilepsy affecting mainly women are usually associated with several other clinical manifestations, especially cognitive delay. The majority of the known genes associated with these conditions localize to the X chromosome, and despite genetic heterogeneity, they have a simple Mendelian inheritance. However, random X-chromosome inactivation can significantly alter phenotype severity. Genetics of the more common and pure epilepsy syndrome of JME is much more complex, with unclear mechanisms affecting several genes. To date, there is no specific treatment for these genetically determined seizures in women, although favorable results have been demonstrated with fenfluramine, ganaxolone, and cannabidiol in some of these conditions. The knowledge of these genetic etiologies is important for genetic counseling, especially for affected individuals and their unaffected family members who plan to have children. In some cases, if the risks of transmission are high, pre-implantation diagnosis can be offered. Furthermore, most of these syndromes present in early childhood, and the long-term outcome is poorly known. Advances in molecular genetics research and diagnosis will lead to a better understanding of pathology, the disease's natural history, and, we hope, to tailored treatment of seizures in these conditions.

References

1. Doose H, Neubauer BA. Preponderance of female sex in the transmission of seizure liability in idiopathic generalized epilepsy. *Epilepsy Res.* 2001;**43**(2):103–14.
2. Christensen J, Kjeldsen MJ, Andersen H, Friis ML. Gender differences in epilepsy. *Epilepsia.* 2005;**46**(6):956–60.
3. Pal, D. K., Durner, M., Klotz, I., et al. Complex inheritance and parent-of-origin effect in juvenile myoclonic epilepsy. *Brain Dev.* 2006;**28**(2):92–8.
4. Loddenkemper T, Sheidley BR, Poduri A. Diagnostic yield of genetic tests in epilepsy. *Neurology.* 2019;**92**(5):e418–e428.
5. Svenstrup D, Jørgensen HL, Winther O, et al. Rare disease diagnosis: A review of web search, social media and large-scale data-mining approaches. *Rare Dis.* 2015;**3**(1):e1083145. https://doi.org/10.1080/21675511.2015.1083145.
6. Schultz RJ, Glaze DG, Motil KJ, et al. The pattern of growth failure in Rett syndrome. *Am J Dis Child.* 1993;**147**(6):633–7. https://doi.org/10.1001/archpedi.1993.02160300039018.
7. Fu C, Armstrong D, Marsh E, et al. Consensus guidelines on managing Rett syndrome across the lifespan. *BMJ Paediatr Open.* 2020;**4**(1):e000717. https://doi.org/10.1136/bmjpo-2020-000717.
8. Brunetti S, Lumsden DE. Rett syndrome as a movement and motor disorder: A narrative review. *European Journal of Paediatric Neurology*, 2020;**28**:29–37. https://doi.org/10.1016/j.ejpn.2020.06.020.
9. Glaze DG. Epilepsy and the natural history of Rett syndrome. *Neurology.* 2010;**74**(11):909–12. https://doi.org/10.1212/WNL.0b013e3181d6b852.
10. Pintaudi M, Grazia M, Vignoli A, et al. Epilepsy in Rett syndrome: Clinical and genetic features. *Epilepsy Behav.* 2010;**19**(3):296–300. http://dx.doi.org/10.1016/j.yebeh.2010.06.051.
11. Operto FF, Mazza R, Maria G, Pastorino G. Epilepsy and genetic in Rett syndrome: A review. *Brain Behav.* 2019;**9**(5):e01250. https://doi.org/10.1002/brb3.1250.
12. Nissenkorn A, Gak E, Vecsler M, et al. Epilepsy in Rett syndrome: The experience of a national Rett center. *Epilepsia.* 2010;**51**(7):1252–8. https://doi.org/10.1111/j.1528-1167.2010.02597.x.
13. Glaze DG, Schultz RJ, Frost JD. Rett syndrome: Characterization of seizures versus non-seizures. *Electroencephalogr*

Clin Neurophysiol. 1998;**106**:79–83. https://doi.org/10.1016/s0013-4694(97)00084-9.

14. Vashi N, Justice MJ. Treating Rett syndrome: From mouse models to human therapies. *Mamm Genome.* 2019;**30**(5):90–110. http://dx.doi.org/10.1007/s00335-019-09793-5.
15. Krajnc N. Management of epilepsy in patients with Rett syndrome: Perspectives and considerations. *Ther Clin Risk Manag.* 2015;**11**:925–32. https://doi.org/10.2147/TCRM.S55896.
16. Kirby RS, Lane JB, Childers J, et al. Longevity in Rett syndrome: Analysis of the North American Database. *J Pediatr.* 2010;**156**(1):135–8. http://dx.doi.org/10.1016/j.jpeds.2009.07.015.
17. Armstrong DD, Dunn JK, Schultz RJ, et al. Organ growth in Rett syndrome: A postmortem examination analysis. *Pediatr Neurol.* 1999;**20**(2):125–9. https://doi.org/10.1016/s0887-8994(98)00124-6.
18. Dolce A, Ben-Zeev B, Naidu S, Kossoff EH. Rett syndrome and epilepsy: An update for child neurologists. *Pediatr Neurol.* 2013;**48**(5):337–45. http://dx.doi.org/10.1016/j.pediatrneurol.2012.11.001.
19. Ramocki MB, Tavyev YJ, Peters SU. The *MECP2* duplication syndrome. *Am J Med Genet.* 2010;**152**(5):1079–88. https://doi.org/10.1002/ajmg.a.33184.www.ncbi.nlm.nih.gov/pmc/articles/PMC3624763/pdf/nihms412728.pdf.
20. Müller A, Helbig I, Jansen C, et al. Retrospective evaluation of low long-term efficacy of antiepileptic drugs and ketogenic diet in 39 patients with *CDKL5*-related epilepsy. *Eur J Paediatr Neurol.* 2016;**20**(1):147–51. http://dx.doi.org/10.1016/j.ejpn.2015.09.001.
21. Fehr S, Downs J, Ho G, et al. Functional abilities in children and adults with the *CDKL5* disorder. *Am J Med Genet Part A.* 2016;**170**(11):2860–9.
22. Fehr S, Wong K, Chin R, et al. Seizure variables and their relationship to genotype and functional abilities in the *CDKL5* disorder. *Neurology.* 2016;**87**(21):2206–13.
23. Olson HE, Demarest ST, Pestana-Knight EM, Swanson LC. Cyclin-dependent kinase-like 5 (CDKL%) deficiency disorder: Clinical review. *Pediatr Neurol.* 2019;**97**:18–25.
24. Devinsky O, Verducci C, Thiele EA, et al. Open-label use of highly purified CBD (Epidiolex®) in patients with *CDKL5* deficiency disorder and Aicardi, Dup15q, and Doose syndromes. *Epilepsy Behav.* 2018;**86**:131–7.
25. Devinsky O, King LT, Schwartz D, Conway E, Price D. Effect of fenfluramine on convulsive seizures in *CDKL5* deficiency disorder. *Epilepsia.* 2021;**62**(7):e98–102.
26. Aledo-Serrano Á, Gómez-Iglesias P, Toledano R, et al. Sodium channel blockers for the treatment of epilepsy in *CDKL5* deficiency disorder: Findings from a multicenter cohort. *Epilepsy & Behavior.* 2021;**118**:3–7.
27. Mari F, Azimonti S, Bertani I, et al. *CDKL5* belongs to the same molecular pathway of *MECP2* and it is responsible for the early-onset seizure variant of Rett syndrome. *Hum Mol Genet.* 2005;**14**(14):1935–46.
28. Parrini E, Conti V, Dobyns WB, Guerrini R. Genetic basis of brain malformations. *Mol Syndromol.* 2016;**7**(4):220–33.
29. Poolos NP, Das S, Clark GD, et al. Males with epilepsy, complete subcortical band heterotopia, and somatic mosaicism for DCX. *Neurology.* 2002;**58**(10):1559–62. https://doi.org/10.1212/wnl.58.10.1559. PMID: 12034802.
30. Poolos NP, Das S, Clark GD et al. Males with epilepsy, complete subcortical band heterotopia, and somatic mosaicism for DCX. *Neurology.* 2002;**58**(10):1559–62.
31. Dericioglu N, Oguz KK, Ergun EL, Tezer F, Saygi S Ictal/interictal EEG patterns and functional neuroimaging findings in subcortical band heterotopia: Report of three cases and review of the literature. *Clin EEG Neurosci.* 2008;**39**(1):43–9.

32. Bernasconi A, Martinez V, Rosa-Neto P, et al. Surgical resection for intractable epilepsy in "double cortex" syndrome yields inadequate results. *Epilepsia.* 2001;**42**(9):1124–9.

33. Mann DM. *Greenfield's neuropathology*, 7th edition. *Journal of Neurology, Neurosurgery & Psychiatry.* 2003;**74**:142.

34. Ross ME, Allen KM, Srivastava AK, et al. Linkage and physical mapping of X-linked lissencephaly/SBH (XLIS): A gene causing neuronal migration defects in human brain. *Hum Mol Genet.* 1997;**6**(4):555–62.

35. Gleeson JG, Luo RF, Grant PE, et al. Genetic and neuroradiological heterogeneity of double cortex syndrome. *Ann Neurol.* 2000;**47**(2):265–9.

36. Matsumoto N, Leventer RJ, Kuc JA, et al. Mutation analysis of the *DCX* gene and genotype/phenotype correlation in subcortical band heterotopia. *Eur J Hum Genet.* 2001;**9**(1):5–12.

37. Mei D, Parrini E, Pasqualetti M, et al. Multiplex ligation-dependent probe amplification detects *DCX* gene deletions in band heterotopia. *Neurology.* 2007;**68**(6):446–50.

38. Caspi M, Atlas R, Kantor A, Sapir T, Reiner O. Interaction between LIS1 and doublecortin, two lissencephaly gene products. *Hum Mol Genet.* 2000;**9**(15):2205–13.

39. Guerrini R, Moro F, Andermann E, et al. Nonsyndromic mental retardation and cryptogenic epilepsy in women with doublecortin gene mutations. *Ann Neurol.* 2003;**54**(1):30–7.

40. Khoo HM, Gotman J, Hall JA, Dubeau F. Treatment of epilepsy associated with periventricular nodular heterotopia. *Curr Neurol Neurosci Rep.* 2020;**20**(12):59. https://doi.org/10.1007/s11910-020-01082-y.

41. Lange M, Kasper B, Bohring A, et al. 47 patients with FLNA associated periventricular nodular heterotopia. *Orphanet J Rare Dis.* 2015;**10**(1):1–11. http://dx.doi.org/10.1186/s13023-015-0331-9.

42. Battaglia G, Chiapparini L, Franceschetti S, et al. Periventricular nodular heterotopia: Classification, epileptic history, and genesis of epileptic discharges. *Epilepsia.* 2006;**47**(1):86–97.

43. D'Orsi G, Tinuper P, Bisulli F, et al. Clinical features and long term outcome of epilepsy in periventricular nodular heterotopia: Simple compared with plus forms. *J Neurol Neurosurg Psychiatry.* 2004;**75**(6):873–8.

44. Clapham KR, Yu TW, Ganesh VS, et al. FLNA genomic rearrangements cause periventricular nodular heterotopia. *Neurology.* 2012;**78**(4):269–78.

45. Liu W, Yan B, An D, et al. Sporadic periventricular nodular heterotopia: Classification, phenotype and correlation with filamin A mutations. *Epilepsy Res.* 2017;**133**:33–40. http://dx.doi.org/10.1016/j.eplepsyres.2017.03.005.

46. Cellini E, Vetro A, Conti V, et al. Multiple genomic copy number variants associated with periventricular nodular heterotopia indicate extreme genetic heterogeneity. *Eur J Hum Genet.* 2019;**27**(6):909–18. http://dx.doi.org/10.1038/s41431-019-0335-3.

47. Rezazadeh A, Bercovici E, Kiehl TR, et al. Periventricular nodular heterotopia in 22q11.2 deletion and frontal lobe migration. *Ann Clin Transl Neurol.* 2018;**5**(11):1314–22.

48. Chen MH, Walsh CA. FLNA-related periventricular nodular heterotopia. In Adam MP, Ardinger HH, Pagon RA, et al., eds. *GeneReviews®*. Seattle: University of Washington Press; 1993–2021. www.ncbi.nlm.nih.gov/sites/books/NBK1213.

49. Juberg RC, Hellman CD. A new familial form of convulsive disorder and mental retardation limited to females. *J Pediatr.* 1971;**79**(5):726–32.

50. Samanta D. *PCDH19*-related epilepsy syndrome: A comprehensive clinical review. *Pediatr Neurol.* 2020;**105**:3–9. https://doi.org/10.1016/j.pediatrneurol.2019.10.009.

51. Hynes K, Tarpey P, Dibbens LM, et al. Epilepsy and mental retardation limited to females with *PCDH19* mutations can present de novo or in single generation families. *J Med Genet.* 2010;**47**(3):211–16.

52. Vlaskamp DRM, Bassett AS, Sullivan JE, et al. Schizophrenia is a later-onset feature of *PCDH19* girls clustering epilepsy. *Epilepsia*. 2019;**60**(3):429–40.
53. Scheffer IE, Turner SJ, Dibbens LM, et al. Epilepsy and mental retardation limited to females: An under-recognized disorder. *Brain*. 2008;**131**(4):918–27.
54. Trivisano M, Specchio N. The role of *PCDH19* in refractory status epilepticus. *Epilepsy Behav*. 2019;**101**(xxxx):106539. https://doi.org/10.1016/j.yebeh.2019.106539
55. Higurashi N, Takahashi Y, Kashimada A, et al. Immediate suppression of seizure clusters by corticosteroids in *PCDH19* female epilepsy. *Seizure*. 2015;**27**:1–5. http://dx.doi.org/10.1016/j.seizure.2015.02.006.
56. Lappalainen J, Chez M, Sullivan J, et al. A multicenter, open-label trial of ganaxolone in children with *PCDH19* epilepsy (P5.236). *Neurology*. 2017;**88**(16 Supplement):P5.236. http://n.neurology.org/content/88/16_Supplement/P5.236.abstract.
57. Sadleir LG, Kolc KL, King C, et al. Levetiracetam efficacy in *PCDH19* girls clustering epilepsy. *Eur J Paediatr Neurol*. 2020;**24**:142–7. https://doi.org/10.1016/j.ejpn.2019.12.020.
58. Dibbens LM, et al. X-linked protocadherin 19 mutations cause female-limited epilepsy and cognitive impairment. *Nat Genet*. 2008;**40**(16):776–81.
59. Wong BKY, Sutton VR. Aicardi syndrome, an unsolved mystery: Review of diagnostic features, previous attempts, and future opportunities for genetic examination. *Am J Med Genet Part C Semin Med Genet*. 2018;**178**(4):423–31.
60. Sutton VR, Hopkins BJ, Eble TN, et al. Facial and physical features of Aicardi syndrome: Infants to teenagers. 2005;**258**:254–8.
61. Grosso S, Farnetani MA, Bernardoni E, Morgese G, Balestri P. Intractable reflex audiogenic seizures in Aicardi syndrome. *Brain Dev*. 2007;**29**(4):243–6.
62. Bernstock JD, Olsen HE, Segar D, et al. Corpus callosotomy for refractory epilepsy in Aicardi syndrome: A case report and focused review of the literature. *World Neurosurg*. 2020. https://doi.org/10.1016/j.wneu.2020.06.230.
63. Glasmacher MAK, Sutton VR, Hopkins B, et al. Phenotype and management of Aicardi syndrome: New findings from a survey of 69 children. *J Child Neurol*. 2007;**22**(2):176–84.
64. Hopkins B, Sutton VR, Lewis RA, Van den Veyver I. Neuroimaging aspects of Aicardi syndrome. *Am J Med Genet*. 2008;**146A**(22):2871–8.
65. Ohtsuka Y, Oka E, Terasaki T, Ohtahara S. Aicardi syndrome: A longitudinal clinical and electroencephalographic study. *Epilepsia*. 1993;**34**(4):627–34.
66. Brodie MJ. Modern management of juvenile myoclonic epilepsy. *Expert Rev Neurother*. 2016;**16**(6):681–8.
67. Martínez-Juárez IE, Alonso ME, Medina MT, et al. Juvenile myoclonic epilepsy subsyndromes: Family studies and long-term follow-up. *Brain*. 2006;**129**(5):1269–80.
68. Camfield CS, Camfield PR. Juvenile myoclonic epilepsy 25 years after seizure onset: A population-based study. *Neurology*. 2009;**73**(13):1041–5.
69. Woermann FG, Free SL, Koepp MJ, Sisodiya SM, Duncan JS. Abnormal cerebral structure in juvenile myoclonic epilepsy demonstrated with voxel-based analysis of MRI. *Brain*. 1999;**122**(11):2101–7.
70. O'Muircheartaigh J, Vollmar C, Barker GJ, et al. Focal structural changes and cognitive dysfunction in juvenile myoclonic epilepsy. *Neurology*. 2011;**76**(1):34–40.
71. Alfradique I, Vasconcelos MM. Juvenile myoclonic epilepsy. *Arq Neuropsiquiatr*. 2007;**65**(4 B):1266–71.
72. Baykan B, Wolf P Juvenile myoclonic epilepsy as a spectrum disorder: A focused review. *Seizure*. 2017;**49**:36–41. http://dx.doi.org/10.1016/j.seizure.2017.05.011.

73. Berkovic SF, Howell RA, Hay DA, Hopper JL. Epilepsies in twins: Genetics of the major epilepsy syndromes. *Ann Neurol.* 1998;**43**(4):435–45.

74. Dos Santos BP, Marinho CRM, Marques TEBS, et al. Genetic susceptibility in juvenile myoclonic epilepsy: Systematic review of genetic association studies. *PLoS One*. 2017;**12**(6):1–17.

75. Haug K, Warnstedt M, Alekov AK, et al. Mutations in *CLCN2* encoding a voltage-gated chloride channel are associated with idiopathic generalized epilepsies. *Nat Genet*. 2003;**33**(4):527–32.

76. Helbig I, Hartmann C, Mefford HC. The unexpected role of copy number variations in juvenile myoclonic epilepsy. *Epilepsy Behav*. 2013;**28**(1):S66–8. http://dx.doi.org/10.1016/j.yebeh.2012.07.005.

77. Qaiser F, Yuen RKC, Andrade DM Genetics of epileptic networks: From focal to generalized genetic epilepsies. *Curr Neurol Neurosci Rep*. 2020;**20**(10):46. https://doi.org/10.1007/s11910-020-01059-x.

Chapter 7

Gender Issues in Childhood- and Adolescence-Onset Epilepsies

Arezoo Rezazadeh, Katherine Muir, and Tadeu Fantaneanu

Key Points

- Epilepsy remains one of the most common neurological disorders in childhood and adolescence.
- Attention deficit hyperactivity disorder and autism spectrum disorder are prevalent comorbidities in children with epilepsy.
- Stigma, bullying, and violence remain important neurodevelopmental disrupters for girls and adolescent women with epilepsy (WWE).
- Transitional care requires a coordinated effort from multiple healthcare professionals to provide uninterrupted holistic care to adolescent WWE.
- Practitioners need to remain sensitive to the needs of girls and adolescent WWE of culturally diverse, Indigenous, and 2SLGBQTIA+ backgrounds.

Introduction

The care of girls and young women with epilepsy (WWE) has grown more complex over the past decades. More emphasis has been placed on identifying psychiatric comorbidities early while psychosocial issues of stigma, bullying, and violence remain potent disrupters of patients' development at this stage in their lives. As adolescence is a time of self-emergence and sexual awakening, understanding how epilepsy impacts patients from diverse backgrounds, including those from 2SLGBTQIA+ populations, is paramount in ensuring they receive timely and appropriate services. Expansion of virtual care as well as globalization also means that practitioners can now assume care for girls and young WWE from diverse cultural backgrounds, including Indigenous cultures, and must develop a broader understanding of their needs if they are to provide them with holistic care. In this chapter, we highlight some important aspects of caring for girls and young WWE in the twenty-first century.

Psychiatric Comorbidities in Childhood

Psychiatric disorders are a common comorbidity in children with epilepsy with a prevalence of 37%, fourfold higher than the general population prevalence of 9% [1]. Two conditions most relevant to this developmental age are attention deficit hyperactivity disorder (ADHD) and autism spectrum disorder.

Attention deficit hyperactivity disorder is one of the most common comorbidities in children with epilepsy. The rate of ADHD is two and a half times higher in children with epilepsy compared to children without seizures. In the general population, ADHD is three to seven times more common in boys than girls. This sex difference has not been shown in children with epilepsy, where most studies report an equal sex distribution [2]. In this context, girls with epilepsy have a much higher risk of developing ADHD than girls in the general population. Attention deficit hyperactivity disorder in children can have a significant effect on health-related quality of life, especially if they have comorbid psychiatric disorders or learning disorders [3]. The International League Against Epilepsy Task Force on Comorbidities recommends screening for ADHD be performed in all children with epilepsy from 6 years of age onward or at the time of diagnosis and repeated annually. Methylphenidate is the most used and studied therapy for ADHD and epilepsy. In their systematic review, Auvin et al. [2] concluded that although seizure exacerbation was reported in 0–18% of studies, most were mild and transient. Also, because studies are not placebo controlled, it is not possible to tell how much of this effect was due to natural fluctuations in seizures. The impact of ADHD on quality of life for children is so significant that treatment of this condition should not be limited by fears of seizure exacerbations.

Autism spectrum disorder is also a common comorbidity in children with epilepsy. The prevalence of autism spectrum disorder has been reported as 6.3% of individuals with epilepsy, compared to 2% in the general population [4]. Autism is more common in males within the population, with a National Health Statistics Report in 2014 showing an estimated lifetime prevalence of 3.29% in males compared to 1.15% in females [5]. Strasser et al. reported male sex to be a risk factor in the development of autism spectrum disorders in individuals with epilepsy [4]. A meta-analysis by Lax-Pericall et al. also showed that the risk of autism spectrum disorders was slightly higher in males with epilepsy (RR = 1.67). Although males with epilepsy have been shown to be at slightly higher risk of autism spectrum disorders compared to females with epilepsy, this difference in risk is not as significant as what is seen in the general population [6]. This once again highlights that girls with epilepsy are at much higher risk of being diagnosed with this condition.

There are many potential reasons that rates of ADHD and autism have a more equal sex-specific prevalence in children with epilepsy compared to children in the general population. These include the fact that seizures may be damaging to neurologic pathways necessary for social skills and attention or that there is a common genetic predisposition for both seizures and these neuropsychiatric syndromes. It is also possible that children seen by epilepsy specialists are more likely to have their neurodevelopment further evaluated. Practitioners caring for children with epilepsy should screen for and identify both conditions as early as possible in order to address potential neurocognitive sequelae in a timely manner.

Adolescence and Lifestyle Changes in Youth with Epilepsy

Adolescence is a time for normative developmental milestones to be reached, the most important of which is identity formation – the sense of self. This is a fundamental stage during which adolescents begin to define who they are and how they fit into their wider family unit and community and look for approval from their peer social groups. It is of importance that they are not perceived as "different" from their peers. Adolescence is also a time of transition when teenagers strive for independence and autonomy. For adolescents with a chronic medical condition, this usually means that they must transition from their medical care being managed by their parents to being responsible for their own medical condition. These unique features of adolescence result in the emergence of many new considerations, including problems with medication compliance or being unable to participate in some of the normal adolescent milestones like getting a driver's license, which may put them at even greater risk of worsening overall quality of life and increased psychiatric comorbidities.

Compliance

Compliance with medication is an issue for any chronic disease population. Parents are responsible for overseeing their children's use of antiseizure medications (ASMs). Adolescents must transition to being responsible for their own compliance. Adolescents have been shown in multiple studies on epilepsy to be less compliant with their medication regimens then adults with epilepsy [7]. No sex difference has been reported in these rates of compliance Teens can use technology such as setting alarms on their phones or using apps to track medications to improve their compliance.

Driving

Adolescence is a time when teenagers begin to seek more independence. One important milestone to many teenagers is obtaining their driver's license. Active seizures often prevent adolescents with epilepsy from obtaining their driver's license. But they are still less likely to obtain their driver's licenses, even if their seizures are controlled. Sillanpää and Shinnar studied adolescents with a history of childhood-onset epilepsy who were eligible based on seizure control to obtain their driver's license and found that only 64% compared to 90% of control subject had obtained their license [8]. Females with epilepsy were even less likely to do so compared to their male counterparts. The reason for this sex difference is not clear from the research, but it may be related to the increased anxiety and negative attitudes toward their illness preventing them from moving forward with normal teenage milestones. A lack of driver's license as a teenager can affect an adolescent's ability to further foster their independence and access employment.

Seizure Triggers

Adolescence is a high-risk period for sleep deprivation due to increased time spent out of the house as well as increased time pressures such as school examinations. Sleep deprivation is known to precipitate seizures, especially in idiopathic generalized epilepsies such as juvenile myoclonic epilepsy (JME), common in adolescent women. The adolescent period is also characterized by risk-taking and experimentation. This often includes the use of alcohol and recreational drugs. Alcohol withdrawal, benzodiazepine withdrawal, stimulant use including amphetamine, methamphetamine, 3,4-methylenedioxymethamphetamine (MDMA, Ecstasy) and cocaine use can all trigger seizures [9].

Self-Image, Sexual Awakening, and Adolescence

When young WWE enter adolescence they are, like many of their peers, entering a stage when they are beginning to establish their self-identity. This is a fundamental stage of their development, shaped in part by their social networks and family values. Their emerging identities will eventually nurture their social connectedness and sense of belonging, strengthening their self-esteem while also establishing their autonomy [12]. This process is impacted in no small part by physical transformations (with the onset of menarche and breast development) but also by the chronic illness of epilepsy, where recurrent and unexpected seizures can lead to negative judgments from peers, a greater sense of embarrassment, and degradation of self-esteem [13].

Sexual awakening and the first sexual experiences can be defining for young women; they may face additional potential hardships during this time. Many studies have shown that patients with epilepsy and, by extension, WWE suffer from more frequent sexual problems, including reduced libido, than their peers [14]. This can be from a number of sources, including the seizures themselves or antiseizure drug side effect profiles, to name but a few. When this occurs in the context of the first sexual experiences, it can contribute to a lowered self-esteem.

Furthermore, the experiences themselves can be traumatic. In the United States, adolescent interpersonal violence victimization remains concerning, with recent data showing that 8.2% of high school students reported both physical dating and sexual dating violence and that female students, among other groups, were disproportionately affected [15]. This finding appears consistent in youth with epilepsy with a younger mean age of first sexual intercourse (14 years) and up to 10% reporting feeling forced in their first sexual intercourse (compared to 2% of controls) [16].

This highlights the importance of addressing these issues early on, especially in children and adolescents with a chronic illness such as epilepsy. Parents may feel uncomfortable broaching these topics, partly because they themselves may have been taught that sexuality is bad [17]. Developing a safe and nurturing environment in which to discuss these topics may fall in part on the clinician. Addressing issues of defined roles during the first sexual encounters, and consent in particular, are paramount while taking a detailed sexual and gynecological history where appropriate. In youth with epilepsy and intellectual disabilities, the issue of consent is even more important to discuss, if the level of cognitive impairment does not preclude it, of course. Youth with epilepsy and mild intellectual disability may often be perceived as asexual, but the clinician should carefully and respectfully address sexuality during the patient's visits, involving the family when appropriate. Importance should also be given to preconception planning and contraception selection, especially given the potential for interactions with ASMs; this is covered more extensively in Chapter 10. It remains important as well for youth with epilepsy to consider additional barrier methods to help prevent sexually transmitted diseases (STDs).

Quality of Life

Quality of life overall is decreased in adolescents with chronic disease, with adolescents with epilepsy reporting poorer quality of life compared to youth with other chronic diseases like asthma [10]. Devinsky et al. reported age, increased seizure severity, neurotoxicity, and low socioeconomic status to be risk factors for poor health-related quality of life in adolescents overall. Female adolescents with epilepsy have been shown to have lower health-related quality of life compared with adolescent males, especially in the areas of attitudes toward illness and health perceptions [11]. This may be related to the fact that female adolescents with epilepsy have been shown to have more self-anxiety, unhappiness, and negative attitudes toward their illness when compared to males [10].

Stigma, Bullying, and Violence

Unfortunately, at the time of this writing, matters of gender equality remain far from settled. According to global health observatory data, on average, one in three women have experienced intimate partner violence in their lifetime [18]. A United Nations (UN) report highlighted that a sustainable development goal toward gender equality was the elimination of all forms of violence against women and girls [19]. Having a chronic illness or caring for someone with a chronic illness such as epilepsy can exacerbate the abuse women experience, and at least one study has shown that adolescents with non-visible chronic illnesses such as epilepsy have proportionately higher rates of sexual abuse [20]. Few studies in the past have explored the prevalence of abuse, physical or otherwise, in patients with epilepsy and fewer still in WWE in particular. In one study the proportion of patients with epilepsy who had been sexually abused was 9.3% [21], though that study could not resolve gender disparities owing to sample size. Another cross-sectional study, matched for age and gender with a non-stigmatized medical condition, in Zambia, found that WWE had higher rates of rape compared to the control group (20% vs. 3%) [22]. The clinician should be sensitive to this reality and respectfully screen youth with epilepsy for violence in the home and abuse, to ensure they are safe and cared for appropriately.

Stigma is defined as "an attribute which is deeply discrediting" [30]. This undesired attribute of the stigmatized person results in social rejection. Perceived stigmatization is a significant part of the hidden psychosocial burden of epilepsy that is tightly associated with low self-esteem, depression, anxiety, negative feelings, and impaired social skills. Furthermore, social disqualification and discrimination are the other consequences of stigmatization that lead to a decline in quality of life.

Stigmatization in patients with epilepsy is well characterized, owing mostly to perceived negative societal attitudes. This social exclusion begins early for children and adolescents with epilepsy and is covered in broader detail in the "Psychosocial and Cultural Considerations" section of this chapter. Patients often bear the added hardship of having seizures in front of their peers or suffering from neurobehavioral comorbidities, partly in relation to their ASM regimens. This can lead to a fraying of their social networks or, worse, peer harassment and bullying. Literature supports that children with epilepsy are more frequently victims of bullying when compared to peers with other chronic conditions or healthy controls [23]. Youth with epilepsy and intellectual disabilities are even more at risk of peer harassment and discrimination. The occurrence of harassment and discrimination can lead to increased rates of anxiety, depression, and, occasionally, suicide, all three of which are already quite prevalent in people living with epilepsy.

A careful inquiry into patients' relationships at school is important in shedding light on potential situations of peer harassment or abuse. Documenting the events when they arise and involving caregivers, school authorities, and other healthcare professionals such as community educators are paramount in attempting to break the cycle of harassment when one exists. The practitioner should also seek access to mental health resources at school and in the community to address comorbid psychiatric conditions.

Transitional Care

A significant proportion of young adults with childhood-onset epilepsy may require ongoing long-term epilepsy care as adults. Transition from pediatric to adult care systems is a major challenge in the management of adolescents with epilepsy. By definition, transition is the purposeful, planned movement from pediatric to adult-oriented healthcare systems where the medical, psychosocial, and educational/vocational needs of adolescents and young adults with long-term medical conditions are actively managed [24].

Young WWE not only suffer from recurrent epileptic seizures that can change over time, but they can also struggle with behavioral, academic, and social predicaments [25]. Therefore, "transition of care" in youth with epilepsy should be considered a "process," not simply a "transfer of care." This can be a very stressful time for both the individuals and their families.

There are limited studies on differences between transition of care in medical conditions including epilepsy in females and males. In one center's transition clinic experience, young WWE were more likely to participate in their healthcare. It was proposed that females were able to communicate more effectively. In addition, the motivation to participate in their care and adaptability skills was comparable to male youth [26]. Compared to males, young women demonstrated a stronger preference for same-sex healthcare professionals. Young women had positive experiences and believed that their families provided social support and encouraged independence in their care.

Studies conducted on the behavioral problems of youth during their transition into adolescence indicate some differences between genders. Behavioral challenges, specifically social problems, attention problems, aggressive behaviors, and anxiety/depression, in girls with high seizure burdens at both baseline and follow-up aggravated substantially over a 4-year period while there was an improving trend in behaviors in boys over the same period [27]. Increased psychological vulnerability has been reported in adolescent girls with other medical conditions such as cerebral palsy [28]. Social stigma and differences in coping strategies between boys and girls, which seem to be less effective in girls, were the proposed reasons. In contrast with adolescent boys, particularly older adolescents aged 16–17 years, adolescent girls had significantly more negative attitudes toward having epilepsy. This gender difference was attributed to the lower self-esteem found pervasively and more commonly in girls than boys. Therefore, their care mandates closer clinical supervision and screening for behavioral issues; this is particularly true of adolescent girls with severe epilepsies during their transition to the adult stream of care.

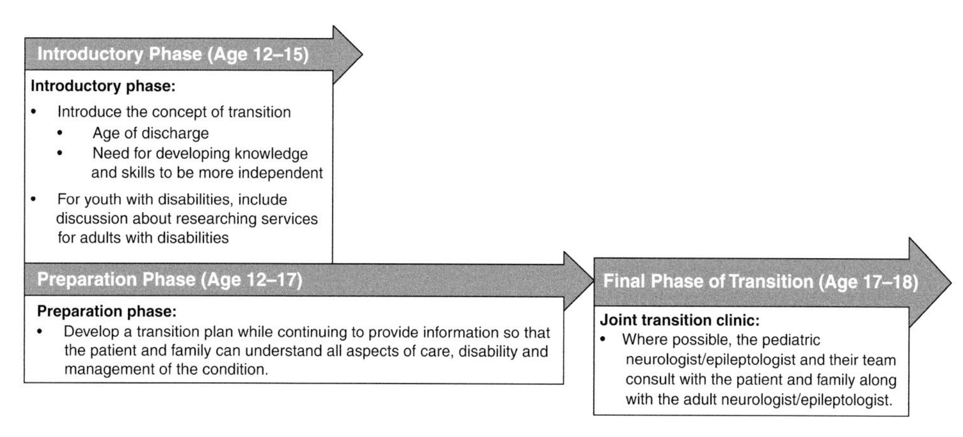

Figure 7.1 Chronological model for transition and transfer of care for epilepsy patients [44]

The other concerns influencing the behaviors of young WWE during their transition from pediatric to adult care were sexual activity, birth control, pregnancy, and raising children. A lower mean age of first intercourse, a failure to use contraception at last intercourse and "forced sex" appeared to be more likely in these individuals [16]. Attention deficit hyperactivity disorder, cognitive problems, low self-esteem, social isolation, and stigma were put forth as contributing factors in one study [29]. Therefore, appropriate education and awareness on various aspects such as the significance of contraception, teratogenicity of ASMs, and the need for folate supplementation should be provided to adolescent WWE during transition.

Psychosocial and Cultural Considerations

As outlined previously, girls and young WWE are exposed to stigmatization early on during the course of their epilepsies. This can lead to a negative impact later on in life in different facets of their social structures, including employment, education, and social activities, as well as their marital prospects [31].

This can be further compounded by cultural practices where girls' access to education is compromised or where young or arranged marriages remain commonplace. While less a reality in developed countries, migration patterns over the past decades mean that today's epilepsy specialist can care for children and young WWE brought up within these structures. It is incumbent on the physician to remain culturally aware and sensitive to these realities and approach these topics respectfully with patients and their families where appropriate.

Education

From an educational perspective, the data remain inconsistent; however, women tend to be more affected. While under-education and even "illiteracy" have been reported in WWE regardless of country of study, epilepsy in and of itself did not deter women from achieving higher levels of education (40.4% females vs. 27.9% males) in one Indian study [32].

Marriage

Studies consistently show reduced marriage rates in both men and women with epilepsy [23, 24]. However, the psychosocial consequences of the stigmatization in epilepsy are more evident in WWE in the marital domain. Both lower rates of marriage and increase in the age of marriage have reported across the world [32–34]. In a Norwegian study, single parenting was linked to epilepsy in young pregnant females [34]. Earlier age of epilepsy onset (before 20 years) was significantly associated with a lower marriage rate [33].

With respect to divorce, a striking difference was also noted between men and women with epilepsy. Women with epilepsy were at increased risk of divorce (4.3%) whereas no such association was reported in men.

These discriminating social consequences of epilepsy could be attributed to the negative attitude of communities toward people with epilepsy. While a large proportion of the general population endorsed that people with epilepsy are entitled to marry, the vast majority (93.2%) acknowledged that they would not marry them or would not allow their children to marry people with epilepsy [35].

The social stigmatization of epilepsy not infrequently may lead to concealment of epilepsy prior to marriage. Up to 90% of WWE may encounter stigma enacted by their societies. The tendency to conceal epilepsy was not significantly different between males and females (e.g., 91.66% of males vs. 98.44% of females in an Indian study) [36]. Likely related, the prevalence of divorce, separation, and disturbed marriages are significantly higher among WWE.

Considerations in Indigenous Girls and Adolescent Women with Epilepsy

Caring for girls and young WWE requires the epilepsy specialists to assume care for individuals from a wide range of backgrounds, including Indigenous backgrounds. The North American Commission of the International League Against Epilepsy has identified Aboriginal status as a risk factor for inequities in epilepsy care; however, research into the causes of these inequities in care is limited [45].

Aboriginal peoples (First Nations, Inuit, and Metis) in Canada suffer from increased rates of chronic disease compared to non-Aboriginal Canadians [37]. Epilepsy falls into this category of chronic disease and has been shown to be more prevalent in Aboriginal people in Canada. Self-declared registered Aboriginal peoples in Saskatchewan were 1.6 times more likely to be newly diagnosed with epilepsy between 2005 and 2010, with no difference found in the rates in men versus women [38].

Aboriginal peoples have lower life expectancy compared to non-Aboriginal peoples. For women, this difference is driven by higher rates of chronic disease and higher rates of death from disease [39]. No data are available on rates of epilepsy in Aboriginal women in Canada.

A population health study in Alberta showed that Aboriginal people with epilepsy were less likely to see a neurologist and more likely to visit the emergency department or be admitted to the hospital [40]. Similar disparities are seen in Indigenous Australians, with Indigenous Australians with epilepsy more likely to present to hospital and to present with more severe disease [46]. The increased hospitalizations suggest that primary preventative care may not be as effective in this population. There are many reasons for this, starting with the disparities in their social determinants of health. In a 2009 publication, Loppie Reading and Wein explored the varied determinants of health and showed that Aboriginal peoples experience inequalities in their physical environments such as overcrowding, in their social environments such as education and employment opportunities, and in their health behaviors such as the misuse of alcohol [37]. They experience inequalities in intermediate determinants of health, including community infrastructures, resources, and systems. They also experience inequalities in distal determinants of health such as racism and social exclusion. Different social determinants of health may also have different impacts in distinct Aboriginal groups. Some of these social determinants of health are specific to Aboriginal women. For example, Aboriginal women are more likely to have been victims of violence or crime and to have received treatment for a drug or alcohol problem compared to non-Aboriginal women [41].

As discussed in the rest of this chapter, many significant considerations need to be addressed in adolescents, and especially adolescent females with epilepsy. No data are available on how these issues affect Aboriginal teenagers with epilepsy, though the astute practitioner should remain vigilant and aware of the disparities outlined earlier in this chapter and address these topics during patient encounters when appropriate.

Although there is a definite increase in prevalence of epilepsy in Aboriginal peoples in Canada, very little literature is available into why this discrepancy exists. There are also clearly described disparities in the health of Aboriginal women and likely adolescent women in particular, but this has not been explored in the context of epilepsy. Very little has been published about the experience of Aboriginal peoples in other countries with a similar history of colonization, though undoubtedly the challenges are similar. These areas will require further research for clinicians to better support this population.

Sex and Gender Differences and Considerations in 2SLGBTQIA+ Populations

Very little has been written about the experiences of people with epilepsy who identify as two spirit, lesbian, gay, bisexual, transgender, queer, intersex, or asexual and people with other sexual orientations and forms of gender expression (2SLGBTQIA+). Poor knowledge, bias, and prejudice from their care providers can contribute to the health disparities 2SLGBTQIA+ people experience [42]. As questions of gender identity and sexual orientation may emerge early on in children and youth with epilepsy, having a cursory knowledge and understanding of these issues is paramount for the practitioner to create a safe and welcoming space for patients with epilepsy and their caregivers in which to discuss their journey.

Transgender people with epilepsy have a special set of medical considerations due to the interaction between many ASMs and sex hormones. Johnson and Kaplan describe how the effects of ASMs on sex steroid levels as well as the effect of hormones on ASM levels must be considered when managing transgender people with epilepsy [43]. Transwomen (male-to-female transgender persons) in adolescence often use GnRH analog-assisted pubertal suppression. Progestin may also be used for this purpose. Cross-sex steroids (estradiol) can then be used to induce female puberty. Non-enzyme-inducing ASMs should be used, if possible, in transwomen using cross-sex steroids. Estrogen itself can have a proconvulsant effect; therefore, when a transwoman begins to take estrogen, she should be counseled about the possibility of increased seizures. Transmen (female-to-male transgender person) in adolescence often also use GnRH analog-assisted pubertal suppression. Depot medroxyprogesterone can also be used to suppress ovulation and progesterone. Male puberty can then be induced with testosterone. Enzyme-inducing ASMs may decrease the level of free testosterone and therefore should be avoided in this group of patients. Refer to Chapter 5 for a detailed discussion of the interaction between ASMs and sex hormones.

Summary

Caring for girls and young adolescents with epilepsy requires a multifaceted and holistic approach in the twenty-first century. While the neurobiological aspects such as hormonal influences and preconception planning need to be taken into consideration (and are reviewed in detail elsewhere in this work), the psychosocial aspects are arguably even more important. These include screening for autism spectrum disorder and ADHD, screening for violence and abuse, and supporting young WWE of diverse, multicultural, and Indigenous backgrounds through their transition into adulthood. In the end, the practitioner's goal remains the same: improving the health and quality of life of this dynamic population.

References

1. Davies S, Heyman I, Goodman R. A population survey of mental health problems in children with epilepsy. *Dev Med Child Neurol.* 2003;**45**(5):292–5.
2. Auvin S, Wirrell E, Donald KA, et al. Systematic review of the screening, diagnosis, and management of ADHD in children with epilepsy: Consensus paper of the Task Force on Comorbidities of the ILAE Pediatric Commission. *Epilepsia.* 2018;**59**(10):1867–80.
3. Klassen AF, Miller A, Fine S. Health-related quality of life in children and adolescents who have a diagnosis of attention-deficit/hyperactivity disorder. *Pediatrics.* 2004;**114**(5): e541–7.
4. Strasser L, Downes M, Kung J, Cross JH, De Haan M. Prevalence and risk factors for autism spectrum disorder in epilepsy: A systematic review and meta-analysis. *Dev Med Child Neurol.* 2018;**60**(1):19–29.
5. Zablotsky B, Black LI, Maenner MJ, Schieve LA, Blumberg SJ. Estimated prevalence of autism and other developmental disabilities following questionnaire changes in the 2014 national health interview survey. *Natl Health Stat Report.* 2015;**2015**(87):1–20.
6. Lax-Pericall MT, Bird V, Taylor E. Gender and psychiatric disorders in children with epilepsy: A meta-analysis. *Epilepsy Behav.* 2019;**94**:144–50.
7. Kyngäs H. Compliance with health regimens of adolescents with epilepsy. *Seizure.* 2000;**9**(8):598–604.
8. Sillanpää M, Shinnar S. Obtaining a driver's license and seizure relapse in patients with childhood-onset epilepsy. *Neurology.* 2005;**64**(4):680–6.
9. Leach JP, Mohanraj R, Borland W. Alcohol and drugs in epilepsy: Pathophysiology, presentation, possibilities, and prevention. *Epilepsia.* 2012;**53**(Suppl. 4):48–57.
10. Austin JK, Huster GA, Dunn DW, Risinger MW. Adolescents with active or inactive epilepsy or asthma: A comparison of quality of life. *Epilepsia.* 1996;**37**(12):1228–38.
11. Devinsky O, Westbrook L, Cramer J, et al. Risk factors for poor health-related quality of life in adolescents with epilepsy. *Epilepsia.* 1999;**40**(12):1715–20.
12. Pfeifer JH, Berkman ET. The development of self and identity in adolescence: Neural evidence and implications for a value-based choice perspective on motivated behavior. *Child Dev Perspect.* 2018;**12**(3):158–64.
13. Zheng K, Bruzzese JM, Smaldone A. Illness acceptance in adolescents: A concept analysis. *Nurs Forum.* 2019;**54**(4):545–52.
14. Morrell MJ, Guldner GT. Self-reported sexual function and sexual arousability in women with epilepsy. *Epilepsia.* 1996;**37**(12):1204–10.
15. Centers for Disease Control and Prevention. Youth risk behavior surveillance: United States, 2019. 2020;**69.**
16. Lossius MI, Alfstad K, Van Roy B, et al. Early sexual debut in Norwegian youth with epilepsy: A population-based study. *Epilepsy Behav.* 2016;**56**:1–4.
17. Mims J. Sexuality and related issues in the preadolescent and adolescent female with epilepsy. *Journal of Neuroscience Nursing.* 1996;**28**:102–6.
18. United Nations. *Understanding and addressing violence against women.* New York: United Nations; 2012.
19. United Nations. *Turning promises into action: Gender equality in the 2030 Agenda for Sustainable Development.* New York: United Nations; 2018.
20. Surís JC, Resnick MD, Cassuto N, Blum RW. Sexual behavior of adolescents with chronic disease and disability. *J Adolesc Heal.* 1996;**19**(2):124–31.
21. Davies FG, Manchanda R, Schaefer B, Blume WT, McLachlan RS. Sexual abuse and psychiatric symptoms in an epileptic population. *Seizure Eur J Epilepsy.* 1992;**1**(4):263–7.
22. Birbeck G, Chomba E, Atadzhanov M, Mbewe E, Haworth A. The social and

economic impact of epilepsy in Zambia: A cross-sectional study. *Lancet Neurol.* 2007;**6**(1):39–44.

23. Hamiwka LD, Yu CG, Hamiwka LA, et al. Are children with epilepsy at greater risk for bullying than their peers? *Epilepsy Behav.* 2009;**15**(4):500–5.
24. Camfield PR, Andrade D, Camfield CS, et al. How can transition to adult care be best orchestrated for adolescents with epilepsy? *Epilepsy Behav.* 2019;**93**:138–47.
25. Rodenburg R, Wagner JL, Austin JK, Kerr M, Dunn DW. Psychosocial issues for children with epilepsy. *Epilepsy Behav.* 2011;**22**(1):47–54.
26. Cui C, Li SZ, Zheng XL, Cheng WJ, Ting W. Participation in healthcare behavior by adolescents with epilepsy and factors that influence it during the transition period: A cross-sectional study in China. *Epilepsy Behav.* 2020;**113**:107576.
27. Austin JK, Dunn DW, Huster GA. Childhood epilepsy and asthma: Changes in behavior problems related to gender and change in condition severity. *Epilepsia.* 2000;**41**(5):615–23.
28. Manuel JC, Balkrishnan R, Camacho F, Smith BP, Koman LA. Factors associated with self-esteem in pre-adolescents and adolescents with cerebral palsy. *J Adolesc Heal.* 2003;**32**(6):456–8.
29. Boislard MA, Bongardt D, Van de Blais M. Sexuality (and lack thereof) in adolescence and early adulthood: A review of the literature. *Behav Sci* (Basel). 2016;**6**(1):8.
30. Aydemir N, Kaya B, Yildiz G, Öztura I, Baklan B. Determinants of felt stigma in epilepsy. *Epilepsy Behav.* 2016;**58**:76–80.
31. Ak PD, Atakli D, Yuksel B, Guveli BT, Sari H. Stigmatization and social impacts of epilepsy in Turkey. *Epilepsy Behav.* 2015;**50**(8):50–4.
32. Gopinath M, Sarma PS, Thomas SV. Gender-specific psychosocial outcome for women with epilepsy. *Epilepsy Behav.* 2011;**20**(1):44–7.
33. Dansky LV, Andermann E, Andermann F. Marriage and fertility in epileptic patients. *Epilepsia.* 1980;**21**(3):261–71.
34. Reiter SF, Veiby G, Daltveit AK, Engelsen BA, Gilhus NE. Psychiatric comorbidity and social aspects in pregnant women with epilepsy: The Norwegian Mother and Child Cohort Study. *Epilepsy Behav.* 2013;**29**(2):379–85.
35. Ezeala-Adikaibe BA, Achor JU, Nwabueze AC, et al. Knowledge, attitude and practice of epilepsy among community residents in Enugu, south east Nigeria. *Seizure.* 2014;**23**(10):882–8.
36. Agarwal P, Mehndiratta MM, Antony AR, et al. Epilepsy in India: Nuptiality behaviour and fertility. *Seizure.* 2006;**15**(6):409–15.
37. Loppie Reading C, Wein F. *Health Inequalities and Social Determinants of Aboriginal Peoples' Health.* Prince George, BC: National Collaborating Centre for Aboriginal Health; 2009.
38. Hernández-Ronquillo L, Thorpe L, Pahwa P, Téllez-Zenteno JF. Secular trends and population differences in the incidence of epilepsy: A population-based study from Saskatchewan, Canada. *Seizure.* 2018;**60**:8–15.
39. Tjepkema M, Wilkins R, Senécal S, Guimond É, Penney C. Mortality of Métis and Registered Indian Study. *Heal Reports.* 2009;**20**(4):1–21.
40. Jetté N, Quan H, Faris P, et al. Health resource use in epilepsy: Significant disparities by age, gender, and aboriginal status. *Epilepsia.* 2008;**49**(4):586–93.
41. Hamdullahpur K, Jacobs KJ, Gill KJ. A comparison of socioeconomic status and mental health among inner-city Aboriginal and non-Aboriginal women. *Int J Circumpolar Health.* 2017;**76**(1):1340693.
42. Moreno A, Laoch A, Zasler ND. Changing the culture of neurodisability through language and sensitivity of providers: Creating a safe place for LGBTQIA+ people. *NeuroRehabilitation.* 2017;**41**(2):375–93.
43. Johnson EL, Kaplan PW. Caring for transgender patients with epilepsy. *Epilepsia.* 2017;**58**(10):1667–72.

44. Andrade DM, Bassett AS, Bercovici E, et al. Epilepsy: Transition from pediatric to adult care. Recommendations of the Ontario Epilepsy Implementation Task Force. *Epilepsia.* 2017;**58**(9):1502–72. https://doi.org/10.1111/epi.13832.

45. Burneo JG, Jette N, Theodore W, et al. Disparities in epilepsy: Report of a systematic review by the North American Commission of the International League Against Epilepsy. *Epilepsia.* 2009;**50**(10):2285–95. https://doi.org/10.1111/j.1528-1167.2009.02282.x.

46. Plummer C, Cook MJ, Anderson I, D'Souza WJ. Australia's seizure divide: Indigenous versus non-Indigenous seizure hospitalization. *Epilepsy Behav.* 2014;**31**:363–8. https://doi.org/10.1016/j.yebeh.2013.09.042.

Catamenial Epilepsy

Alexa King and Elizabeth E. Gerard

Key Points

- Catamenial epilepsy is a pattern of seizure exacerbation throughout the menstrual cycle.
- One-third of women with epilepsy have a catamenial pattern of seizures.
- There are three patterns of catamenial epilepsy: perimenstrual (C1) and periovulatory (C2) patterns occur in women with normal cycles, and a luteal phase pattern (C3) may occur during anovulatory cycles.
- The pathophysiology of catamenial epilepsy may be related to a loss of balance between the proconvulsant effect of estrogen and the anticonvulsant effect of progesterone at certain times in the menstrual cycle. It is also possible that metabolic differences in antiseizure medications throughout the menstrual cycle play a role.
- Standard epilepsy treatment, including optimizing antiseizure medications or surgical management, should be the first line of care for women with catamenial epilepsy.
- Supplementary treatment options for refractory catamenial epilepsy include hormonal and nonhormonal strategies, though more research is needed to find highly effective treatment options.
- Women with catamenial epilepsy may experience an improvement in seizure frequency during pregnancy, worsening during perimenopause, and an improvement during menopause. However, further prospective studies are need to verify these findings.

Introduction

The term *catamenial* is derived from the Greek word *katamenios*, which means monthly. Catamenial epilepsy is a monthly pattern of seizure exacerbation due to fluctuations in the sex hormones throughout the menstrual cycle. Sir Charles Locock first published the relationship between menstruation and seizures. The first case series on the subject was published in 1881 by Dr. Gowers, who stated "the attacks were worse at the monthly periods" in more than half of women he treated with epilepsy [1]. We now have a better understanding of the pathophysiology and classification of catamenial epilepsy, though evidence-based treatment options remain limited.

The Hypothalamic-Pituitary-Ovarian Axis and the Menstrual Cycle

The hypothalamic-pituitary-ovarian axis is a complex feedback system that is responsible for the cyclical pattern of female sex hormones and the normal menstrual cycle. The normal menstrual cycle lasts 24–35 days, with 28 days being average. The menstrual cycle has three phases: the follicular phase, ovulation, and the luteal phase. Day 1 begins on the first day of menses, corresponding to the onset of the follicular phase (days 1–14). Gonadotropin-releasing hormone (GnRH) from the hypothalamus stimulates follicular-stimulating hormone (FSH) and luteinizing hormone (LH) to be released from the anterior pituitary gland. Follicular-stimulating hormone and LH in turn stimulate the follicles in the ovaries. A dominant follicle develops into the oocyte that releases estradiol (a form of estrogen). Estrogen causes negative feedback that reduces FSH but stimulates GnRH, resulting in a relative LH surge. This causes ovulation, which occurs around day 14. The luteal phase (days 14–28) occurs as the oocyte matures into the corpus luteum, which releases progesterone. In the absence of pregnancy, the corpus luteum regresses, progesterone and estrogen fall, and menses occurs. At times a follicle does not fully develop and the corpus luteum does not stimulate ovulation. Therefore, progesterone levels remain low. This is called an inadequate luteal phase and is associated with irregular cycle length (see Figure 8.1).

Pathophysiology of Catamenial Epilepsy

Several mechanisms for cyclical seizure exacerbations have been hypothesized over time, including water balance, metabolism of antiseizure medication, and hormonal influences. Current knowledge supports that seizure threshold is modulated by the variation in the neuroactive sex hormones throughout the normal menstrual cycle. Estrogen and progesterone are both important modulators of neuronal excitability and play a role in catamenial epilepsy. In general, estrogen has been shown to be proconvulsant while progesterone has anticonvulsant effects.

Estrogen

There are three biologically active estrogens: 17β-estradiol (E2), estriol, and estrone. Estrogens are highly lipophilic and can cross the blood–brain barrier. The principal estrogen in premenopausal women is E2; estrone predominates in the postmenopausal period and estriol predominates during pregnancy. Estrogens have been shown to be proconvulsant in human and animal studies. Intravenous injection of a water-soluble estrogen led to increased frequency and amplitude of epileptiform discharges in 68% of a group of 16 women with epilepsy. Seizures occurred in 25% of the women within 24 hours of the estrogen injection [2]. Estradiol facilitates pentyletetrazol (PTZ) and kainic acid-induced seizures and accelerates kindling following limbic network stimulation in animal models of epilepsy [3, 4]. A significant positive correlation between focal-to-bilateral tonic-clonic seizures and an elevated estrogen-to-progesterone (E/P) ratio was found, peaking in the premenstrual and preovulatory periods in ovulatory cycles and declining in the midluteal phases of six women with epilepsy. In three anovulatory cycles, seizure frequency correlated positively with E2 levels but no progesterone levels, highlighting the importance of estrogen in seizure exacerbation [5].

The mechanism by which estrogen exerts proconvulsant effects is incompletely elucidated. While E2 enhances glutamate receptor-mediated excitatory neurotransmission and decreases GABAergic inhibition [6], other work suggests that estrogen has anticonvulsant properties through transcriptional regulation of neuropeptides [7]. Therefore, the effect of estrogen on the seizure threshold may depend on factors not yet fully understood.

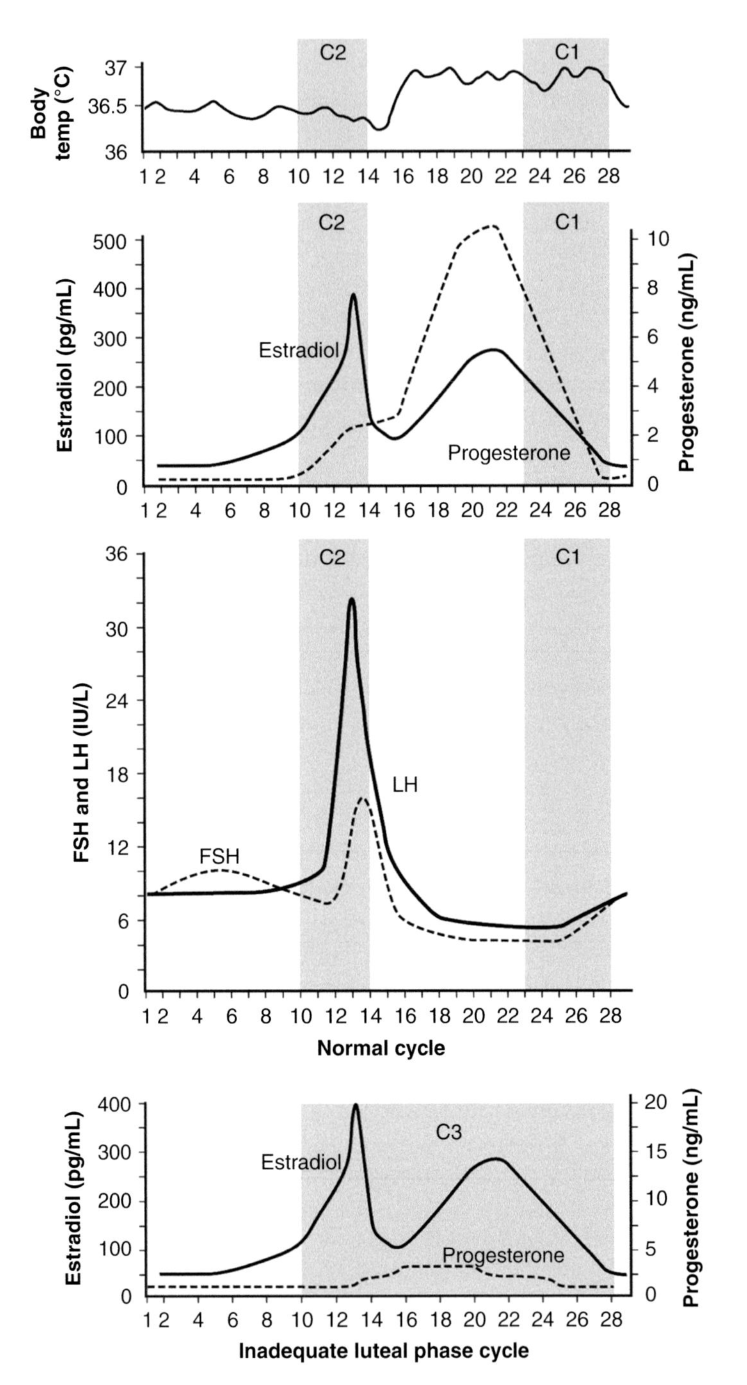

Figure 8.1 Schematic of the menstrual cycle and the three patterns of catamenial epilepsy. The top panel depicts basal body temperature across the normal menstrual cycle. The second two panels depict hormonal patterns during a normal menstrual cycle. The inadequate luteal phase cycle (lower panel) is defined by progesterone levels less than 5 ng/mL. Patterns of seizure expression include the perimenstrual (C1), periovulatory (C2), and inadequate luteal phase (C3) types. The inadequate luteal phase is depicted in the last panel.

Progesterone

Progesterone plays a critical role in the pathophysiology of catamenial epilepsy. The anticonvulsant effects of progesterone are primarily attributed to its metabolite, allopregnanolone [8]. Progesterone is first metabolized to 5α-dihydroprogestrone by the enzyme 5α-reductase, then to allopregnanolone by 3α-hydroxysteroid oxidoreductase. The rate-limiting step in the conversion of progesterone to allopregnanolone depends on the enzyme 5α-reductase. The use of a 5α-reductase inhibitor in an animal model of catamenial epilepsy demonstrated that the anticonvulsant effect of progesterone depends on the conversion of progesterone to allopregnanolone. Both progesterone and allopregnanolone potentiate GABA-A-mediated inhibition of neurons by increasing the frequency and duration of chloride channel opening at GABA-A receptors. At physiologic and pharmacologic levels, allopregnanolone is a more potent modulator of GABA-A receptors than progesterone [9, 10]. Elevated concentrations of allopregnanolone and progesterone increase the seizure threshold in kainic acid, PTZ, and pilocarpine animal models [9]. In mice, a precipitous drop in progesterone using a 5α-reductase inhibitor can simulate menses and creates an animal model of catamenial epilepsy [11]. Many investigators attribute the perimenstrual seizure susceptibility in women with catamenial epilepsy to the precipitous drop in progesterone and the rise in the E/P ratio at the end of the luteal phase [5, 9].

These studies have led to a leading theory of progesterone withdrawal as the major factor in catamenial epilepsy. Recent work, however, has raised the possibility that the progesterone has excitatory as well as inhibitory properties, making the catamenial model more complex. Kapur and colleagues propose that progesterone has immediate inhibitory effects due to the effect of allopregnenalone on GABA-A receptors, but also has secondary excitatory effects due to the binding of the progesterone receptors, which leads to longer-term seizure-promoting effects [12]. The authors reported that both endogenous and exogenous progesterone upregulate α-amino-3-hydroxy-5-methyl-4-isoxazolepropionic acid (AMPA) receptors and AMPA receptor synaptic transmission. This effect was modulated by the binding of progesterone receptors [13]. They then used RU-486, which blocks progesterone receptors, in the 5α-reductase inhibitor animal model of catamenial epilepsy. Their first study found that co-treatment with RU-486 during the hormone priming phase significantly mitigated seizures occurring during the period when progesterone levels fall [13]. In a follow-up study, they found similar effects in a model of progesterone withdrawal where epileptic rats were treated with exogenous progesterone followed by a period of withdrawal. Again, RU-486, when administered along with the progesterone, attenuated seizures seen after progesterone withdrawal [14]. Finally, nestrone, a progesterone receptor agonist, exacerbated seizures in female rats [14]. The authors suggest that this bidirectional effect of progesterone may be one of the reasons it has been hard to find a highly effective progesterone-based treatment for catamenial epilepsy [12]. This is discussed in greater detail in Chapter 4.

Water Balance

In the early twentieth century, observations of the association between cerebral edema and convulsions led to a series of experiments investigating the effect of water ingestion on seizures. In patients with epilepsy, the antidiuretic hormone vasopressin and excessive water ingestion provoked seizures, while negative water balance produced by fluid restriction had the opposite effect. It was proposed that water retention during menstruation might be an underlying mechanism of the perimenstrual seizure exacerbation in some women with epilepsy [15]. However, no significant difference in sodium metabolism, total body water, or body weight was found between women with perimenstrual seizures and healthy controls, or between epileptic women with and without catamenial epilepsy [16].

Antiseizure Medications and Hormone Interaction

Another proposed mechanism of catamenial epilepsy is the interaction between the metabolism of antiseizure medications and neuroactive sex hormones, leading to perimenstrual lowering of antiseizure medication concentrations. Many antiseizure medications are metabolized by the hepatic cytochrome P450 enzymes, sharing a common pathway with neuroactive hormones. Furthermore, enzyme-inducing antiseizure medications increases the serum concentration of sex hormone–binding globulin. This may lead to a reduction in the available free sex hormones in women with epilepsy [8, 17].

In a study investigating these relationships in women taking phenytoin (PHT) monotherapy or in combination with phenobarbital, despite higher daily dosage, women with perimenstrual seizures had lower PHT serum concentrations and greater fluctuations in concentrations across the cycle than women without catamenial seizures. Women with perimenstrual seizures were more likely to have a 30% or greater reduction in PHT concentration on day 28 of the cycle. Phenobarbital concentrations did not significantly vary. The reduced PHT concentration corresponded to an increase in seizure frequency in the perimenstrual period in this study [18]. Several similar studies on PHT confirm the finding of decreased serum concentration around menses in women with catamenial seizure exacerbation [19, 20]. In contrast, there was a smaller decrease [19] or no difference [20] in PHT concentration perimenstrually in women without catamenial epilepsy. In another group of women with perimenstrual seizures, fluctuations in salivary PHT and carbamazepine concentrations were found with lower concentrations during the period of seizure susceptibility [21].

Variations in lamotrigine and valproic acid serum concentrations secondary to endogenous steroid fluctuations across the menstrual cycle have also been investigated. Twelve women with epilepsy on each of these medications had serum concentration levels drawn at different points throughout a single menstrual cycle. There was a 31% and 8% decrease in lamotrigine and valproic acid concentrations, respectively, in the midluteal phase compared to the midfollicular phase, though neither of these changes was statistically significant [22]. This study was done with a limited sample size, but highlights the need for further work to better elucidate the pharmacokinetic relationships between endogenous steroids and antiseizure medications.

Definition and Prevalence

Catamenial epilepsy is the preponderance of seizures to occur during certain points of the menstrual cycle, but it is often ambiguously defined as worsening of seizures around menses. Foldvary-Schaefer and Falcone reviewed the incidence and found that a catamenial pattern is reported in 10–78% of women with epilepsy, varying wildly throughout the literature depending on methodology and clinical criteria used [23]. The most widely accepted definition of catamenial epilepsy was proposed by Herzog and colleagues and consists of a twofold increase in seizure frequency during a vulnerable portion of the menstrual cycle [24]. Using this definition, about one-third of women with epilepsy qualify as having catamenial epilepsy [24, 25].

Three distinct patterns of seizure exacerbation throughout the menstrual cycle have emerged: perimenstrual (C1), periovulatory (C2), and the luteal phase in anovulatory cycles (C3) (see Figure 8.1). Herzog, Klein, and Rand studied seizure frequency across a single menstrual cycle in 184 women with refractory focal epilepsy, with mid-cycle progesterone levels measured to distinguish ovulatory (progesterone > 5 ng/mL) from anovulatory cycles. In this cohort, 98 ovulatory cycles and 86 anovulatory cycles were studied. The most common pattern was perimenstrual (C1), which consists of increased seizure frequency in the 3 days prior through 3 days following onset of menses. This occurred in 35% of women with epilepsy with ovulatory cycles. The periovulatory pattern (C2) has seizure exacerbation in the 4 days leading up to ovulation to the day following ovulation and occurred in 26% of ovulatory cycles. In anovulatory cycles, there was a significantly reduced frequency of seizures in the follicular phase relative to the remainder of the cycle, which is called the C3 pattern. The C3 pattern was seen in around 40% of the anovulatory cycles monitored in this study. Of note, seizure frequency was nearly 1.5 times greater in cycles with an inadequate luteal phase [24]. Around 10% of patients will have both C1 and C2 patterns of seizure exacerbation [25].

Of note, catamenial epilepsy can occur in patients with focal or generalized epilepsy. In focal epilepsy, temporal lobe epilepsy has been shown to be more frequently associated with a catamenial epilepsy pattern than extratemporal or multifocal epilepsy [26]. Moreover, left temporal epilepsy is more frequently associated with catamenial epilepsy than right temporal lobe epilepsy [26, 27]. Women with genetic generalized epilepsies were found to have higher odds of being medically refractory if they have catamenial epilepsy [28]. This finding is not yet fully understood.

Diagnosis

The diagnosis of catamenial epilepsy requires careful collaboration between the patient and healthcare provider. Careful review of seizure frequency in relation to menses should be tracked, as research has shown that women tend to overestimate the relationship of seizures to menstruation from memory alone [29]. The patient should document menses, ovulatory status, and seizure for at least three cycles for review [30]. This can be done using a calendar or newer seizure-tracking applications. Ovulatory status can be measured at home with several methods. Monitoring morning basal body temperature can be done daily, with a rise of 0.7° Fahrenheit signaling ovulation due to the presence of progesterone [23]. Alternatively, over-the-counter ovulation kits are available for purchase. These kits typically measure the LH surge in urine that occurs around the time of ovulation.

Management Strategies

Though the incidence of catamenial epilepsy is high, treatment regimens targeted at this specific pattern are largely based on small-series, anecdotal case reports. Randomized controlled trials have failed to show a significant impact of progesterone formulations on catamenial seizures [31]. To date there is not a specific treatment option proven to be more effective than standard epilepsy therapy. Hormonal therapies should not be offered as first-line treatment options for catamenial epilepsy. First and foremost, typical antiseizure medication appropriate for seizure type should be initiated. In the case of medically refractory epilepsy, surgical evaluation should be pursued [30]. If conventional epilepsy management strategies are ineffective, other therapies that may be considered include hormonal or nonhormonal treatments (see Table 8.1).

Table 8.1 Studies of catamenial epilepsy

Treatment	Study type and citation	Dosage	Sample size/efficacy	Additional comments
Progesterone lozenges	Prospective, double blind, placebo-controlled study Herzog et al. 2012 [33]	200 mg 3 times daily on days 14–25 of menstrual cycle	No difference in seizure decrease from placebo (n = 85)	Primary endpoint not met, but subset of women with perimenstrual (C1) pattern of catamenial epilepsy had significant seizure reduction
Progesterone tablets	Prospective, placebo controlled study Najafi et al. 2013 [34]	80 mg on days 15–25 of menstrual cycle	Decrease seizure frequency in progesterone group (n = 38)	Individual change from baseline, responder rates and seizure freedom rates were not available
Medroxyprogesterone acetate	Prospective study (not placebo controlled) Mattson et al. 1984 [38]	Medroxyprogesterone 10 mg orally, 2–4 times daily or medroxyprogesterone acetate 120–150 mg IM every 6–12 weeks	Average 39% seizure reduction occurred in >50% of women and 63% who achieved amenorrhea (n = 14 total; n = 11 achieved amenorrhea)	Dosage was increased to goal of amenorrhea. Side effects included breast tenderness, spotting and weight gain
Combined oral contraceptive pills	No data available for efficacy	Estrogen and progesterone combination; dosage varies by formulation		May consider continuous dosing (skipping placebo week)
Ganaxolone	2 case reports McAuley et al. 2001 [36]	300 mg twice daily on days 21–23 of menstrual cycle	Moderate reduction in seizure frequency (n = 2)	

Clomiphene citrate	Prospective study (not placebo controlled) Herzog 1988 [41]	25–100 mg daily on days 5–9; dose increase until regular menstrual cycle	50% reduction in seizures in 66% of patients Average seizure reduction 87% (n = 12)	Side effects included breast tenderness, pelvic pain, ovarian cysts
Triptorelin (gonadotropin-releasing hormone analog)	Prospective study (not placebo controlled) Bauer et al. 1992 [42]	3.75 mg IM once per month	Seizure freedom in 30% of patients Seizure improvement in 80% of patients (n = 10)	Side effects included headaches, weight gain and hot flushes
Clobazam	Prospective placebo-controlled cross over study Feely et al. 1982 [45]	20–30 mg daily for 10 days beginning 2–4 days before menses	Seizure reduction in 80% of patients >50% reduction in seizures in 44% of patients (n = 18)	Side effects included sedation and depression
Pulse dose benzodiazepines	No data available for efficacy	Clonazepam Ativan		Consider several days before and during menses
Acetazolamide	Retrospective review Lim et al. 2001 [48]	4 mg/kg daily (can be titrated up to 1 g daily) starting 5 days before menses for 5–7 days	>50% seizure reduction occurred in 40% of women	Side effects include dizziness and polyuria Tolerance develops over time in ~15% of patients

Hormonal Strategies

Progesterone Therapies

Given the known anticonvulsant effects of progesterone and its metabolites, progesterone formulations have been tried as a treatment for catamenial seizures. In 1983, Dana-Haeri and Richens published a randomized trial of nine women with catamenial seizures and focal epilepsy. The women were assigned to high-dose or low-dose oral norethisterone or placebo to be taken beginning on the fifth day of the menstrual cycle for 21 days and then crossed over to the other arm. No difference in seizure frequency was noted [32].

An investigation of natural oral progesterone was performed more recently. This was a multicenter prospective randomized clinical trial that evaluated 200 mg progesterone lozenges given three times daily on days 14-28 of the menstrual cycle versus placebo. Nearly 300 women with focal epilepsy were randomized, and they were stratified by catamenial or non-catamenial status. Unfortunately, this study did not find a significant difference in seizure frequency or severity for women treated with progesterone compared to placebo. Of note, post hoc analysis did find that a subgroup of women with a C1 (perimenstrual) pattern of catamenial epilepsy did have improved seizure frequency rate in the progesterone group, indicating that there may be a role for progesterone therapy in a select group of patients [33].

A smaller prospective placebo-controlled trial from Iran looked at the effect of 80 mg of oral progesterone in 38 women with catamenial epilepsy. Participants had either a C1 pattern or a luteal pattern uniquely defined as day 2 to day 10 along with a low progesterone level. The women were treated from day 15 to day 25. The mean number of seizures significantly decreased in the treatment group but not in the control group. However, individual changes from baseline, responder rates, and seizure-freedom rates were not available [34].

A recent Cochrane review of these three studies and a norethisterone trial published in abstract form concluded that there is low-certainty evidence of no treatment effect of norethisterone. For natural progesterone, they cited moderate-to-low certainty evidence of no treatment effect in catamenial epilepsy. The authors indicated that all studies were underpowered to detect a treatment effect, so it is not possible to definitively exclude a clinical effect of oral progesterone [31].

Ganaxolone (3α-hydroxy-3β-methyl-5α-pregnane-20-one) is an orally active synthetic analog of allopregnanolone. This modulates $GABA_A$ receptors, which has an anticonvulsant effect. Importantly, the 3β subunit prevents conversion to a hormonally active metabolite, so ganaxolone limits hormonal activity and therefore side effects when compared to natural steroids [11]. In a rat model of pseudopregnancy to simulate catamenial progesterone withdrawal, ganaxolone had enhanced anticonvulsant potency. In contrast, valproate and diazepam had reduced efficacy during steroid withdrawal [35]. While this animal study supports ganaxolone as a specific treatment for catamenial epilepsy, few studies have investigated this in humans. A moderate reduction in seizures was achieved in two women with perimenstrual seizures treated with ganaxolone 300 mg twice daily on days 21–23 of treatment cycles [36]. Larger-scale investigations into this treatment option for catamenial epilepsy are needed. Recently, ganaxolone for the adjunctive treatment of focal seizures was studied in a 10-week placebo-controlled phase II trial [37]. In this study, mean percent change from baseline was significantly greater in the treatment arm (17.6% vs. 2%, P = 0.0144) but there was no significant difference in responder rates (≥50% reduction in seizure frequency). The majority of the participants in this trial were women (68%), which the authors noted might be due to the perceived benefit of ganaxolone for catamenial epilepsy. The effect of treatment on catamenial seizures in this trial has not been reported, however [37].

Medroxyprogesterone acetate (MPA) is a progesterone derivative that can be administered orally or as a depot injection given every 3 months. In 1984, Mattson and colleagues studied the effectiveness of this hormone as an adjunct to traditional antiseizure medication on seizure control in 14 women with epilepsy. Initially, the women were treated with the oral preparation, but 6 women moved on to depot injection after failing to develop amenorrhea. On average, medroxyprogesterone acetate yielded a 39% reduction in seizure frequency, with no patients becoming seizure free [38]. More recently there has been an isolated case report noting seizure reduction with this therapy [39].

Other Hormonal Therapies

Oral contraceptives are typically composed of a combination of synthetic estrogen and progesterone. These contraceptives are sometimes used in clinical practice to reduce the effect of the cyclic hormonal fluctuations. Theoretically, elimination of menstruation through continuous dosing of oral contraceptives may be advantageous, but clinical evidence is lacking on the efficacy of this approach [40]. In addition, there are complex interactions between antiseizure medications and oral contraceptives with the potential for contraceptive failure or lower serum lamotrigine levels. Therefore, careful patient counseling must be undertaken if this treatment approach is being considered.

There have been isolated reports of improvement of catamenial epilepsy with a number of other hormonal agents, including clomiphene citrate, the synthetic androgen danazol, and synthetic gonadotropin analogs triptorelin or goserelin. Clomiphene is an estrogen analog which has estrogenic and antiestrogenic effects which is primarily used to modulate the release of gonadotropins for fertility purposes. Twelve women with focal epilepsy and abnormal menstrual cycles were treated with clomiphene citrate pulses during days 5–9 of the menstrual cycle. Ten of these women (83%) experienced a reduction in seizure frequency with an average of 87% improvement, and normalization of the luteal phase of menses. The two patients who did not respond had doses limited by the side effects of pelvic pain, and around half of all patients reported pelvic pain, breast tenderness, or were found to have ovarian cyst formation [41]. A series of ten women with catamenial epilepsy were treated with the synthetic GnRH triptorelin in a depot injection. Three patients became seizure free and another four patients had seizure reductions of more than 50%. Side effects including hot flushes, weight gain or headaches occurred in the majority of patients [42].

A single case report of a woman with catamenial epilepsy attributed to cerebral endometriosis documents seizure freedom with 6-month treatment with danazol, a synthetic androgen [43]. Similarly, another woman with presumed cerebral endometriosis became seizure free with goserelin treatment followed by oophorectomy [44]. It is unclear if these cases can be generalized to all women with epilepsy occurring without cerebral endometriosis, which is a rare cause of catamenial seizure exacerbation. It is important to mention that outside of these case reports of cerebral endometriosis, surgical hysterectomy or oophorectomy have not been studied in the management of catamenial seizures. Hormone-sensitive seizures are not considered a reasonable indication for surgical menopause in most cases.

Hysterectomy would not prevent the hormonal fluctuations thought to contribute to catamenial seizures and oophorectomy has significant side effects without known efficacy.

Nonhormonal Strategies

Given the cyclical nature of catamenial epilepsy, intermittent increase or addition of antiseizure medications may be considered at the time of seizure exacerbation. Benzodiazepines in particular are commonly prescribed in this manner. Clobazam is a 1–5 benzodiazepine with a long half-life that is approved by the US Food and Drug Administration (FDA) as an adjunctive treatment for Lennox–Gastaut syndrome and refractory seizures. Feely, Calvert, and Gibson evaluated the efficacy of intermittent clobazam in a small (N = 18) placebo-controlled crossover study. Doses of 20–30 mg daily were given for 10 days around the time of menstruation. Clobazam was superior in reducing seizure frequency in nearly 80% of women in this study [45].

When a subgroup (N = 14) of these same patients was monitored over time, the treatment effect was maintained over the observation period (4 months to nearly 3.5 years) in most cases. Nine of the women were maintained on clobazam for more than a year without the development of tolerance. Of note, two women were found to have improvement of catamenial seizures but increased seizure frequency in later stages of the menstrual cycle, which raises the concern of a withdrawal effect [46]. Sedation and depression were the most encountered side effects and were at times dose-limiting. The typical dosage for off-label use of clobazam for catamenial epilepsy is 20–30 mg daily for 10 days during the premenstrual period [46].

Clonazepam, a shorter-acting benzodiazepine, is also sometimes used intermittently around menses, but there is no literature to support this practice currently. An increase in a patient's baseline antiseizure medication doses is also sometimes tried, but there is no clear evidence to support this. In addition, this may lead to dose confusion in both patients and healthcare providers, thus requiring careful consideration and counseling should this be tried.

Acetazolamide is a sulfonamide and carbonic anhydrase inhibitor. Acetazolamide raises the seizure threshold in rats in an electroshock model [47]. This has been used to treat catamenial epilepsy for years based on anecdotal reports, though data of efficacy are lacking. Lim and colleagues conducted a retrospective review of 20 women with epilepsy using acetazolamide (mean daily dose 347 mg). Women in this study had either a perimenstrual (C1) or a periovulatory (C2) catamenial pattern. Around 40% of women in this study reported moderate (>50%) improvement in seizure frequency, though none were seizure free. This study included a mix of women taking acetazolamide continuously or intermittently around menses, which is often done to limit tolerance over time. No difference in efficacy was found between intermittent or continuous use. Nearly one-third of women reported side effects, including dizziness and polyuria. If employing this strategy, the recommended dose is to start with 4 mg/kg per day in one to four divided doses, not to exceed 1 gm per day [48]. This is often started 5–7 days before and continued through menstruation.

Before beginning any plan for pulse-dosed therapy, the potential that a patient could become pregnant when using these therapies should be considered and the patient should be counseled appropriately. Safety data on acetazolamide, benzodiazepines, and clobazam are limited [49, 50]. Some recent data suggest that clobazam may be associated with relatively high major congenital malformation rates, and it is known that higher doses of several antiseizure medications at conception may be associated with higher rates of structural and cognitive teratogenesis [36, 50].

Pregnancy and Catamenial Epilepsy

Women with catamenial epilepsy commonly worry that hormonal changes during pregnancy will worsen their seizure control [51]. Cagnetti and colleagues investigated seizure control throughout pregnancy in a prospective study of women with (N = 59) or without (N = 215) catamenial epilepsy. The catamenial pattern was established in women after following them for 24 months. Only those with a perimenstrual pattern (C1) were included. Nearly 80% of women with catamenial epilepsy remained seizure free throughout pregnancy, compared to only 22% of women without catamenial epilepsy. In addition, 50% of women with catamenial epilepsy had reduced seizure frequency compared to 8% of women without catamenial epilepsy throughout pregnancy. The greater than 50% seizure reduction rate showed a similar pattern. Logistic regression models confirmed that catamenial epilepsy is associated with improved seizure outcomes during pregnancy. The decrease in monthly hormonal fluctuations and increased progesterone is hypothesized to be the mechanism of improved seizure control throughout pregnancy [52]. It is notable that, in general, the seizure frequency in this study was higher than in most other prospective series [51]. This raises the question of whether the same difference would be seen in pregnancies in women with relatively well-controlled seizures.

A recent publication from the prospective Maternal Outcomes and Neurodevelopmental Effects of Antiepileptic Drugs (MONEAD) study demonstrated that, in general, control of seizures in women with epilepsy in the pregnancy and peripartum period relative to an epoch of time 7.5 months after pregnancy did not differ from a comparison of two similar epochs in nonpregnant women with epilepsy. The seizures studied were seizures that impaired awareness. In this study, the effect of a reported history of catamenial epilepsy on the difference between seizure frequency in pregnancy and the postpartum epoch was evaluated in a sensitivity analysis and was not statistically significant (OR 1.27 [0.60–2.67]) [53]. These studies are helpful in advising women with catamenial epilepsy that pregnancy likely does not exacerbate seizures for women with catamenial epilepsy; however, neither should not be used to argue against continued medical management in pregnancy for women with a catamenial pattern.

Menopause and Catamenial Epilepsy

Given the influence of sex hormones on seizure susceptibility, it is reasonable to believe that menopause will alter the course of catamenial epilepsy. Harden and colleagues performed a retrospective questionnaire study of the seizure course of women with epilepsy during perimenopause and menopause. A total of 42 menopausal women participated, with 38% reporting a catamenial seizure pattern prior to perimenopause. In women with catamenial epilepsy, seizures significantly increased during perimenopause and decreased during menopause [54]. Use of hormonal replacement therapy was associated with seizure worsening at menopause, in women both with and without catamenial epilepsy [54]. Further studies are needed to better understand this relationship.

Conclusion

Catamenial epilepsy is a pattern of seizure exacerbation from sensitivity to hormonal changes throughout the menstrual cycle and is common in women with epilepsy. There are three patterns of catamenial epilepsy, with the perimenstrual (C1) pattern the most frequent. The pathophysiology of catamenial epilepsy is not fully understood, but studies suggest that it is due to the fluctuations in the ratio of progesterone to estrogen throughout the menstrual cycle. Despite the prevalence of this disorder, evidence for highly effective treatments remains limited.

The term *catamenial epilepsy* can imply that this is a unique type of epilepsy. Given its prevalence, it is sometimes helpful to explain it to patients as a hormonal sensitivity rather than a specific condition. For many women, hormonal fluctuations are a trigger for seizures in much the same way as sleep deprivation is a trigger for some patients. Patients may benefit from an understanding of the periods of time when they are more vulnerable to seizures. Charting seizures can help manage the unpredictable nature of epilepsy that has a significant impact on quality of life. A common misunderstanding among patients and healthcare providers, however, is that patients with catamenial epilepsy will not benefit from standard epilepsy therapies. In fact, standard therapies should still be the first line of treatment for these women with hormone-sensitive seizures before attempting less evidence-based approaches.

References

1. Foldvary-Schaefer N, Harden C, Herzog A, et al. Hormones and seizures. *Cleveland Clinic Journal of Medicine*. 2004;**71**(2): S11–S8.
2. Logothetis J, Harner R, Morrell F, Torres F. The role of estrogens in catamenial exacerbation of epilepsy. *Neurology*. 1959;**9**(5):352–60.
3. Woolley CS. Estradiol facilitates kainic acid-induced, but not flurothyl-induced, behavioral seizure activity in adult female rats. *Epilepsia*. 2000;**41**(5):510–15.
4. Hom AC, Butterbough GG. Estrogen alters the acquisition of seizures kindled by repeated amygdala stimulation or pentylenetetrazol administration in ovariectomized female rats. *Epilepsia*. 1986;**27**:103–8.
5. Backstrom T. Epileptic seizures in women related to plasma estrogen and progesterone during the menstrual cycle. *Acta Neurologica Scandinavia*. 1976;**54**(4):321–47.
6. Woolley CS, McEwen BS. Estradiol regulates hippocampal dendritic spine density via an N-methyl-D-aspartate receptor-dependent mechanism. *Neuroscience*. 1994;**14**(12):7680–7.
7. Veliskova J, De Jesus G, Kaur R, et al. Females, their estrogens, and seizures. *Epilepsia*. 2010;**51**(3):141–4.
8. Reddy DS. Neuroendocrine aspects of catamenial epilepsy. *Hormones and Behavior*. 2013;**63**(2):254–66.
9. Reddy DS. Role of neurosteroids in catamenial epilepsy. *Epilepsy Research*. 2004;**62**(2–3):99–118.
10. Herzog, AG. Hormonal therapies: Progesterone. *Neurotherapeutics*. 2009;**6**(2):383–91.
11. Reddy DS, Rogawski MA. Neurosteroid replacement therapy for catamenial epilepsy. *Epilepsy*. 2010;**6**:501–13.
12. Kapur J, Joshi S. Progesterone modulates neuronal excitability bidirectionally. *Neuroscience Letters*. 2021;**744**:135619.
13. Joshi S, Sun H, Rajasekaran K, et al. A novel therapeutic approach for treatment of

catamenial epilepsy. *Neurobiology of Disease*. 2018;**111**:127–37.

14. Shiono S, Sun H, Batabyal T, et al. Limbic progesterone receptor activity enhances neuronal excitability and seizures. *Epilepsia*. 2021; **62**(8):1946–59.
15. Ansell B, Clarke E. Epilepsy and menstruation: The role of water retention. *Lancet*. 1956;**271**(6955):1232–5.
16. de Wildt SN, Kearns GL, Leeder JS, van den Anker JN. Glucuronidation in humans: Pharmacogenetic and developmental aspects. *Clin Pharmacokinet*. 1999;**36**(6):439–52.
17. Isojärvi JIT, Tauboll E, Herzog AG. Effect of antiepileptic drugs on reproductive endocrine function in individuals with epilepsy. *CNS Drugs*. 2005;**19**(3):207–23.
18. Rosciszewski D, Buntner B, Guz I, et al. Ovarian hormones, anticonvulsant drugs, and seizures during the menstrual cycle in women with epilepsy. *J Neurol Neurosurg Psychiatry*. 1986;**49**(1):47–51.
19. Kumar N, Behari M, Ahuja GK, Jailkhani BL. Phenytoin levels in catamenial epilepsy. *Epilepsia*. 1988;**29**(2):155–8.
20. Shavit G, Lerman P, Korczyn AD, et al. Phenytoin pharmacokinetics in catamenial epilepsy. *Neurology*. 1984;**34**(7):959–61.
21. Herkes G, Eadie MJ. Possible roles for frequent salivary AED monitoring in the management of epilepsy. *Epilepsy Res Suppl*. 1990;**6**:146–54.
22. Herzog AG, Fowler KM, Smithson SD. Valproate and lamotrigine level variation with menstrual cycle phase and oral contraceptive use. *Neurology*. 2009;**72**:911–14.
23. Foldvary-Schaefer N, Falcone T. Catamenial epilepsy: Pathophysiology, diagnosis, and management. *Neurology*. 2003;**61**:S2–15.
24. Herzog AG, Klein P, Rand BJ. Three patterns of catamenial epilepsy. *Epilepsia*. 1997;**38**(18):1082–8.
25. Herzog AG, Harden CL, Liporace J, et al. Frequency of catamenial seizure exacerbation in women with localization-related epilepsy. *Annals of Neurology*. 2004;**56**(3):431–4.
26. Quigg M, Smithson SD, Fowler KM, Susal T, Herzog AG. Laterality and location influence catamenial seizure expression in women with partial epilepsy. *Neurology*. 2009;**73**:224–7.
27. Kalinin VV, Zheleznova EV . Chronology and evolution of temporal lobe epilepsy and endocrine reproductive dysfunction in women: Relationships to side of focus and catameniality. *Epilepsy & Behavior*. 2007;**11**:185–91.
28. Kamitaki BK, Janmohamed M, Kandula P, et al. Clinical and EEG factors associated with antiseizure medication resistance in idiopathic generalized epilepsy. *Epilepsia*. 2022;**63**:150–61.
29. Duncan S, Read CL, Brodie MJ. How common is catamenial epilepsy? *Epilepsia*. 1993;**34**(5):827–31.
30. Gerard EE, Meador KJ. Managing epilepsy in women. *Continuum*. 2016;**22**:204–26.
31. Maguire MJ, Nevitt SJ. Treatments for seizures in catamenial (menstrual-related) epilepsy. *Cochrane Database of Systematic Reviews*. 2019;**9**(9):CD013225.
32. Dana-Haeri J, Richens A. Effect of norethisterone on seizures associated with menstruation. *Epilepsia*. 1983;**24**(3):377–81.
33. Herzog AG, Fowler KM, Smithson SD, et al. Progesterone vs. placebo therapy for women with epilepsy: A randomized clinical trial. *Neurology*. 2012;**78**(24):1959–66.
34. Najafi M, Sadeghi MM, Mehvari J, Zare M, Akbari M. Progesterone therapy in women with intractable catamenial epilepsy. *Advanced Biomedical Research*. 2013;**2**(1):P8.
35. Reddy DS, Rogawski MA. Enhanced anticonvulsant activity of neuroactive steroids in a rat model of catamenial epilepsy. *Epilepsia*. 2001;**42**(3):337–44.
36. McAuley J, Moore JL, Reeves AL, et al. A pilot study of the neurosteroid ganaxolone in catamenial epilepsy: Clinical experience in two patients. *Epilepsia*. 2001;**42**:P85.

37. Sperling MR, Klein P, Tsai J. Randomized, double-blind, placebo-controlled phase 2 study of ganaxolone as add-on therapy in adults with uncontrolled partial-onset seizures. *Epilepsia*. 2017;**58**(4):558–64.

38. Mattson RH, Cramer JA, Caldwell BV, Siconolfi BC. Treatment of seizures with medroxyprogesterone acetate: Preliminary report. *Neurology*. 1984;**34**(9):1255–8.

39. Phan T, Nur M. Improvement in seizure control after initiation of depot medroxyprogesterone acetate. *Journal of Pediatric and Adolescent Gynecology*. 2017;**30**(2):325–6.

40. Pennell PB. Hormonal aspects of epilepsy. *Neurologic Clinics*. 2009;**27**(4):941–65.

41. Herzog AG. Clomiphene therapy in epileptic women with menstrual disorders. *Neurology*. 1988;**38**(3):32–434.

42. Bauer J, Wild L, Flügel D, Stefan H. The effect of a synthetic GnRH analogue on catamenial epilepsy: A study in ten patients. *Journal of Neurology*. 1992;**239**(5):284–6.

43. Ichida M, Gomi A, Hiranouchi N, et al. A case of cerebral endometriosis causing catamenial epilepsy. *Neurology*. 1993;**43**(12):2708–9.

44. Vilos GA, Hollett-Caines J, Abu-Rafea B, Ahmad R, Mazurek MF. Resolution of catamenial epilepsy after goserelin therapy and oophorectomy: Case report of presumed cerebral endometriosis. *Journal of Minimally Invasive Gynecology*. 2011;**18**(1):128–30.

45. Feely M, Calvert R, Gibson J. Clobazam in catamenial epilepsy: A model for evaluating anticonvulsants. *Lancet*. 1982;**2**(8289):71–3.

46. Feely M, Gibson J. Intermittent clobazam for catamenial epilepsy: Tolerance avoided. *Journal of Neurology, Neurosurgery and Psychiatry*. 1984;**47**(12):1279–82.

47. Anderson RE, Howard RA, Woodbury DM. Correlation between effects of acute acetazolamide administration to mice on electroshock seizure threshold and maximal electroshock seizure pattern, and on carbonic anhydrase activity in subcellular fractions of brain. *Epilepsia*. 1986;**27**(5):504–9.

48. Lim LL, Foldvary N, Mascha E, Lee J. Acetazolamide in women with catamenial epilepsy. *Epilepsia*. 2001;**42**(6):746–9.

49. Falardeau J, Lobb BM, Golden S, Maxfield SD, Tanne E. The use of acetazolamide during pregnancy in intracranial hypertension patients. *Journal of Neuro-ophthalmology*. 2013;**33**(1):9–12.

50. Thomas SV, Jose M, Divakaran S, Sankara Sarma P. Malformation risk of antiepileptic drug exposure during pregnancy in women with epilepsy: Results from a pregnancy registry in south India. *Epilepsia*. 2017;**58**(2):274–81.

51. Pack AM. Having catamenial epilepsy equals fewer seizures in pregnancy. *Epilepsy Currents*. 2015;**15**(3):124–5.

52. Cagnetti C, Lattanzi S, Foschi N, Provinciali L, Silvestrini M. Seizure course during pregnancy in catamenial epilepsy. *Neurology*. 2014;**83**(4):339–44.

53. Pennell PB, French JA, May RC, et al. Changes in seizure frequency and antiepileptic therapy during pregnancy. *New England Journal of Medicine*. 2020;**383**(26):2547–56.

54 Harden CL, Pulver MC, Ravelin L, Jacobs AR. The effect of menopause and perimenopause on the course of epilepsy. *Epilepsia*. 1999;**40**(10):1402–7.

Chapter 9

Fertility in Women with Epilepsy

Lidia Di Vito, Mark Quigg, and Barbara Mostacci

Key Points

- Women with epilepsy (WWE) have lower fertility rates compared to the general population, though this likely applies to only a subset of women.
- Infertility in WWE is likely multifactorial. Psychosocial factors, hyposexuality, and neuroendocrine alterations secondary to seizures and to some antiseizure medications (ASMs) have been implicated.
- The hypothalamic-pituitary-gonadal axis (HPG axis) and feedback inhibitory mechanisms play a key part in infertility among WWE.
- Counseling and evaluation focused on sexuality and fertility are key to address potentially reversible or treatable causes of infertility.

Introduction

According to the World Health Organization (WHO), infertility is the failure to conceive after regular unprotected sexual intercourse in 1 year or longer [1]. However, in clinical practice, women aged 35 years or older are often evaluated and treated for infertility after 6 months of unprotected intercourse. It has been estimated that infertility affects one in every seven couples in the Western world and one in every four couples in developing countries [2].

Since 1950, it has been suggested that persons with epilepsy might be disadvantaged with respect to reproduction. Both social and biological risk factors might be implicated in reducing fecundity in this population. Historically, constraints on reproductive rights – bans on marriage and having children – were important factors in the ability of women with epilepsy (WWE) to bear children. For example, state laws in the United States allowed forcible sterilization of WWE until 1956, while in the United Kingdom, people with epilepsy were not allowed to marry until 1970 [3]. Until 1999, epilepsy was grounds for annulment of marriage in India [4].

Although these laws are obsolete, reduced marriage rates are still reported in people with epilepsy, at least partly due to persisting social isolation and stigmatization. Moreover, attitudes toward childbearing and childrearing might be influenced by the presence of comorbidities and/or disabilities and by the fear of increased risk to offspring. On the other hand, hyposexuality and impaired reproductive function may be a consequence of seizures themselves or adverse events of some antiseizure medications (ASMs). The purpose of this chapter is to summarize the epidemiological data on infertility in WWE, to explore social and biologic culprits, and to review aspects of the evaluation and treatment of infertility in this population.

Box 9.1 Causes of reduced fertility rates in women with epilepsy

Law constraints (probably influencing early studies figures)
Social issues (isolation, stigmatization)
Comorbidities limiting attitudes toward parenthood
Concerns of risk to offspring from intrauterine exposure to ASMs/disease transmission
Hyposexuality/impaired reproductive function due to seizures and/or ASMs

Epidemiology of Infertility in Women with Epilepsy

Table 9.1 summarizes data from the main epidemiological studies of fertility in WWE. Studies vary in the measurements of fertility, with some reporting the number of children (live births per woman or by patient-years) and others the proportion of women successfully achieving or, more often, concluding a pregnancy (proportion of women with at least one birth). To standardize the different studies, whenever possible, Table 9.1 and the discussion that follows use a normalized "fertility rate" – the proportion of observed fertility expected in the units – as defined by each study.

Most studies that assess fertility in WWE use public health databases. These studies were conducted in Northern Europe or North America [5–11] and most of them demonstrate decreased fertility among WWE with a range of 59–95% compared to controls. One national healthcare system-based study from Iceland conflicts with these findings, reporting that, between 1960 and 1964, 209 WWE had two live births per patient, no different from age-matched controls [6]. Similarly to the majority of registry-based studies, studies based on clinic samples show ranges of fertility, among WWE, of 55–95% compared to controls [12–19].

A prospective clinical-based study, which followed WWE through a period of time to directly observe birth rates, showed a fertility rate of 55–60% compared to controls, when WWE with "epilepsy-only," including idiopathic or cryptogenic epilepsy without cognitive impairment or symptomatic cause, were selected [12]. A US study surveyed a group of WWE about their overall pregnancy history compared to a control group of their oldest female siblings. Women were included only if they had been married at least once. Women with epilepsy had a fertility rate of 70% compared to their sisters without epilepsy [13].

Two studies focused only on WWE attempting to conceive. A prospective study performed in India tracked a group of nulliparous WWE anticipating pregnancy: 38% of women remained infertile, a rate nearly double that of a non-epileptic comparison obtained from the same region's census board [16]. Interestingly, a multicenter US study, which for the first time prospectively compared WWE with women without epilepsy willing to become pregnant, showed a similar likelihood of pregnancy, time to pregnancy, and live birth rates in the two groups. However, women with known infertility diagnosis or diagnoses associated with reproductive disorders were excluded [17]. Of note, as detailed in the following sections, in the Indian study, infertility was mainly associated with the use of phenobarbital and polytherapy, which concerned a significant number of the studied women. Conversely, most women in the US study were on monotherapy with either levetiracetam (LEV) or lamotrigine (LTG), medications that have not been associated with diminished sexuality or fertility.

Table 9.1 Studies of fertility rates in women with epilepsy

First author	Year	Country	Design	N	Duration of sample or study (years)	WWE sample	Control sample	Fertility rate WWE	Fertility rate controls	Fertility rate ratio
Dansky [14]	1980	Canada	Retro	100	na	Clinic sample, age > 15	Regional demographics	1.7 LB per woman	2.9 LB per woman	0.59
Webber [5]	1986	USA	Retro	220	40	All WWE between 1935 and 1974 Rochester, MN	All women without epilepsy	71.0 LB per 1,000 person-years	82.9 LB per 1,000 person-years	0.86
Schupf and Ottman [13]	1996	USA	Retro	581	3	Sample from people with epilepsy organizations	Siblings without epilepsy (n 170)	1.4 LB per woman	2 LB per woman	0.70
Jalava [12]	1997	Finland	Pro	100	35	Clinic sample (pts with epilepsy only)	age-matched National health survey N 99, Age-matched employee survey N 100	0.97 LB per woman	1.77 LB per woman, 1.61 LB per woman	0.55 0.60
Olafsson [6]	1998	Iceland	Retro	75	5	All WWE Iceland National Health	Age-matched non-epileptic sample N 150	2.0 LB per woman	2.1 LB per woman	1.00
Wallace [7]	1998	UK	Retro	7,626	5	All women with treated epilepsy, age 15–44 National Health	All women without epilepsy age 15–44	47.1 LB per 1,000 women	62.1 LB per 1,000 women	0.75

Table 9.1 (cont.)

First author	Year	Country	Design	N	Duration of sample or study (years)	WWE sample	Control sample	Fertility rate WWE	Fertility rate controls	Fertility rate ratio
Artama [8]	2004	Finland	Retro	6,535	17	All WWE 1985–2001 age 15–45 National Health	All women without epilepsy age 15–45	0.54 LB per woman	0.88 LB per woman	0.61
Artama [9]	2006	Finland	Retro	Na	10	All WWE 1985–1994 age 15–49 With/without ASMs use National Health	Stratified age-matched random sample without epilepsy	Untreated 41.7–44.6 On ASMs 33.7–40.7 per 1,000 person-yrs	56.3–57.4 per 1,000 person-yrs	0.60–69 on ASMs 0.83–1.01 on ASMs
Viinikainen [10]	2007	Finland	Retro	286	1	All women using ASMs age 16–39 National Health	Public health database	2.1 LB +/−1.3	2.2 LB+/−1.2	0.95
Kariuki [15]	2008	Kenya	Retro	175	4	Clinic sample	National demographic	45.87 LB per 1,000 women-yrs	na	0.75
Sukumaran [16]	2010	India	Pro	375	1–10	Clinic sample	Public health database	61.8% with at least 1 LB	84.9% with at least 1 LB	0.73
Farmen [11]	2016	Oppland County, Norway	Retro	303 pregnancies	23	All WWE in the perinatal database who gave consent (166/176) comparing with the estimated prevalence of epilepsy	All women without epilepsy in the perinatal database (95% LB of the county)	na	na	Na

Pennell [17]	2018	US	Pro	89	5	Clinic sample: WWE seeking a pregnancy, 18–40 yrs	Women without epilepsy seeking a pregnancy, age 18–40	60.7% achieved pregnancy in 1 year	60.2%	1
Starck [18]	2018	Finland	Retro	143	1980–92	Clinical sample (all persons with childhood-onset epilepsy)	1/4 matching controls from Public health database			
Li [19]	2019	China	Cross-sec	972	4	Clinic sample	National population census	41.8% with at least 1 LB		

Fertility ratio: fertility rate of WWE/controls; design: retro(spective) or pro(spective); LB: live birth; na: not available, yrs: years

As fertility is measured mainly by the number of live births, it is worth mentioning that there are some conflicting data on the risk of spontaneous abortions and intrauterine deaths in WWE, or women taking ASMs, with most studies indicating a substantially un-increased risk. Data on termination of pregnancies in WWE are scanty. In an Indian study, terminations of pregnancies were not increased in WWE compared to the general population figures [20]. In a Canadian study, female patients had a significantly increased frequency of one or more induced abortions compared to male patients' wives (13.8% vs. 0). Interestingly, the same study found approximate doubling of illegitimate children in WWE compared to the expected rate (6.8% vs. 3.8%) [14]. We speculate this could be a further indirect proof that marriage was a less frequent option for WWE, probably due to social stigma. Mostacci and colleagues also observed an almost doubled frequency of induced abortion (21% vs. 12%) in women taking ASMs compared to controls in a population study in northern Italy [21].

Etiology and Characteristics of Infertility in Women with Epilepsy

Social Factors and Stigma

Several hints suggest that social factors may at least partly underlie the reduced fertility found in WWE. Two Indian studies examined perceptions of epilepsy and marriage. From interviews of 400 WWE in rural India, researchers determined the onset of epilepsy before 20 years of age reduces the chances of patients finding a spouse among those who disclose their diagnosis to family or community members [22]. This relationship between age of onset and delay in marriage (and hence possibly reduced fertility) was confirmed in the Indian population in a second study that showed WWE are less likely to get married, are more likely to be older when married, and have higher rates of "withheld marriage" (spinsterhood). On the other hand, the large majority of women (95%) do not disclose their diagnosis before marriage. Perhaps lack of disclosure is one factor that accounts for higher rates of divorce compared to national means as observed in this study [20].

Decreased marriage rates have been observed in other cultures. In a survey of 100 WWE in Canada [14], the marriage rate was 83% of the expected rate. Early onset of seizures was the main demographic factor noted to worsen the chance of marriage. The stigma against marriage was the main finding in a Hong Kong survey; in a sample of persons without epilepsy, 94% of respondents thought it appropriate for people with epilepsy to marry; however, one-third thought it inappropriate to marry a person with epilepsy if the proposed spouse was their child [23]. The rates of marriage were also evaluated in a Finnish study [12]. Compared to controls with an 83% marriage or significant cohabitation rate, only 60% of WWE achieved marriage or cohabitation over the duration of the study; WWE were 3.6 times more likely to remain single. In contrast, the Icelandic study – in which fertility of WWE was not impaired compared to controls – found no disadvantage in rates of marriage of WWE [6].

Several studies pointed out that a subset of patients might be more disadvantaged with respect to fertility, showing much lower rates of marriage and live births. This subset includes people with cognitive impairment and disabilities, but also with childhood-onset epilepsy, a condition likely to have a heavier, long-lasting impact on social life [6, 10, 16, 18].

Furthermore, in a Rochester study in which birth rates were compared in different decades of the past century, the largest fertility gap between WWE and controls occurred during the period of peak population reproductivity (1945–64), while during low-population fertility periods (1965–74), the deficit was less marked or absent. The authors speculated that, albeit capable of conceiving, WWE choose less often to give birth to many children and therefore live births per woman are comparably lower when the general population tends more to large families [5]. Similar findings were seen in a cohort study by Schupf and Ottman [13]. However, it should be noted that the gap reduction could also reflect the improved social conditions of WWE, including changes in laws, which previously allowed forced sterilization in this condition.

In a Norwegian study assessing age-specific birth rates, fertility was reduced in WWE older than 20 years, but not in the younger ones, an interesting result that, however, according to the authors, is open to different interpretations. As a matter of fact, young adults with epilepsy could be more prone than their peers to risk-taking behavior, including early sexual debut and reduced use of contraceptives. Fears of risk to the offspring may be less prominent in younger WWE, though, while these concerns may increase with age as executive functions mature, suggesting that reduced fecundity might be driven at least in part by the deliberate avoidance of pregnancy in older women [11]. Consistently, in a UK survey, 33% of WWE were not considering motherhood because of their epilepsy [24].

Box 9.2 Psychosocial issues associated with reduced fertility in women with epilepsy

Cultural aspects, stigma
Comorbidities/disability
Childhood-onset epilepsy
Age (different perception of risk to the offspring?)

Sexual Desire and Mood

Problems with mood and libido may affect fertility in WWE. For example, even WWE who have the appropriate social possibility of conceiving children may do so less frequently because of decreased sexual desire or depressed mood.

Morrell and colleagues studied sexual function and hormones in WWE aged 18–40 with focal or generalized epilepsies compared to non-epileptic controls [25]. Questionnaires examined sexual experience, arousability, anxiety, and depression; the questionnaires were then compared to endocrine assessments. Compared to controls, women with focal epilepsy had significantly impaired sexual function, lower degrees of self-reported arousal, and worse depression scores. Women with generalized epilepsy were less impaired overall, but still reported decreased arousal. Women taking enzyme-inducing ASMs were most affected. Hormonal measurements that correlated with sexual dysfunction were estradiol (negatively correlated with sexual anxiety) and dehydroepiandrosterone (negatively correlated with sexual dysfunction and lack of arousal).

Furthermore, the associations among low libido, low testosterone, and the use of enzyme-inducing ASMs are also observed in men with epilepsy [26]. Tao and colleagues compared 112 married WWE who were taking ASMs for ≥ 1 year and 120 healthy controls without epilepsy, all of Chinese Han nationality. They found a high rate of sexual dysfunction in WWE (70.5%) and a higher serum prolactin level and estradiol-to-progesterone ratio in the WWE compared to the control group. [27].

In addition to hormonal abnormalities and ASM effects, epilepsy itself may contribute to sexual dysfunction in WWE. Among epilepsies, sexual dysfunction is more frequently reported in temporal lobe epilepsy (TLE) [28]. Hyposexuality seems to be more prominent in women with right TLE than with left temporal foci [29]. Morrell and colleagues observed different patterns of sexual dysfunction depending on the type of epilepsy; women with idiopathic generalized epilepsy (IGE) experienced anorgasmia and sexual dissatisfaction, while women with focal epilepsy reported more sexual anxiety, dyspareunia, vaginismus, and arousal insufficiency [30].

Box 9.3 Sexual dysfunction in women with epilepsy

Reduced arousal, anorgasmia, sexual dissatisfaction, sexual anxiety, dyspareunia, and vaginismus are reported in WWE.

Depression, focal epilepsy (particularly temporal epilepsy), and enzyme-inducing ASMs are associated factors.

Sex hormones levels are frequently altered and may be implicated in sexual dysfunction in WWE.

Direct Biological Effects

The interactions between epilepsy, neuroendocrine regulation of the hypothalamic-pituitary-gonadal axis (HPG axis), and ASMs are complex (see Figure 9.1). A direct role for epilepsy in the pathogenesis of infertility is suggested by the differences in fertility according to epilepsy syndrome, the high rate of reproductive disorders in those with epilepsy irrespective of ASMs, the acute disruption of normal hypothalamic-pituitary activity by seizures and interictal discharges, the physiologic and clinical effects of laterality of epileptic foci [31–33], and the resolution of menstrual disturbances after successful epilepsy surgery [34]. Regions of the hypothalamus involved in the regulation, production, and secretion of gonadotropin-releasing hormone (GnRH) receive extensive direct connections from the cerebral hemispheres, especially from temporolimbic structures commonly involved in epilepsy, particularly the amygdala [35].

Type and Etiology of Epilepsy

Several of the surveys in Table 9.1 evaluated the effects of epilepsy type, syndrome, or etiology on fertility. Some show that fertility is most affected in case of remote symptomatic epilepsy compared to idiopathic/cryptogenic epilepsy. Schupf and Ottman in their study of WWE compared to their healthy sisters [13] found that the effects of infertility were higher in focal rather than generalized epilepsies, a difference that was most marked before the diagnosis of epilepsy. Similar findings were seen in the large population study by Webber and colleagues [5].

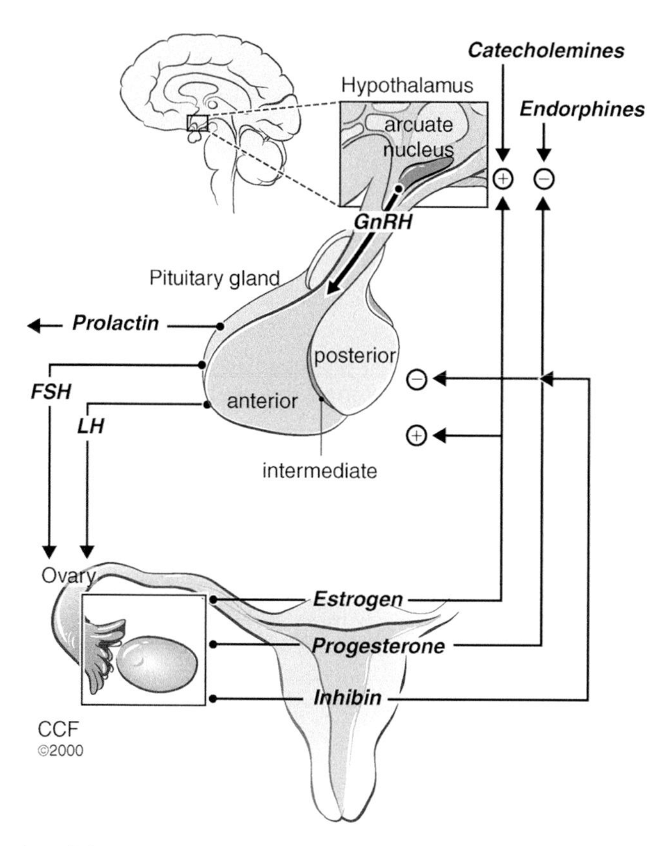

Figure 9.1 The hypothalamic-pituitary-ovarian axis regulates the interactions between neurohormones, gonadotropin-releasing hormone, pituitary gonadotropins, and the gonadal steroids through a feedback loop mechanism.

In comparison, the Icelandic survey, in addition to finding no disadvantage in fertility in WWE, also found no differences between those with focal versus generalized epilepsies [6]. When WWE with idiopathic/cryptogenic epilepsy were compared with controls, there was no difference in the number of children or number of partners overall, nor were there differences when stratified by seizure type or age at diagnosis. Patients with remote symptomatic epilepsy, when cognitive impairment or cerebral palsy were excluded, also had an equal rate of live births to controls. Differences from controls only emerged in patients with cognitive impairment or cerebral palsy, from which only 8% of women bore children [6]. A large effect of cognitive impairment on infertility was also seen in the Finnish population (type of epilepsy was not measured) [10].

A prospective study of an Indian cohort similarly found that the type of epilepsy had no significance in fertility rates [16]. Demographic factors associated with infertile WWE included older age and lower educational status (perhaps reflective of the severity of epilepsy rather than a direct effect of education).

Other studies have documented reproductive endocrine disorders in women with IGE: in a study conducted over a population of 148 WWE, Lofgren and colleagues found that women with IGE tended to have menstrual disorders and hyperandrogenism more often than women with focal epilepsy, both in women taking valproate (VPA) and in women not taking VPA, concluding that IGE is one of the factors predicting anovulatory cycles in WWE [36–38].

Reproductive Disorders in Women with Epilepsy

Women with epilepsy have higher than expected rates of disorders that directly affect fertility, and these disorders have been either directly linked to or have enough evidence to infer that they are present largely because of disruption of normal function due to the epileptic condition (including ASMs use) or epileptic seizures. These disorders include polycystic ovary syndrome, hypothalamic hypogonadism, sex hormones changes, functional hyperprolactinemia, and premature menopause [35].

Polycystic Ovary Syndrome

Polycystic ovary syndrome (PCOS) is a multifactorial and complex disease characterized by some combination of androgen excess, ovulatory dysfunction, and polycystic ovaries frequently associated with obesity. It is the main cause of anovulatory infertility in women, with a prevalence of 5–15%, depending on the criteria used and population studied, but in most studies comprised 4–7% in the general population. In a series of 50 consecutive women with temporal-limbic epilepsy, Herzog and colleagues found that 20% were affected with PCOS [39]. Another study of women with generalized epilepsy found an incidence of 15% of combined hyperandrogenism and ovulatory dysfunction in 15 of 101 consecutive patients with epilepsy with similar frequencies of menstrual disorders and PCOS in women with primary generalized and focal epilepsy [40]. Overall, in populations of WWE, PCOS occurs in 13–25%.

Although ASM treatment may be an important factor in the development of PCOS as detailed later in this chapter, seizure activity itself may lead to neuroendocrine dysfunction depending on the area of the brain from which seizures originate. In particular, women with left TLE show increased rates of PCOS. Epileptic discharges from the amygdala to the hippocampus might impair the secretion of GnRH and therefore the ratio of luteinizing hormone (LH) to follicle-stimulating hormone (FSH), promoting ovarian dysfunction [31, 41–45]. However, different studies have reported [38] that women with IGE are more likely to have anovulatory cycles, especially those who have been using VPA treatment, and polycystic-appearing ovaries, probably in relation to a dysfunction of the hypothalamic-pituitary axis due to frequent generalized epileptiform discharges [37, 38].

Hypothalamic Hypogonadism

Hypothalamic hypogonadism, or inadequate stimulation of ovarian function due to insufficient or disordered secretion of gonadotropins, results in infertility and amenorrhea or oligomenorrhea and has been reported to occur in 12% of a sample of women with TLE, compared to a rate of 1.5% in the general population [39]. Laterality and focality of epilepsy seem to be important determinants of endocrine function: distinct reproductive endocrine disorders may be related to the area of the brain primarily affected by seizure activity and suggest that specific neural pathways act as substrates to drive altered endocrine functions [46].

Both generalized and focal epilepsy may affect the function of the hypothalamic-pituitary axis: elevation of FSH serum levels and disturbed LH secretion have been described in women with IGE [36]. In left TLE, higher-pulse frequencies of GnRH secretion and consequently higher LH/FSH ratios and higher serum testosterone levels have been reported [35]. On the other hand, in right TLE, lower GnRH pulse frequency and higher rates of hypothalamic amenorrhea have been observed [31, 41–45].

Sex Hormones Alterations

Serum levels of sex hormones are commonly altered in people with epilepsy, as an effect of ASMs, particularly valproic acid and enzyme inducers, or of epilepsy and seizure activity themselves [47–50].

As mentioned, seizures may affect the hypothalamic-pituitary axis and elevated testosterone is often observed in WWE, in cases of focal epilepsy [45] or IGE [37]. Among patients with TLE, women with left-sided TLE show higher testosterone compared with women with right-sided TLE [45], the latter showing significantly decreased estradiol levels compared to left-sided TLE [31, 46].

Hyperprolactinemia

Hyperprolactinemia theoretically may be a factor in infertility in active epilepsy. Hyperprolactinemia suppresses the GnRH-LH axis, causing polymenorrhea, oligomenorrhea, or amenorrhea, as well as poor fertility, galactorrhea, and hirsutism. As noted, the blood level of prolactin rises immediately after seizures, sometimes four or five times from preictal levels, and stays elevated for about 1 hour postictally [32]. Prolactin rise is more likely to occur after generalized tonic-clonic seizures, but it has been also reported after focal seizures with impaired awareness, possibly related to the intensity and duration of the seizure [33, 51]. Herzog demonstrated that small prolactin surges can occur as the result of interictal discharges in the case of TLE, predominantly after right temporolimbic discharges [35]. Although theoretically important from a temporolimbic interaction perspective, hyperprolactinemia from a clinical standpoint may be rare in WWE. An evaluation of reproductive disorders in WWE disclosed that out of 238 Finnish women treated for epilepsy, none had hyperprolactinemia [48].

Premature Menopause

Premature menopause (primary gonadal failure with amenorrhea and high gonadotropin levels at age < 40) occurs more frequently in WWE than in the general population. The highest rate of premature menopause was seen in a study of 50 WWE whose rate of 14% stood far above the control rate of 4% [52].

In their study of the distribution of reproductive disorders in TLE, Herzog and colleagues found that 4% had early menopause compared with an expected general rate of about 1% [39]. A Finnish cohort, however, found a rate of premature menopause in only 1.4% [48].

Other studies confirmed the occurrence of premature menopause in WWE [53, 54], especially when associated with the use of multiple ASMs and high seizure frequency [55]. Gold and colleagues in their study demonstrated a negative correlation between the age at menopause and the lifetime number of seizures, once again possibly due to the seizures' disruption of hypothalamic and pituitary functions [54].

Box 9.4 Reproductive disturbances in women with epilepsy

Polycystic ovarian syndrome is up to four times more common in WWE compared to the general population.
Both TLE and IGE were associated with PCOS.
Antiseizure medications might be implicated in promoting (VPA) or counteracting (enzyme-inducers) PCOS.
Both focal and generalized epilepsies may affect the hypothalamic-pituitary axis, promoting hypogonadism.
Premature menopause is more common in WWE.

Effects of Chronic Epilepsy and Acute Seizures

Several considerations suggest a direct influence of epilepsy on reproductive disturbances: an acute change in serum prolactin and gonadotropin levels may be acutely observed following seizures, and a relation between the laterality of temporolimbic epileptiform discharges and the specific type of disturbance has been reported. Finally, menstrual disorders can reverse after epilepsy surgery [34].

The physiological means by which epilepsy affects the HPG axis are discussed in what follows. Both interictal and ictal discharges affect the function of the HPG axis at the hypothalamic level [31, 32]. In a study of HPG function in men with TLE (in this case used as a "model" for WWE not susceptible to menstrual effects), Quigg and colleagues evaluated the pattern of pulsatile LH secretion for 24-hour periods with two comparisons [32]. First, to evaluate the effects of interictal dysfunction (the effect of the chronic epileptic lesion), interictal LH secretion of men with TLE was compared to age-matched healthy controls. Second, to evaluate postictal effects, LH secretion patterns from the first 24 hours after a seizure were matched with each patient's interictal sample. Chronic epilepsy, or interictal function in people with epilepsy compared to healthy controls, was associated with changes in LH pulse frequency, amplitude, and amount per pulse. Acute seizures induced timing irregularity – a degradation in pulse rhythm – in LH secretion. Clinical effects, however, were not measured in this study.

Even interictal discharges may acutely disrupt normal hypothalamopituitary endocrine function as suggested by the possible elevation of prolactin pulse after right temporolimbic discharges or by the suppression of LH pulsatility with higher LH baseline values after left temporolimbic discharges [35]. However, comparing WWE who had seizures within the prior 9 months with seizure-free WWE seeking a pregnancy, Pennel and colleagues did not find any difference in pregnancy outcomes [17].

Laterality of the Epileptic Lesion

Another example of the direct effects of the epileptic lesion on the HPG axis, and by extension, fertility, is the unexpected influence of epileptic laterality on HPG dysfunction. Quigg and colleagues' study of male LH secretion found that the rate of pulses of LH was faster in men with right-sided temporal foci than in those with left-sided foci. Lateralization of LH pulsatile secretion was also seen in women with TLE [41].

Herzog and colleagues linked physiologic lateralization to clinical phenotype, noting that sexual dysfunction scores and accompanying low testosterone levels were more often present in women with right-sided rather than left-sided TLE [31]. Furthermore, as regards reproductive disorders aggregated by side of the epileptic lesion, those with PCOS tended to have left-sided epileptic foci, and those with hypogonadotropic hypogonadism, right-sided. Kalinin and colleagues conducted a study over 80 women with TLE and found that a catamenial pattern was more common in the women with left TLE as compared to the women with right TLE; furthermore, catamenial right TLE was associated with a longer duration of epilepsy [42].

Epilepsy Surgery

The argument for the direct effects of epilepsy on HPG axis function has been investigated in studies of WWE after epilepsy surgery. Bauer and colleagues [34] assessed menstrual function before and 1 year after either temporal lobectomy or selective amygdala hippocampectomy for 16 women. Eight patients achieved seizure remission, and all remained on their ASMs. Documentation of menstrual cycles in addition to laboratory parameters revealed postsurgical changes in the menstrual cycle in eight patients. Four patients had a change in menstrual periodicity: in two patients who became seizure-free after surgery, regular cycles instead of oligomenorrhea occurred, whereas two patients with incomplete seizure control presented with oligomenorrhea instead of regular cycles after surgery.

In contrast to cycle changes, no definitive changes were seen in postsurgical concentrations of testosterone, prolactin, dehydroepiandrosterone sulfate (DHEAS), growth hormone, cortisol, and sex hormone-binding globulin (SHBG). There was, however, a significant increase in serum androstenedione concentrations 6 months postsurgically, mainly in those patients achieving seizure remission. The authors interpreted the study as demonstrating that successful epilepsy surgery can alter menstrual cycle function. Although no gross serum changes in sex hormones occurred, one can hypothesize that other physiologic changes – such as in the aforementioned pulsatile secretion patterns – may have occurred after surgery and seizure remission.

Fabris and colleagues conducted a study on 113 WWE of childbearing age with drug-resistant focal epilepsy who had undergone a focal cortical resection between 1997 and 2008 at the Mayo Clinic in Rochester. The authors did not find a direct effect of postoperative seizure outcome, nor seizure onset localization and lateralization on pregnancies and births after surgery. However, they did find an increase in pregnancies and births in women who were younger and received fewer ASMs at the time of surgery. They speculated that surgery might have an indirect effect on fertility while increasing social integration and marriage rates and underlined the importance of earlier surgical intervention in drug-resistant focal epilepsy [56].

Some studies reported a postoperative improvement of sexual dysfunction in patients who underwent right anterior temporal lobectomy (ATL) as compared to left ATL surgery [29, 57]. A study conducted by Baird and colleagues demonstrated that sexual outcome after ATL correlates with the volume of the amygdala contralateral to the side of surgery, with patients reporting postoperative sexual increase having a larger amygdala volume as compared to those reporting sexual worsening or no change [58].

Antiseizure Medications

The studies from India [16], Finland [10], and Iceland [6] emphasize that ASMs may contribute to infertility. In particular, in the Indian prospective study of WWE that compared those who bore children and those who did not, ASM exposure was the most important factor in infertility. The proportion of infertile women was highest (60%) for those on three or more ASMs and decreased with the number of ASMs (2 ASMs – 41%; 1 ASM – 32%). It was also significantly increased in women taking phenobarbital. Although a similar trend was noted for phenytoin usage, this was not observed when monotherapy alone was considered [16]. However, another Finnish population study did not show any difference among women treated with oxcarbazepine (OXC), carbamazepine (CBZ), or VPA, and epilepsy appeared as a more important factor than ASM in influencing fertility [9].

Potential interactions between ASMs and fertility could arise from their effects on direct disruption of the HPG axis and gonadal function, on hormonal metabolism or serum binding (which in turn may induce changes in hypothalamic regulation/feedback), and from secondary interactions with weight/appetite regulation or insulin sensitivity.

One of the most discussed and controversial interactions between infertility and ASMs is the contribution of VPA to the pathogenesis of PCOS or to one of its isolated components (polycystic ovary or hyperandrogenism) in WWE. Isojärvi and colleagues described for the first time the reproductive phenotypes of 238 WWE taking different ASM combinations, with 12% on VPA monotherapy, 50% on CBZ monotherapy, 31% on combination or other monotherapy, and 6% untreated. They evaluated ovary status with ultrasound, menstrual cycles, and hormonal levels. Whereas 45% of the women taking VPA had menstrual disturbances and 43% had polycystic ovaries, patients on other ASMs had less than one-half the rate of menstrual problems or polycystic ovaries. Some patients on VPA had no polycystic ovaries but did have hyperandrogenism. Overall, 60% of women on VPA had polycystic ovaries and hyperandrogenism (80% of women who started VPA before the age of 20 years) [48]. These results were supported by other studies and discontinuation of VPA, and shifting to LTG led to normalization in 12 women with PCOS prospectively followed up for 1 year [59].

However, other studies did not find any association between menstrual disturbance and any ASM. Moreover, long-term VPA treatment in healthy monkeys did not result in any ovarian dysfunction. Interestingly, a reduced incidence of PCOS in WWE treated with enzyme inducers compared with untreated WWE (13% vs. 30%) has been shown [39]. Hence it was hypothesized that epilepsy itself may cause a disruption of the hypothalamic-pituitary axis and therefore menstrual disturbance and anovulatory cycles, whereas VPA may cause hyperandrogenism and possible metabolic derangement with carbohydrate intolerance and obesity. It was also speculated that enzyme-inducing ASMs might treat PCOS by enzyme induction that increases the synthesis of SHBG and the metabolism of testosterone, resulting in lower levels of bioavailable testosterone [35].

On the other hand, enzyme inducers have been implicated in reproduction disturbances as well. They interfere with the normal function of sex steroid-binding proteins, which in turn reduces the amount of available sex steroids in serum. A menstrual disturbance characterized by low estradiol and a low estradiol-to-SHBG ratio was observed [60]. Furthermore, although a drop in testosterone with treatment of epilepsy with CBZ in some instances appears to be a "benefit," as noted earlier, low testosterone associated with the use of enzyme-inducing ASMs may cause depressed libido [25, 26].

A cross-sectional survey conducted in Norway and Austria explored sexual complaints, menstrual disorders, and hormonal changes in people with epilepsy at fertile age taking LEV, LTG, or CBZ as monotherapy without endocrine disturbances or recent hormonal treatment. Menstrual disturbances were more frequent in all treatment groups compared with controls, but the differences were not significant. No statistically significant hormonal changes were observed in the women being treated with LEV. Progesterone levels were significantly lower and SHBG levels were significantly higher in women treated with CBZ. Women treated with LTG had significantly higher DHEAS and lower androstenedione (a result of uncertain clinical meaning). Scores in the survey on sexual function indicated a greater degree of satisfaction among women taking LEV and LTG [61]. See Chapter 5 for additional discussion on the effects of ASMs on reproductive function.

Box 9.5 Antiseizure medications and fertility

Valproate promotes insulin resistance and weight gain and could promote hyperandrogenism and PCOS in WWE.

Enzyme inducers could counteract PCOS, reducing bioavailable (free) testosterone.

Enzyme inducers, lowering free sex steroids, may affect sexuality and promote menstrual disturbances.

Levetiracetam and LTG do not seem to affect hormone blood levels or sexuality.

Counseling, Evaluation, and Treatment

An important feature in evaluating infertility in WWE is that the factors associated with epilepsy – from social to biological – occur in the context of reproductive health in general. In other words, WWE who are infertile may have the same reproductive problems as women without epilepsy. Though ovulatory disorders were observed with a higher frequency in WWE, as detailed in the preceding paragraphs, endometriosis, tubal abnormalities, and other causes of infertility may occur as well in WWE. Hence, investigations of reproductive dysfunction must be remanded to gynecologists or fertility specialists and a multidisciplinary approach is an important part of the workup.

However, a detailed history of menstrual characteristics, hormonal intake, and contraception should be taken on every fertile WWE by the neurologist, who should also inquire about weight or, better, weigh the patient at every visit. Hirsutism and acne should be noted at inspection.

Counseling on contraception and pregnancy should be given to every WWE and reinforcement of this information should be made at every visit. Counseling on pregnancy must not be perceived only as a way to warn about risks related to ASMs, but it should also allow WWE to look at motherhood as a possible achievement. Sharing information on seizures and epilepsy with the woman's partner, including first aid maneuvers, may also improve the couple's confidence and lessen the fear of a seizure during sexual intercourse.

Assisted reproduction technology treatment has the same rate of success in women with and without epilepsy, irrespective of ASM use, according to a large registry-based Danish study [62]. Of note, ovarian stimulation and endometrial preparation, which are generally performed in this setting, imply administration of estradiol and gonadotropins, and the latter in turn lead to a surge in estrogen blood levels. A significant increase in exogenous or endogenous estrogens might lead to seizure worsening in WWE by lowering the seizure threshold. Furthermore, estrogens induce glucuronidation in women taking LTG and OXC.

We have observed several cases of a reduction of LTG blood levels and three cases of seizure exacerbation (we previously reported two of them) [63] during hormonal treatment for assisted reproduction. In the case of administration of estradiol and gonadotropins, we suggest performing serial blood levels testing of possibly affected medication, and, at least in selected cases, considering a proactive adjustment of doses.

Box 9.6 Counseling and evaluating women with epilepsy of childbearing age

Always get a detailed history of menstrual characteristics, hormone intake, contraception, and pregnancies.

Weigh the patient at every visit and check for hirsutism and acne.

Provide tailored information on contraception and pregnancy at every visit.

Provide information on epilepsy (including first aid), contraception, and pregnancy to the couple, if appropriate.

If infertility is diagnosed, consider type and severity of epilepsy and type of ASMs. However, the diagnostic workup dedicated to all infertile couples should be performed.

If infertility is diagnosed, reassure the couple that assisted reproduction treatments have the same rates of success in WWE.

If hormone treatments are prescribed, consider adjusting the dose of ASMs metabolized via glucuronidation (i.e., LTG and OXC).

Conclusions

In most epidemiological studies, fecundity in WWE is lower than in controls. Several biological factors have been implicated that could be only partly modifiable. However, in the authors' opinion, the problem of infertility in WWE may have been overstated due to outdated laws and social limitations that are hopefully currently being overcome. Furthermore, the ever-increasing use of newer ASMs with a lesser impact on reproduction issues could provide a benefit to WWE.

Several other factors could be addressed to reduce the gap and improve the lives of WWE. First of all, giving correct information to WWE and the public is key in abating stigma and unjustified excessive fear of childbearing. Second, provided that the appropriate ASMs should always be chosen considering the type of epilepsy and that maintaining control of seizures should be the utmost priority, possible adverse neuroendocrine effects should not be overlooked. To do so, a comprehensive anamnesis on menstrual characteristics and sexual life and a search for potential signs of hyperandrogenism are crucial. The partner's involvement and a multidisciplinary approach, including gynecologists, are key for the good care of WWE of fertile age.

Acknowledgments

We thank Stefania Mazzoni for helping with the table and Cecilia Baroncini for editing the English text.

References

1. World Health Organization (WHO). *International classification of diseases, 11th Revision (ICD-11)*. Geneva: World Health Organization; 2018.

2. Vander Borght M, Wyns C . Fertility and infertility: Definition and epidemiology. *Clin Biochem*. 2018;**62**:2–10. https://doi.org/10.1016/j.clinbiochem.2018.03.012.
3. World Health Organization (WHO). *Epilepsy: Social consequences and economic aspects: Fact sheet 166*. Geneva: World Health Organization; 2001.
4. D'Souza C. Epilepsy and discrimination in India. *Neur Asia*. 2004;**9**:53–4.
5. Webber MP, Hauser WA, Ottman R, et al. Fertility in persons with epilepsy: 1935–1974. *Epilepsia*. 1986;**27**(6):746–52.
6. Olafsson E, Hauser WA, Gudmundsson G. Fertility in patients with epilepsy: A population-based study. *Neurology*. 1998;**51**(1):71–3.
7. Wallace H, Shorvon S, Tallis R. Age-specific incidence and prevalence rates of treated epilepsy in an unselected population of 2,052,922 and age-specific fertility rates of women with epilepsy. *Lancet*. 1998;**352**(9145):1970–3.
8. Artama M, Isojärvi JI, Raitanen J, et al. Birth rate among patients with epilepsy: A nationwide population-based cohort study in Finland. *Am J Epidemiol*. 2004;**159**(11):1057–63.
9. Artama M, Isojärvi JI, Auvinen A. Antiepileptic drug use and birth rate in patients with epilepsy: A population-based cohort study in Finland. *Hum Reprod*. 2006;**21**(9):2290–5.
10. Viinikainen K, Heinonen S, Eriksson K, et al. Fertility in women with active epilepsy. *Neurology*. 2007;**69**(22):2107–8.
11. Farmen AH, Grundt JH, Tomson T, et al. Age-specific birth rates in women with epilepsy: A population-based study. *Brain Behav*. 2016;**6**(8):e00492.
12. Jalava M, Sillanpaa M. Reproductive activity and offspring health of young adults with childhood-onset epilepsy: A controlled study. *Epilepsia*. 1997;**38**(5):532–40.
13. Schupf N, Ottman R. Reproduction among individuals with idiopathic/cryptogenic epilepsy: Risk factors for reduced fertility in marriage. *Epilepsia*. 1996;**37**(9):833–40.
14. Dansky LV, Andermann E, Andermann F. Marriage and fertility in epileptic patients. *Epilepsia*. 1980;**21**(3):261–71.
15. Kariuki JG, Joshi MD, Adam AM, et al. Fertility rate of epileptic women at Kenyatta National Hospital. *East Afr Med J*. 2008;**85**(7):341–6.
16. Sukumaran SC, Sarma PS, Thomas SV. Polytherapy increases the risk of infertility in women with epilepsy. *Neurology*. 2010;**75**(15):1351–5.
17. Pennell PB, French JA, Harden CL, et al. Fertility and birth outcomes in women with epilepsy seeking pregnancy. *JAMA Neurol*. 2018;**75**(8):962–9.
18. Starck C, Nevalainen O, Auvinen A, Eriksson K. Fertility and marital status in adults with childhood onset epilepsy: A population-based cohort study.*Epilepsia*. 2019;**60**(7):1438–44.
19. Li S, Chen J, Abdulaziz ATA, et al. Epilepsy in China: Factors influencing marriage status and fertility. *Seizure*. 2019;**71**:179–84.
20. Agarwal P, Mehndiratta MM, Antony AR, et al. Epilepsy in India: Nuptiality behaviour and fertility. *Seizure*. 2006;**15**(6):409–15.
21. Mostacci B, Esposto R, Lello S, et al. Estrogen-related seizure exacerbation following hormone therapy for assisted reproduction in women with epilepsy. *Seizure*. 2018;**61**:200–2.
22. Pal SK, Sharma K, Prabhakar S, et al. Psychosocial, demographic, and treatment- seeking strategic behavior, including faith healing practices, among patients with epilepsy in northwest India. *Epilepsy Behav*. 2008;**13**(2):323–32.
23. Fong CY, Hung A. Public awareness, attitude, and understanding of epilepsy in Hong Kong Special Administrative Region, China. *Epilepsia*. 2002;**43**:311–16.
24. Crawford P, Hudson S. Understanding the information needs of women with

epilepsy at different life stages: Results of the "Ideal World" survey. *Seizure*. 2003;**12**(7):502–7.

25. Morrell MJ, Flynn KL, Done S, et al. Sexual dysfunction, sex steroid hormone abnormalities, and depression in women with epilepsy treated with antiepileptic drugs. *Epilepsy Behav*. 2005;**6**(3):360–5.
26. Herzog AG, Drislane FW, Schomer DL, et al. Differential effects of antiepileptic drugs on sexual function and hormones in men with epilepsy. *Neurology*. 2005;**65**(7):1016–20.
27. Tao L, Duan Z, Liu Y, Hou H, Zhang X. Correlation of sexual dysfunction with sex hormone and estrogen receptor gene polymorphism in Chinese Han women with epilepsy. *Epilepsy Res*. 2021;**169**:106527.
28. Ramesha KN, Radhakrishnan A, Jiayaspathi A, et al. Sexual desire and satisfaction after resective surgery in patients with mesial temporal lobe epilepsy with hippocampal sclerosis. *Epilepsy Behav*. 2012;**25**(3):374–80.
29. Daniele A, Azzoni A, Bizzi A, et al. Sexual behavior and hemispheric laterality of the focus in patients with temporal lobe epilepsy. *Biol Psychiatry*. 1997;**42**:617–24.
30. Morrell MJ, Guldner GT. Self-reported sexual function and sexual arousability in women with epilepsy. *Epilepsia*. 1996;**37**:1204–10.
31. Herzog AG, Coleman AE, Jacobs AR, et al. Relationship of sexual dysfunction to epilepsy laterality and reproductive hormone levels in women. *Epilepsy Behav*. 2003;**4**(4):407–13.
32. Quigg M, Kiely JM, Shneker B, et al. Interictal and postictal alterations of pulsatile secretions of luteinizing hormone in temporal lobe epilepsy in men. *Ann Neurol*. 2002;**51**(5):559–66.
33. Chen DK, So YT, Fisher RS. Use of serum prolactin in diagnosing epileptic seizures: Report of the Therapeutics and Technology Assessment Subcommittee of the American Academy of Neurology. *Neurology*. 2005;**65**(5):668–75.
34. Bauer J, Stoffel-Wagner B, Flugel D, et al. The impact of epilepsy surgery on sex hormones and the menstrual cycle in female patients. *Seizure*. 2000;**9**(6):389–93.
35. Herzog AG. Disorders of reproduction in patients with epilepsy: Primary neurological mechanisms. *Seizure*. 2008;**17**(2):101–10.
36. Bilo L, Meo R, Nappi C, et al. Reproductive endocrine disorders in women with primary generalized epilepsy. *Epilepsia*. 1988.
37. Löfgren E, Mikkonen K, Tolonen U, et al. Reproductive endocrine function in women with epilepsy: The role of epilepsy type and medication. *Epilepsy Behav*. 2007;**10**(1):77–83.
38. Morrell MJ, Giudice L, Flynn KL, et al. Predictors of ovulatory failure in women with epilepsy. *Ann Neurol*. 2002;**52**(6):704–11.
39. Herzog AG, Seibel MM, Schomer DL, et al. Reproductive endocrine disorders in women with partial seizures of temporal lobe origin. *Arch Neurol*. 1986;**43**:341–6.
40. Murialdo G, Galimberti CA, Magri F, et al. Menstrual cycle and ovary alterations in women with epilepsy on antiepileptic therapy. *J Endocrinol Invest*. 1997;**20**(9):519–26.
41. Drislane FW, Coleman AE, Schomer DL, et al. Altered pulsatile secretion of luteinizing hormone in women with epilepsy. *Neurology*. 1994;**44**(2):306–10.
42. Kalinin VV, Zheleznova EV, Chronology and evolution of temporal lobe epilepsy and endocrine reproductive dysfunction in women: Relationships to side of focus and catameniality. *Epilepsy Behav*. 2007;**11**:185–91.
43. Quigg M, Smithson SD, Fowler KM, et al. Laterality and location influence catamenial seizure expression in women with partial epilepsy. *Neurology*. 2009;**73**(3):223–7.
44. Herzog AG. A relationship between particular reproductive endocrine disorders and the laterality of epileptiform

discharges in women with epilepsy. *Neurology*. 1993;**43**(10):1907–10.

45. Herzog AG, Coleman AE, Jacobs AR, et al. Interictal EEG discharges, reproductive hormones, and menstrual disorders in epilepsy. *Ann Neurol*. 2003; **54**(5):625–37.
46. Christian CA, Reddy DS, Maguire J, Forcelli PA. Sex differences in the epilepsies and associated comorbidities: Implications for use and development of pharmacotherapies. *Pharmacol Rev*. 2020;**72**(4):767–800.
47. Harden CL. Polycystic ovaries and polycystic ovary syndrome in epilepsy: Evidence for neurogonadal disease. *Epilepsy Curr*. 2005;**5**(4):142–6.
48. Isojärvi JI, Laatikainen TJ, Pakarinen AJ, et al. Polycystic ovaries and hyperandrogenism in women taking valproate for epilepsy. *N Engl J Med*. 1993;**329**(19):1383–8.
49. Isojärvi JI, Löfgren E, Juntunen KS, et al. Effect of epilepsy and antiepileptic drugs on male reproductive health. *Neurology*. 2004;**62**(2):247–53.
50. Isojärvi J. Disorders of reproduction in patients with epilepsy: Antiepileptic drug related mechanisms. *Seizure*. 2008;**17**(2):111–19.
51. Collins WC, Lanigan O, Callaghan N. Plasma prolactin concentrations following epileptic and pseudoseizures. *J Neurol Neurosurg Psychiatry*. 1983;**46**(6):505–8.
52. Klein P, Serje A, Pezzullo JC. Premature ovarian failure in women with epilepsy. *Epilepsia*. 2001;**42**(12):1584–9.
53. Harden CL, Koppel BS, Herzog AG, et al. Seizure frequency is associated with age at menopause in women with epilepsy. *Neurology*. 2003;**61**:451.
54. Gold EB, Bromberger J, Crawford S, et al. Factors associated with age at natural menopause in a multiethnic sample of midlife women. *Am J Epidemiol*. 2001;**153**:865.
55. Herzog AG. Menstrual disorders in women with epilepsy. *Neurology*. 2006;**66**(6 Suppl 3): S23–8.
56. Fabris RR, Cascino TG, Mandrekar J, et al. Drug-resistant focal epilepsy in women of childbearing age: Reproduction and the effect of epilepsy surgery. *Epilepsy Behav*. 2016;**60**:17–20.
57. Baird AD, Wilson SJ, Baldin PF, et al. Sexual outcome after epilepsy surgery. *Epilepsy Behav*. 2003;**4**:268–78.
58. Baird AD, Wilson SJ, Bladin PF, et al. The amygdale and sexual drive: Insights from temporal lobe epilepsy surgery. *Ann Neurol*. 2005;**55**:87–96.
59. Isojärvi JI, Rattya J, Myllylä VV, et al. Valproate, lamotrigine, and insulin-mediated risks in women with epilepsy. *Ann Neurol*. 1998;**43**(4):446–51.
60. Isojärvi JI, Laatikainen TJ, Pakarinen AJ, Juntunen KT, Myllylä VV. Menstrual disorders in women with epilepsy receiving carbamazepine. *Epilepsia*. 1995;**36**(7):676–81.
61. Svalheim S, Taubøll E, Luef G, et al. Differential effects of levetiracetam, carbamazepine, and lamotrigine on reproductive endocrine function in adults. *Epilepsy Behav*. **16**(2):281–7.
62. Larsen MD, Jølving LR, Fedder J, Nørgård BM. The efficacy of assisted reproductive treatment in women with epilepsy. *Reprod Biomed Online*. 2020;**41**(6):1015–22.
63. Mostacci B, Esposto R, Lello S, et al. Estrogen-related seizure exacerbation following hormone therapy for assisted reproduction in women with epilepsy. *Seizure*. 2018;**61**:200–2.

Chapter 10

Contraception and Prepregnancy Counseling

Naveed Chaudhry and Emily Johnson

Key Points

- Enzyme-inducing antiseizure medications (EI-ASMs) such as phenytoin, carbamazepine, oxcarbazepine, and phenobarbital may decrease contraceptive efficacy.
- The intrauterine device (IUD) is a first-line contraceptive choice for all women with epilepsy (WWE).
- Hormonal contraception with estrogenic components induces the metabolism of lamotrigine.
- Preconception counseling should be started early and revisited frequently for WWE of childbearing age.
- The majority of WWE are likely to have a safe pregnancy and a healthy newborn.
- Prepartum optimization of ASMs ideally should be done 9–12 months before a planned pregnancy.

Introduction

While several consensus opinions have agreed upon the importance of preconception counseling for women with epilepsy (WWE) [42–44], there are no evidence-based guidelines on how to effectively counsel patients [42]. This chapter will present an approach to counseling WWE of reproductive age and summarize the information required to effectively counsel most patients. Some of the essential components to effective counseling in this unique population are listed next, using the SAFER approach:

Start early. Preconception counseling should start as early as possible, often at a woman's first visit. It is important to note that teen pregnancies also can occur among WWE. Deferring counseling until a woman knows she wants to become pregnant is unrealistic as 50% of pregnancies in WWE are not planned [38, 45], a rate similar to that of the general population [46]. In addition, most useful interventions take more than 1 year to implement.

Ask and listen. The preconception discussion should be tailored to the patient's personal goals, concerns, and risks. A prior history of irregular menses or miscarriages, or a family history of fetal malformations may affect an individual's risk for complications and certainly her anxiety about pregnancy. It is also important to understand the patient's sexual history as well as her personal goals and timeline. In most circumstances, counseling should be an interactive encounter between the patient and her physicians. There is tremendous individual variability in the concerns that patients find most important to their reproductive decisions.

Facts can reassure. Among WWE, 23–33% report that they would likely refrain from having children on account of their epilepsy [40, 47]. Many WWE are under the impression that it is unwise or irresponsible for them to become pregnant because of their seizures or medications. For many patients, advice about the pregnancy and ASM-related risks may be frightening. Reassuringly, more than 94% of pregnancies exposed to ASMs and maternal epilepsy are *not* complicated by major congenital malformations. Exposure to ASMs is almost never an indication to terminate a pregnancy. It is important to emphasize that the risks related to ASMs and seizures during pregnancy can be reduced in many circumstances by careful and early planning.

Expert referral. The responsibility of preconception counseling for WWE should be shared among all her physicians, including her neurologist, gynecologist, and internist. In practice, however, the principal responsibility usually falls on the neurologist who is prescribing the antiepileptic drug. In most cases, it is appropriate for a neurologist to refer a patient for an early subspecialty opinion regarding preconception counseling for WWE.

Repeat. Thorough and comprehensive reproductive health counseling frequently need to be reinforced. In one survey of British WWE, Fairgrieve and colleagues reviewed the medical charts of women who did not recall receiving preconception counseling [38]. The medical records indicated that in 32% of these cases, the patient's physician had documented that counseling had occurred. This indicates that even when physicians attempt to counsel their patients, the initial message does not always get through.

Selecting Contraception for Women with Epilepsy

Effective and safe contraceptive options are important for all women, but are arguably even more essential and more complicated for WWE. Avoiding unplanned pregnancies is a key cornerstone to improving outcomes for children born to WWE. Using an ASM with a favorable risk profile for structural and neurodevelopmental teratogenicity, at the lowest effective dose for that patient, and the use of periconceptional supplemental folic acid can help optimize pregnancy outcomes [1–3]. When a pregnancy is unplanned, WWE can miss the opportunity to benefit from these modifiable aspects of care.

The average woman will require some form of contraception for about three decades during her childbearing years. In the United States, of the 43 million fertile and sexually active women not seeking pregnancy, 89% use contraception [4]. Nationally representative surveys show that 63% of those who use contraception rely on reversible methods, most often the oral contraceptive pill and male condom, whereas 37% rely on the permanent methods of tubal sterilization or vasectomy [4]. Notably, use of long-acting reversible methods in the United States (intrauterine device [IUD] or implant) increased to 11.6% by 2012, but remains uncommon compared to European countries, where sterilization is much less common and use of the IUD is widespread [5].

Contraceptive Use in Women with Epilepsy

Data from existing, large contraception surveys cannot be used to estimate contraception use among WWE because such surveys do not collect information on coexistent chronic illness. Data from small samples of women suggest contraception remains a challenge for WWE, despite published guidelines [6]. Cross-sectional data from the Epilepsy Birth Control Registry (EBCR) demonstrated that the most common contraception in WWE was systemic hormonal contraception (46.6%), followed by barrier methods (23.2%) and the IUD (17.0%) [7].

Another study at an urban medical center queried 145 WWE regarding current sexual activity and contraception use [8]. Only 53% of those at risk of unplanned pregnancy used the more effective methods (those with typical pregnancy rates of <10% in the first year of use), most often sterilization or oral contraceptives. The rest relied on condoms, spermicide, natural family planning (timed intercourse), or withdrawal, alone or in combination. These methods have typical failure rates of 10–20% per year. Not surprisingly, half of their 181 pregnancies were unplanned. Women with epilepsy of lower socioeconomic status and Hispanic WWE were more vulnerable; they experienced more unplanned pregnancies than did Caucasian women of higher socioeconomic status. This disparity mirrors the US population overall.

Healthy women face barriers to access effective contraception, including prohibitive cost and misperceptions regarding efficacy and safety. Women with epilepsy face another barrier: many physicians responsible for contraceptive counseling are often not adequately knowledgeable about this complicated topic. Surveys of US physicians highlight this gap in treating physicians' knowledge. A 1996 survey queried US obstetricians and neurologists about interactions between oral contraceptives (OCs) and ASMS [9]. They were asked if they knew the interactions between OCs and the six ASMs most commonly used at that time (phenytoin, carbamazepine, valproic acid, phenobarbital, primidone, and ethosuximide). The average percentage correct for the neurologists' knowledge of OC interactions was 61 ± 2.2%, and for obstetricians' knowledge it was 37.8 ± 1.9%. Only 4% of the neurologists and none of the obstetricians answered correctly for all six ASMs.

Another survey, of attendees at the American College of Physicians 2003 annual meeting, showed that most knew EI-ASMs reduce the efficacy of OCs (71%) and women do not need to discontinue all ASMs during pregnancy (75%). However, less than half (47%) of participants knew that women taking ASMs could breastfeed safely [10]. Like many of their healthcare providers, WWE experience confusion about ASMs and contraception. In their questionnaire study of WWE, Pack and Davis found that among 66 women currently using EI-ASMs, 65% did not know whether their ASM changed the effectiveness of OCs [11].

Contraception Methods

For WWE and for women in general, efficacy and safety are primary considerations when selecting a contraceptive method. Pregnancy rates are less than 1% per year for highly effective methods, and these should be considered first line or top tier (Table 10.1). Highly effective methods include permanent contraception via tubal ligation or vasectomy, and long-acting reversible contraceptive (LARC) methods of IUD and the single-rod, 3-year contraceptive implant. Short-term hormonal methods such as OCs remain a good option for many WWE, although unplanned pregnancy is more likely compared to LARCs [12].

Long-Acting Reversible Contraception

Intrauterine Device – The intrauterine device (IUD) is recommended as a contraceptive of choice for all WWE [89]. The progestin (levonorgestrel [LNG])-releasing and the copper T 380A IUDs are widely used around the world. The LNG IUD is approved for 3–6 years of use by the US Food and Drug Administration (FDA); the nonhormonal copper device for 10 years. Both IUDs primarily prevent pregnancy by pre-fertilization mechanisms of interference with sperm transport and function. The IUD is an appropriate choice for women and adolescents who have never been pregnant, as well as for women who have children [13, 14].

Table 10.1 Contraceptives available in the United States

Method	Efficacy*	Reversibility	Menstrual bleeding	Duration of use	Ovulation inhibition
Oral contraceptive pill	88–94%	Immediate	Decreased, regular	Daily	Yes
Transdermal patch	88–94%	Immediate	Decreased, regular	Weekly	Yes
Vaginal ring	88–94%	Immediate	Decreased, regular	Monthly	Yes
Depotmedroxyprogesterone acetate (DMPA)	88–94%	Delayed†	Initially irregular, amenorrhea likely with continuation	Every 3 Months	Yes
Subdermal implant	>99%	Immediate	Decreased, irregular	3 years	Yes
Levonorgestrel IUD	>99%	Immediate	Decreased, initially irregular	5 years	Sometimes
Copper IUD	>99%	Immediate	Sometimes increased, regular	10 years	No

* With typical use, per year, assuming no drug interaction present
† Median return to ovulation more than 6 months from time of last injection

Recent data clearly demonstrate excellent safety and efficacy for nulliparous women [12, 15]. Intrauterine devices are safe with very low rates of complications such as infertility or pelvic inflammatory disease (PID). The risk of PID is highest in the first 20 days after an IUD is inserted, but the overall risk of PID is small at 0–2% [16, 17]. Both IUDs are completely reversible; fertility quickly and completely returns after removal. The IUDs also have the benefit of decreased or lighter menstrual bleeding for many women. A recent study showed that LNG concentrations remain stable in WWE, even in those who are taking EI-ASMs [18], providing evidence that these devices are reliable and recommended as first-line contraception for WWE desiring long-term, reversible birth control.

Drawbacks include temporary pain during IUD insertion and expulsion. Pain and discomfort can be common during IUD insertion, observed in more than 70% of women, though this quickly resolves for most [19]. Expulsion of the IUD is possible, with rates around 2–10%, higher in younger (ages 14–19) women [20].

Intramuscular Injection – Intramuscular depot medroxyprogesterone acetate (DMPA) is also a highly effective method, with a failure rate comparable to the IUD or implant. Unlike those methods, however, the high efficacy of DMPA depends on reinjection every 3 months. Like the contraceptive implant, DMPA reliably inhibits ovulation. Bleeding with DMPA is irregular, but decreases greatly over time. After 1 year, 75% of users experience amenorrhea. Unlike the IUD and all other hormonal methods, DMPA is not immediately reversible. Return to full fertility may be delayed up to 18 months. Overall, intramuscular DMPA is relatively safe; like other progestin-only methods, DMPA does not increase the risk of thrombosis. However, DMPA does cause modest decreases in bone mineral density. In healthy women receiving DMPA, these bone mineral density changes are reversible and do not appear to increase the risk of fracture in the short or long term [22]; therefore, no routine bone density screening is recommended. Since some ASMs may also decrease bone density as discussed in Chapter 19, use of DMPA with these ASMs should be individualized after weighing the risks and benefits, and patients screened for bone density loss when appropriate.

Implant – The contraceptive implant is a 3 cm soft, flexible rod placed subdermally in the upper arm. The device continuously elutes the contraceptive progestin etonogestrel, and is approved for 3 years of use. Neither the IUD nor the implant contain estrogenic components and therefore do not increase the risk of thrombosis. However, studies have shown low serum etonogestrel in WWE on EI-ASMs at levels below those necessary to suppress ovulation, making this a less suitable option for WWE due to potential for contraceptive failure [21].

Oral Contraceptives

Many OCs are available. Combined oral contraceptives (COCs) contain an estrogen (usually ethinyl estradiol) and a synthetic progestin, which differs from natural progesterone. Early progestins include norethindrone and levonorgestrel, whereas newer progestins include desogestrel, norgestimate, and drospirenone. The majority of available OCs contain ethinyl estradiol (EE) or estradiol valerate as the estrogenic component. When choosing a pill for a WWE treated with a strong inducer, a pill with the highest doses should be selected. A formulation with 50 micrograms of EE and relatively high doses of progestin is best [5, 6]; however, these pills are not widely available. While practical and often suggested in the clinical literature, this strategy is unsupported by data proving efficacy. Any woman treated with a strong inducer using a lower-dose OC should use another method such as condoms as well.

The progestin-only pill (POP) formulation available in the United States is a very low-dose pill; it is taken continuously and does not reliably inhibit ovulation. Its primary mechanism is thickening of cervical mucous. Additionally, it is difficult to use, as it must be taken at exactly the same time of day every day, since the progestin dose is low and has a short half-life. Progestin-only pills in those using mild EI-ASMs, lamotrigine in particular, may induce norethindrone metabolism to a degree that allows for ovulation. Prescription of the progestin-only pill in the United States is generally limited to women who are breast-feeding or have other contraindications to the use of EE. Higher-dose progestin-only OCs are available in other parts of the world.

Other Combination Methods – In addition to COCs, which are taken daily, other combined methods include a transdermal patch and a vaginal ring. These are administered weekly and for 4 weeks, respectively. These methods inhibit ovulation and have the noncontraceptive benefit of regular and decreased menstrual bleeding. Oral contraceptive use improves acne and prevents ovarian cysts and, if sustained, greatly decreases the risk of ovarian and uterine cancer. The estrogenic component of combined methods is associated with an increased risk for thrombosis; however, the absolute risk of venous thrombosis for a healthy woman using these methods is very low, about 1 in 1,000 users. Women with risk factors for thrombosis, stroke, or myocardial infarction should not use combined hormonal contraception, including migraine with aura and even migraine without aura if the woman is more than 35 years old. For smokers over age 35, hormonal contraception use is contraindicated because of an increased risk of myocardial infarction and stroke [23]. Similar to COCs, EI-ASMs may lower the effective hormonal levels, and these methods should not be used as the primary method of birth control in WWE on EI-ASMs [21, 25].

Traditional OC formulations as well as the patch and ring are used for 3 weeks then stopped for 1 week to allow for a menstrual withdrawal bleed. Some OC formulations shorten the time off (pill-free interval) to 4 days monthly or 1 week every 3 months, or eliminate the pill-free interval completely. Some of these methods result in very short, infrequent menses or induce complete amenorrhea. This is safe for women; the amenorrhea is due to reversible endometrial thinning and does not impact fertility after discontinuation. Breakthrough bleeding may occur with these extended regimens. Studies of continuous OC use show excellent safety and return to fertility.

Dual-Method Contraception – The term *dual-method use* usually refers to a male barrier method combined with some other method. Most often in healthy women, this strategy is recommended for pregnancy prevention and sexually transmitted infection (STI) prevention, especially for adolescents. In the context of WWE, the usual STI prevention recommendations would apply for those at risk, but condoms could also be recommended as a back-up method to reduce the risk of pregnancy in the context of a drug interaction. If STI prevention is not a concern, dual-method use is not a first-choice strategy for contraception because adherence becomes more complex. Dual-method use would be recommended for strong inducer ASMs coadministered with OCs, ring, patch, or implant. Dual method use would not improve efficacy in a clinically meaningful way for either IUD or DMPA.

Bidirectional Interactions of Hormonal Contraceptives and Antiseizure Medications

Effects of Antiepileptic Drugs on Reproductive Hormones

Oral contraceptives were the first effective reversible method of contraception and became available in the 1960s. Shortly after their introduction, clinicians caring for WWE observed pregnancies during coadministration of certain ASMs, despite the high doses of contraceptive steroids in these early formulations [24]. Since those early observations, ASMs have been systematically studied for how they impact the pharmacokinetic properties of EE and various contraceptive ingredients and grouped as enzyme-inducing or non-enzyme-inducing ASMs. Unfortunately, these groupings based on pharmacokinetic changes do not clearly and directly relate to the risk of ovulation or pregnancy.

Antiepileptic drugs may impact contraceptive pharmacokinetics by several mechanisms. Some induce the hepatic cytochrome P450 system, specifically CYP3A4, the primary metabolic pathway of EE and progestins. Some ASMs also enhance glucuronidation, another hepatic elimination pathway for these sex steroid hormones. More rapid clearance of the sex steroid hormones may allow ovulation in women using hormonal contraceptive agents [25]. In general, ASMs that induce hepatic metabolic enzymes are labeled EI-ASMs and directly alter reproductive hormone levels (Table 10.2). These ASMs also induce production of sex hormone-binding globulin (SHBG), thereby reducing biologically active (free) reproductive hormone serum levels [26].

Hormonal contraceptives work by inhibiting ovulation and changes in cervical mucous. Ovulation inhibition depends largely on the contraceptive progestin, via inhibition of luteinizing hormone (LH) production. This is a threshold effect. If the progestin component remains above the level at which ovulation is inhibited, the contraceptive effect should be preserved even if enzyme induction occurs. Prescribers of hormonal contraception for WWE should be aware that efficacy also depends on adherence. Missed pills or late patches or rings decrease contraceptive effectiveness. These adherence problems are very common in typical users of short-acting hormonal contraception.

Table 10.2 Antiepileptic drugs: Degree of induction of metabolism of hormonal contraceptive agents

Strong inducers*	Weak inducers	Non-inducers
Phenobarbital	Topiramate †	Ethosuximide
Phenytoin	Lamotrigine	Valproate**
Carbamazepine	Felbamate	Gabapentin
Primidone	Rufinamide	Clonazepam
Oxcarbazepine	Perampanel †	Levetiracetam
Clobazam	Eslicarbazepine	Zonisamide
Cenobamate		Pregabalin
		Lacosamide
		Briviracetam

* Avoid concomitant use with the lowest-dose oral contraceptive pills
** Enzyme inhibitor
† At higher doses, are typically strong inducers

Recommendations

Many authors have recommended "high-dose" OCs (50 μg EE) with EI-ASMs, assuming enzyme induction will lower levels to what occurs with an effective lower-dose OC [6]. A few OCs with higher doses of EE and progestin remain available but are infrequently used in practice for healthy women. While reasonable in the context of EI-ASMs, no direct evidence supports efficacy in this situation. The CDC Medical Eligibility Criteria for contraception classifies certain ASMs (PHT, CBZ, PB, PMD, TPM, and OXC) as category 3: the risks generally outweigh the benefits. In this category, the risk refers to birth control failure. The authors clarify that although the interaction of certain ASMs with COCs, POP, or the vaginal ring is not harmful to women, it is likely to reduce the effectiveness. The authors further state that if a COC is chosen, a preparation containing a minimum of 30 μg EE should be used [23].

Oral contraceptives, as well as patches, rings, and the implant, are not first-line contraceptive methods for WWE who use EI-ASMs known to cause substantial changes in progestin levels (Table 10.2). For these women, the copper or LNG IUDs are excellent choices. One caution with the copper IUD is that some radiology departments are not willing to perform a 3 Tesla (or higher) brain MRI on women with a copper IUD in place, potentially compromising the evaluation of WWE. The LNG IUD prevents pregnancy by local hormonally mediated changes in cervical mucous, which are not likely to be impacted by hepatic changes in P450 enzyme induction. One reassuring prospective registry study in the United Kingdom demonstrated a pregnancy rate of 1.1 per 100 women-years for 56 women using the LNG IUD with EI-ASMs, a rate slightly higher than expected but still very low compared to other contraceptive methods available [27]. Another choice with EI-ASMs is DMPA. No direct evidence examines how DMPA metabolism is impacted by EI-ASMs; however, the dose of DMPA even at 12 weeks significantly exceeds the level needed for ovulation inhibition. Use of DMPA must be considered in light of the side effects discussed in this chapter.

Effects of Hormonal Contraceptives on Antiseizure Medications

Estradiol-containing contraceptives induce the metabolism of lamotrigine (LTG). One study in WWE on LTG enrolled 22 COC users and 39 nonusers. The LTG clearance (LTG dose/body weight/plasma concentration) was more than twofold higher in the COC group than in the nonuser group [28]. A study investigating the mechanism of the enhanced clearance measured the main metabolite, lamotrigine-2-N-glucuronide, in WWE taking COC ($n = 31$), in WWE with the LNG IUD ($n = 12$), and in WWE on no contraceptive ($n = 20$) [29]. Compared to controls, the LTG dose/concentration ratio was 56% higher in the COC group, and the N-2-glucuronide/LTG ratio was 82% higher ($p < 0.01$ in both). There were no differences between the control and IUD groups. Findings indicate that the enhanced metabolism of LTG is primarily by induction of the N-2-glucuronide pathway. A small study of 7 women also reported lower plasma concentrations with COC use, but added information about the time course; baseline LTG levels were reached at an average of 8.0 (s. d. 3.69) days after the start of COCs. Two of the 7 women experienced seizure worsening that correlated with reduced LTG concentrations [30, 31].

The CDC Medical Eligibility Criteria specifically labels LTG monotherapy as category 3 (the risks generally outweigh the benefits) for use with COCs, given that pharmacokinetic studies have shown not only decreased LTG levels but also associated increased seizures [23]. However, adjusting the LTG dose after initiation of estrogen can mitigate these effects.

Valproate (VPA) and oxcarbazepine (OXC) also undergo hepatic glucuronidation as a major elimination pathway. Similar pharmacokinetic interaction principles likely apply with estrogens, decreasing ASM concentrations, although surprisingly, this is not reported with OXC in the literature. Enhanced clearance of OXC during pregnancy is reported, however. A later study investigated the effects of OCs on VPA as well as LTG serum concentrations [37–41]. The researchers enrolled four groups of WWE, with 12 women in each group: VPA, VPA plus OC, LTG, and LTG plus COC. The VPA concentrations were lower in the VPA-plus-COC group than in the VPA-only group, with a median decrease of 23.4%. The LTG concentrations were 32.6% lower in the LTG-plus-COC group compared to the LTG-only group.

Potential of Contraceptives as a Therapeutic Tool for Seizure Control

Catamenial epilepsy is the term used for the pattern of seizure worsening associated with different menstrual phases (see Chapter 8). Some WWE tend to have seizure worsening during certain phases of their menstrual cycles: in the perimenstrual, periovulatory, or the second half of the anovulatory cycles. Approximately one-third of reproductive-aged women with focal epilepsy and on no exogenous hormones will meet criteria for at least one catamenial pattern [32]. Animal models and a few human studies suggest that the enhanced seizure susceptibility is related to premenstrual withdrawal of the anticonvulsant effects of progesterone and its neurosteroid metabolite, allopregnanolone, the sudden estrogen peak in the day prior to ovulation, and increased frequency of anovulatory cycles and consequent low progesterone luteal phases [33].

Hormonal contraceptives could potentially be used as a therapeutic tool in women with a catamenial pattern to their epilepsy by providing continuous levels of sex steroid hormones, as opposed to variable levels of estrogen peaks and progesterone withdrawal, or unopposed estrogen during the second phase of an anovulatory cycle. However, synthetic progestins are not metabolized to allopregnanolone, and therefore, there is no binding to the GABA-A-benzodiazepine receptor at the neurosteroid site and likely no direct benefit. There is no evidence from randomized controlled trials that hormonal contraceptives worsen seizure control in WWE, although some women report a worsening in seizures when starting hormonal contraception [34, 35].

Depot medroxyprogesterone acetate is a synthetic progestin that completely inhibits ovulation, which may be beneficial when seizures worsen with peaks of estrogen or progesterone withdrawal in spontaneous cycles. Two small studies investigated the use of medroxyprogesterone acetate (MPA) for "intractable" epilepsy (n = 14 and n = 19) [36]. Participants received both oral and intramuscular MPA in variable doses at variable intervals. Seizure frequency was significantly reduced in both cohorts, with average reductions of 30% and 39%. A more rigorous controlled study is needed to investigate whether intramuscular DMPA affects seizure control. Additionally, after cessation of use, the transition period with erratic endogenous hormone cycling could theoretically cause seizure worsening as well as prolonged return to normal fertility.

As with the contraceptive implant and DMPA, OC formulations at effective doses cause continuous suppression of ovulation and may theoretically benefit WWE sensitive to endogenous fluctuations. Some clinicians may preferentially prescribe continuous OC in women with catamenial epilepsy or women on LTG to provide non-fluctuating hormone levels. However, no published study has yet investigated the use of any OC regimen for seizure control in WWE.

Cyclic administration of progesterone lozenges during the second half of the menstrual cycle has been studied in a multicenter, double-blind, placebo-controlled, randomized trial, but THE results found that adjunctive progesterone was effective only for women with a strong catamenial pattern of seizure worsening during the perimenstrual phase [37]. However, this is not a form of contraception, and its administration can be especially difficult given that the women cannot be on a hormonal contraceptive and need to maintain their natural menstrual cycles.

Preconception Counseling for Women with Epilepsy

Transitioning from contraception to preconception planning provides a valuable window of opportunity for the clinician. Not only does it allow the clinician to reassess the type of ASM(s) prescribed and reinforce supplemental folic acid and prenatal vitamins, but it also provides an opportunity to reassess the dose prescribed. This is especially important for ASMs such as LTG that undergo glucuronidation as a major metabolic pathway of elimination.

When helping WWE prepare for pregnancy, the clinician should try to establish the lowest effective dose of the safest ASM(s) appropriate for the woman's epilepsy type and severity. The clinician cannot wait until a patient is pregnant to determine the optimal lowest dose for the individual patient. Nor should they wait until the decision to become pregnant. It is critical that WWE receive regular counseling about pregnancy and contraception from their physicians. Both seizures and ASMs pose risks to a pregnancy, which must be carefully discussed with WWE. Additionally, the epilepsy and ASM-related risks can be significantly reduced by early and careful planning. Unfortunately, patient surveys demonstrate that less than half of WWE recall being counseled on teratogenic effects of ASMs or the need to plan pregnancy [38, 39], and many are misinformed [40]. Most patients feel that when the topic is discussed, it is more likely to be raised by the patient herself rather than her physician [41]. Without effective counseling, women are liable to either over- or underestimate the risks to a potential pregnancy.

Preconception counseling is not limited to a discussion of pregnancy. It should include all elements of family planning, such as fertility, contraception, prepartum screening, breastfeeding, and social support (Table 10.3). The length of a typical doctor's visit does not allow for a comprehensive review of all these topics, which makes it all the more important that a physician introduce reproductive health early in the patient–physician relationship and revisit the topic regularly.

Common Questions Encountered

This chapter will provide an overview of most of the topics essential to an effective preconception visit. Since fertility, contraception, and obstetrical concerns are reviewed elsewhere, this chapter will focus on other essential components of counseling for WWE of childbearing age. This will provide the information to answer the most common questions regarding pregnancy and epilepsy, including: “Will my child have epilepsy?” “Will my medications or seizures hurt my baby?” “What will happen to my seizures during pregnancy?”

Table 10.3 Essential elements of preconception counseling for women with epilepsy

- Contraceptive options and interactions with antiepileptic medications
- Fertility
- Risk of epilepsy in the child
- Risks of antiepileptic medications in pregnancy
- Folic acid supplementation/prenatal vitamins
- Risks of seizures during pregnancy
- Importance of monitoring drug levels
- Risk of obstetrical complications
- Breastfeeding
- Importance of avoiding sleep deprivation
- Seizure safety and importance of social support in taking care of an infant
- Postpartum depression

Heritability of Epilepsy

While genetic susceptibility clearly plays a role in most epilepsies, only a few have identifiable genes that can be tested, and even fewer have complete or predictable penetrance. A detailed history of the patient's personal and family epilepsy history is critical to assessing a patient's risk of passing epilepsy to her children. An open discussion about these risks is important as a patient's perception of the risk of passing on epilepsy seems to strongly influence her decision to have children [48].

In general, the risk of a parent with epilepsy having a child with epilepsy is approximately 2.4–4.6% [49]. When compared to the lifetime incidence in the general population of 1–3%, epilepsy in one parent increases the risk approximately twofold. Some studies suggest mothers with epilepsy are more likely than fathers to pass on epilepsy, with an absolute risk of 2.8–8.7% in children born to WWE. Risk may be on the higher end of this spectrum for parents in whom epilepsy began before age 20, while it is exceedingly rare for parents whose epilepsy presents after age 35 to have affected children.

A population-based study in Rochester, Minnesota, looked at 660 patients with epilepsy and their 2,439 first-degree relatives to assess the incidence of epilepsy. Among relatives of all patients, risk was increased 3.3 times, to the greatest extent in relatives of patients with idiopathic generalized epilepsies (IGE) and epilepsies associated with intellectual or motor disability. In relatives of patients with IGE, standardized incidence ratios were 8.3 for IGE and 2.5 for focal epilepsy. In relatives of patients with focal epilepsy, standardized incidence ratios were 1.0 for IGE and 2.6 for focal epilepsy [50]. A more detailed discussion regarding the heritability of specific epilepsy syndromes can be found in Chapter 6.

Risk of Antiepileptic Drugs in Pregnancy

Antiepileptic Drugs and Major Congenital Malformations – Prepartum counseling for WWE has changed significantly in the past decade because of data from several international antiepileptic drug pregnancy registries. It is important that patients are provided with a basic understanding of how registry data are acquired and what they mean in order to correctly interpret the risks presented and apply them to their own situation appropriately. The explanation may be tailored to the needs of the individual patient, though every patient should be encouraged to enroll in the appropriate registry.

There are no placebo-controlled studies of ASMs in pregnancy. Pregnancy registries are predominantly prospective, observational studies that enroll WWE early in their pregnancies. The primary endpoint of most registries is risk of major congenital malformations (MCMs) associated with each antiepileptic drug. The patient being counseled should understand that MCMs are defined as structural malformations of development that have functional or cosmetic significance and typically require surgical repair. They range from neural tube defects to hypospadias. Other MCMs associated with ASMs include heart defects and cleft lip/palate. The MCMs typically occur during development before the 8–10th weeks of pregnancy, underscoring the necessity of early preconception counseling and planning. There is an increased risk of MCMs in WWE, which seems to be a consequence of the medication(s) and not epilepsy itself [51].

The baseline risk of MCMs among the general population is 1.5–3%, but varies by country and study. In general, the risk associated with any ASM therapy in pregnancy has been reported to be approximately 4–5% [52]. When possible, this information should be tailored to the patient, addressing her personal risk factors and the medication she is taking. When discussing MCM risk for a given ASM, it is reasonable to summarize the absolute risk data from multiple registries, which have for the most part been congruent (see Chapter 11). However, it is important to recognize the strength of the data for each ASM; clearly 0% risk of MCMs among 50 pregnancies is much less informative than a 3–6% risk among 5,000 enrolled pregnancies (see Figure 10.1).

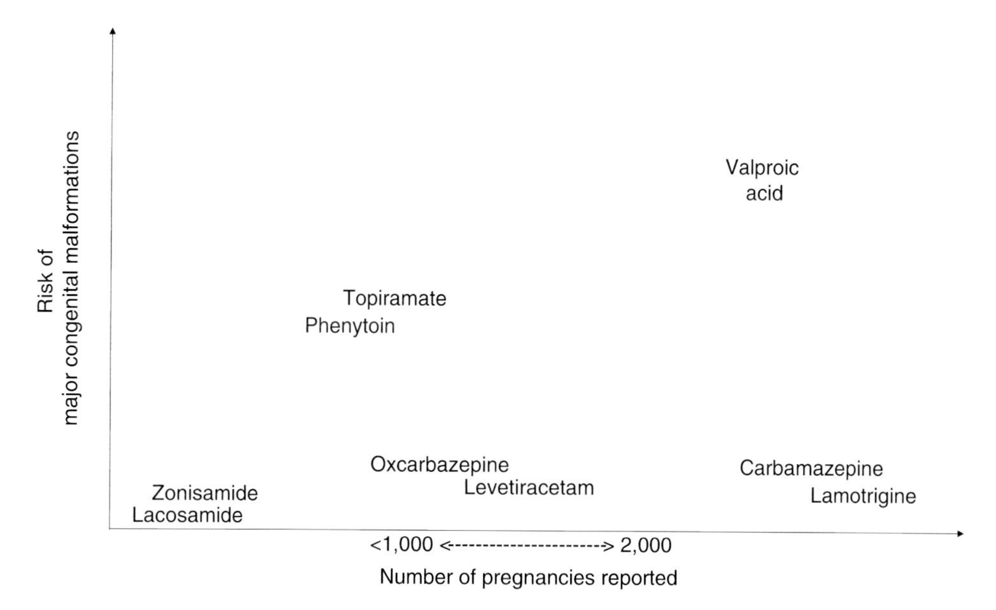

Figure 10.1 Reported risk of major congenital malformations with exposure to individual antiseizure medications in monotherapy versus number of pregnancies reported

The most consistent finding across all antiepileptic drug registries is that VPA significantly increases the risk of MCMs. The absolute risk of MCMs with VPA monotherapy has been reported to range from 6.2% to 14.8% in six registries and over 2,500 pregnancies [52–56]. Drugs with a favorable risk profile include carbamazepine and LTG, both of which have more than 5,000 pregnancies reported. Rates of congenital malformations for these drugs are 2.2–5.9% for carbamazepine and 1.9–4.9% for LTG [52–56]. Data on levetiracetam are also reassuring; the largest study of levetiracetam monotherapy included over 1,200 pregnancies with a malformation rate of 1.8% [53].

Data for both topiramate and phenobarbital suggest that they should be used with caution in women of childbearing age. Phenobarbital has been specifically associated with a risk of congenital heart malformations [57] and the US FDA has recently listed topiramate as a category D drug due to a significant 20-fold increase in the risk of cleft lip and/or palate [58]. A more detailed review on this topic can be found in Chapter 11.

Major Congenital Malformations: Effect of Antiseizure Medication Dose – It has been known for some time that the adverse effects of VPA are clearly dose-related, with a greater risk of malformations at doses of more than 700–1,000 mg a day [53, 55]. A similar dose-related effect has been shown in some, but not all, studies of LTG [50, 53]. A recent publication by the European International Antiepileptic Drug and Pregnancy Registry (EURAP) assessed the rates of MCMs in close to 5,000 pregnancies with monotherapy exposures to carbamazepine, LTG, VPA, or phenobarbital. The authors found that for each of these ASMs, higher doses at the time of conception were associated with a higher rate of MCMs [54]. Additional studies will need to look at the association between MCM and ASM levels, which can vary greatly by individual and may be more likely to influence the effect of the drug on the fetus. A more detailed review on this topic can be found in Chapter 11.

Antiepileptic Drugs and Cognitive Outcomes – Data on the effects of antiepileptic drugs on cognition have been conflicting, which may be due in large part to differences in study design and incomplete control of important variables [57]. Studies of WWE not taking antiepileptic drugs have not shown any significant decrease in the cognitive abilities of their children, suggesting that epilepsy itself does not complicate cognitive development (though this is somewhat confounded by the presumably milder epilepsy syndromes in these patients). On the other hand, several studies have suggested that ASMs can adversely affect developmental outcomes [1]. Despite discrepancies between studies, most have consistently demonstrated an adverse effect of VPA on cognitive development, and some studies have implicated it in behavioral abnormalities and autism spectrum disorder [1, 57–60].

The Neurodevelopmental Effects of Antiepileptic Drugs (NEAD) study is a multicenter, prospective, observational study of children born to WWE taking ASMs. This study has demonstrated a negative effect of in utero VPA exposure on cognitive development in children at up to 6 years of age – specifically in cognitive processing, working memory, and learning deficits – which is dose-dependent [61]. When adjusted for maternal IQ and gestational age, the average IQ of children exposed to VPA was 10 points lower than that of children exposed to phenytoin, LTG, or carbamazepine. This study has also demonstrated that while maternal IQ is a strong predictor of a child's IQ, this correlation is not significant in children exposed to VPA [62, 63]. Several early studies demonstrated potential adverse effects of phenytoin and phenobarbital on cognition, though the phenytoin effect was not substantiated by the NEAD study. A more detailed review on this topic can be found in Chapter 11.

Polytherapy versus Monotherapy – Early studies presented consistent evidence that polytherapy was associated with a greater risk of MCMs compared with monotherapy [1, 64]. One study from the North American ASM Pregnancy Registry, however, suggests that risks related to polytherapy may have been largely driven by the inclusion of VPA in these polytherapy combinations [65]. In this study, pregnancies exposed to LTG and VPA had a 9% rate of MCMs, while combinations of LTG with other ASMs were associated with a rate of 3%. Similarly, carbamazepine and VPA together resulted in a 15% rate of MCMs, while carbamazepine and other ASMs in polytherapy were associated with a 2% risk.

Other registries have also found that VPA was largely responsible for the increased risk of MCMs in polytherapy [52]. These data need to be replicated in other prospective studies but pose an interesting challenge to the prior dogma that monotherapy should be a paramount objective in managing young WWE. Given the established correlation between antiepileptic drug doses and MCMs, perhaps combinations of two drugs at lower doses may prove to be a better strategy for minimizing the risks related to ASMs in pregnancy in some patients who otherwise require high doses of a single agent. An important caveat, however, is that in limited studies, ASM polytherapy has also increased the risk of adverse cognitive outcomes [1]. Thus, future studies on the effect of ASM combinations and cognition will also be needed to determine if this approach is reasonable. A more detailed review on this topic can be found in Chapter 11.

Folic Acid Supplementation – Folic acid supplementation is typically recommended for all women of childbearing age taking ASMs. Historically, the recommendation of folic acid supplementation for WWE is largely extrapolated from studies demonstrating that it is associated with a lower risk of neural tube defects in the general population and in women at risk due to a previously affected pregnancy [66, 67]. Low first-trimester serum folic acid levels have also been associated with an increased risk for congenital malformations in WWE taking certain ASMs [68]. It is not yet clear if folic acid depletion is one of the mechanisms by which antiepileptic medications lead to fetal malformations.

Only a few studies have detected a protective effect of folic acid on MCM rates in women taking ASMs [69]. One study demonstrated a decrease in spontaneous abortions in WWE taking folic acid, particularly those treated with VPA [70]. The majority of studies, however, have not been able to demonstrate a significant effect of folic acid on malformation rates in ASM-exposed pregnancies. The American Academy of Neurology's 2009 Practice Parameter Update on Pregnancy in Epilepsy concluded that these studies were not sufficiently powered to exclude a beneficial effect of folic acid supplementation. The committee concluded that the risk of malformation is "possibly decreased by folic acid supplementation" and "preconceptional folic acid supplementation in WWE may be considered to reduce the risk of MCMs" [71].

Additionally, folic acid may be beneficial for cognitive development: the NEAD study found that preconception folic acid supplementation was associated with higher IQ scores, particularly verbal IQ scores, in children born to WWE [72]. While it is not clear if this is an effect specific to WWE, it provides an additional rationale for folic acid supplementation. Another important finding is that folic acid supplementation can lower risk of autistic traits in children exposed to ASMs in utero [73].

Large epidemiological studies will be needed to thoroughly evaluate the effect of folic acid supplementation on ASM-exposed pregnancies. In the meantime, most clinicians and guidelines agree that folic acid supplementation is an important part of preconception planning for WWE. There are wide variations in the recommended dose, with 0.4–4 mg recommended in the United States and 5 mg recommended in the United Kingdom, Europe, and Canada [44, 69, 74]. Most women's multivitamins include 0.4 mg of folic acid, whereas prenatal vitamins include 0.8 mg. In the United States, folic acid comes in a 1 mg pill by prescription, whereas it is available as a 5 mg pill in most other countries. In the United States, a common practice is to start all WWE on 0.4–1 mg of folic acid and increase the dose to 1–2 mg (1 mg by prescription plus a prenatal vitamin) when the patient is actively trying to conceive. These higher doses should also be considered in women who are at risk for an unplanned pregnancy. A more detailed review on this topic can be found in Chapter 11.

Risk of Seizures during Pregnancy

Seizure Frequency during Pregnancy – The best predictor of seizure occurrence and frequency during pregnancy is a patient's seizure pattern prior to pregnancy [44, 57, 75]. Most studies of WWE demonstrate that seizure frequency typically remains unchanged in the majority of women when compared to their individual prepregnancy baseline (54–80%). It tends to increase in less than a third (17–32%) and decreases in the remainder of cases (3–24%). A recent prospective study showed that WWE who were pregnant did not have a higher likelihood of increased seizures over their baseline seizure frequency than did nonpregnant WWE during a similar time period [76].

Seizure freedom for 9 months prior to conception is associated with an 84–92% likelihood of seizure freedom throughout the pregnancy [75]. Monitoring ASM levels and appropriately adjusting doses during pregnancy is critical to seizure control. This applies to all ASMs, but is best illustrated by LTG, which often needs to be increased by two or threefold over the course of a pregnancy [77, 78]. A more detailed review can be found in Chapter 12.

Risks Related to Seizures during Pregnancy – It is generally accepted that the risks of seizures, particularly tonic-clonic seizures, during pregnancy outweigh the risk of the medications. Seizures can put the patient (and thus her unborn child) at risk for falls and other accidental injuries. Tonic-clonic seizures and complex partial seizures can result in maternal hypoxia and arrhythmias, as well as put the mother at risk for sudden unexpected death in epilepsy (SUDEP). Case reports have documented fetal and maternal deaths with status epilepticus, and fetal intracranial hemorrhage and bradycardia in association with convulsions. One report of a complex partial seizure during pregnancy also documented fetal heart rate changes and prolonged contractions [79].

A study of cognitive development associated the presence of tonic-clonic seizures in pregnancy with lower verbal IQ in exposed children [80]. The EURAP study evaluated seizure frequency and outcomes among 406 WWE. In this cohort, no stillbirths, miscarriages, or maternal deaths were associated with isolated convulsions or nonconvulsive seizures. Among 12 cases of status epilepticus, there was one stillbirth and no maternal deaths [81]. One study from Taiwan and another from Austria demonstrated an association between generalized tonic-clonic seizures during pregnancy and preterm birth [82, 83]. On the whole, the risks of individual seizures to a given pregnancy are not clear. For now, advice about seizure control during pregnancy needs to be practical and cautious, emphasizing the risks of abruptly stopping seizure medications in most patients.

Breastfeeding

Most WWE should be encouraged to breastfeed, as it is largely felt that the important health benefits of breastfeeding outweigh any real or theoretical effects of ASM exposure in the baby [84]. Highly protein-bound ASMs such as phenytoin, carbamazepine, and VPA are expressed in breast milk at very low levels unlikely to affect an infant. Moreover, an NEAD study confirmed that breastfeeding has neurodevelopmental benefits for infants of WWE, regardless of the medication [85]. A more detailed review can be found in Chapter 18.

Putting It All Together: Balancing the Risks of Seizure and Medications before and during Pregnancy

A patient and her physician must balance the potential risks of antiepileptic drugs with her personal risk for seizures. This often requires a highly individualized treatment plan. For example, VPA, despite its known risks for teratogenicity, may be the most effective medication for the patient (especially in cases of juvenile myoclonic epilepsy [JME]). However, since the majority of patients with JME may also respond favorably to another broad-spectrum drug such as LTG or levetiracetam, a young woman with newly diagnosed JME should not be started on VPA as a first-line agent. If, however, the same patient proves refractory to several broad-spectrum antiepileptic medications at reasonable doses, it may be reasonable to use VPA at the lowest dose that controls seizures instead of continuing high doses of multiple other agents that have been ineffective. This should be done with very careful counseling of the patient as to all potential risks.

In choosing a first-line antiepileptic medication for a WWE, it makes sense to start with LTG or levetiracetam. Deciding whether to switch a patient who is already controlled on a different single agent depends on several factors, including the risks related to the present medication and the patient's personal preference and timeline. Some carefully selected patients who have been seizure free for at least 2 years can also consider weaning off of ASMs completely, as they have a reasonable chance of staying seizure free [87]. Whenever possible, it is best to make attempts to optimize therapy for pregnancy more than 9–12 months before the patient plans to conceive, as the seizure frequency in the ensuing year will best predict her pattern in pregnancy. Making medication changes in a patient who is currently pregnant should be done only in exceptional cases where benefits clearly outweigh risks, as changes in medications during pregnancy expose the patient and her fetus to polytherapy and the possibility of worsening seizures. Similar caution is advised in making changes in women who are actively trying to conceive or are not using contraception. There are, however, cases in which these late changes may be merited, such as women on VPA when it is not clearly needed. In these patients, referral to an epileptologist with expertise in the area is highly recommended.

In a woman whose epilepsy has been well controlled, it is reasonable to consider tapering the dose of her medications well in advance of her pregnancy to determine her minimal therapeutic drug level. For this reason, it is important to check ASM levels regularly in WWE as part of their routine care, both when they are doing well and in the event of a seizure. Checking drug levels on a regular basis establishes the patient's individual therapeutic window, which is critical in planning pregnancy and managing ASMs during the pregnancy. For example, a patient who was controlled for many years on 400 mg of LTG

Table 10.4 Timeline: management of women with epilepsy from diagnosis to conception

At diagnosis	- Take a careful history including all seizure types, frequency, risk factors, family history of epilepsy - Take sexual and reproductive history, including family history of fetal malformations - Perform basic epilepsy evaluation, including MRI and EEG - Consider inpatient monitoring prior to AEDs in patients with atypical histories - Start an AED most appropriate for patient AND with low risk of teratogenesis - Discuss available data on teratogenic risk and the AED chosen - Discuss risks of seizures and AED noncompliance in general and in regards to pregnancy - Start folic acid 0.4–5 mg - Ensure adequate contraception - Consider discussion of fertility in epilepsy, social support, and breastfeeding

>1 year preconception	- Recommend inpatient monitoring if seizures have not responded to AEDs
	- Consider epilepsy surgery in appropriate patients
	- Consider medication change in patients taking:
	  - AEDs associated with higher rates of teratogenicity
	  - AEDs that are not controlling seizures
	- Consider trial of AED withdrawal in patients who have been seizure free for > 2–4 years
	- Decrease dose of AEDs in patients whose seizures have been well controlled
	- Establish therapeutic drug levels (ideally troughs) at least twice a year
	- Discuss balancing risks of AEDs and risks of seizures during pregnancy
	- Continue folic acid 0.4–5 mg

<1 year preconception	- Recommend inpatient monitoring if seizures have not responded to AEDs
	- Consider cautious AED adjustment in appropriate patients who are not trying to conceive
	- Check AED levels (ideally troughs) 3–4 times a year and establish target level for pregnancy
	- Discuss genetic screening/counseling with appropriate patients
	- Establish a pregnancy plan with patient:
	  - Patient should notify doctors at first sign of pregnancy
	  - AED levels should be checked more frequently, at least every 4 weeks
	  - Decide which seizure types and/or AED levels will prompt medication adjustment

Table 10.4 (cont.)

	- Increase folic acid to 3–5 mg and start prenatal vitamin - Discuss social support, seizure safety in caring for infants, and need to avoid sleep deprivation - Discuss breastfeeding

Peri- and postconception	- Confirm patient is taking pre-natal vitamin and supplemental folic acid (total 4–5 mg)
	- Establish/review pregnancy plan
	- Adjust or lower AEDs only in exceptional cases where benefits clearly outweigh risks
	- Discuss appropriate prenatal screening with patient and other physicians:
	  - Genetic counseling in appropriate patients
	  - Targeted anatomic ultrasound at 18–20 weeks
	- Discuss social support, seizure safety, sleep deprivation, and breastfeeding

and birth control pills should be able to substantially reduce her LTG dose once she discontinues her oral contraceptive pills (OCPs) and still maintain her previous levels, as the effect of the OCPs on glucuronidation will be reversed. Recognizing this important interaction and adjusting her dose appropriately may reduce the risk of MCMs. Discussing the plan for monitoring drug levels and adjusting medications during pregnancy is also important to set expectations for management during pregnancy. Chapter 18 discusses this in further detail.

Safety and Social Support

In explaining and managing all of the important risks related to ASMs and seizures in pregnancy, it is easy to lose sight of some of the most important considerations, which include the patient's home life and ability to take care of her infant. Women with epilepsy are at increased risk for seizures in the postpartum period due to hormone and ASM fluctuations, as well as sleep deprivation. Even a woman with rare seizures needs to think practically how one of her typical seizures might affect the safety of her child. Worthwhile tips include changing or feeding the baby on the floor, using a stroller around the house, and not bathing the baby alone.

While breastfeeding is encouraged, new mothers need to consider asking for help with night feeding from their partners and/or family to minimize sleep deprivation. In addition, patients should be aware that postpartum depression in women is common and WWE are at even greater risk [88]. These considerations and a patient's social support should be discussed within preconception counseling and revisited during the pregnancy [86]. A detailed review of this can be found in Chapter 16.

Conclusions

Effective contraception in WWE is essential to allow for preconception planning and to implement the measures known to improve pregnancy outcomes. However, concomitant use of ASMs and hormonal contraceptives is complicated because of the bidirectional pharmacokinetic interactions, the pharmacodynamic consequences, and the potential effects on seizure control. The IUD is a safe and effective method of contraception for all WWE. Preconception counseling for WWE should begin as early as possible, usually at the time of initiating an antiepileptic drug in a woman of childbearing age, or near puberty in an adolescent taking seizure medication. While counseling should be tailored to the patient's sophistication and personal timeline, it should be repeated at regular intervals, allowing the patient to ask questions each time. Counseling should include a discussion of the risks related to seizures and ASMs during pregnancy. It should stress that most WWE have healthy pregnancies, but should also emphasize that early prepartum planning can optimize fetal outcomes.

References

1. Harden CL, Meador KJ, Pennell PB, et al. American Academy of Neurology; American Epilepsy Society. Practice parameter update: Management issues for women with epilepsy. Focus on pregnancy (an evidence-based review). Teratogenesis and perinatal outcomes. Report of the Quality Standards Subcommittee and Therapeutics and Technology Assessment Subcommittee of the American Academy of Neurology and American Epilepsy Society. *Neurology*. 2009;**73**(2):133–41.
2. Tomson T, Battino D, Bonizzoni E, et al. for the EURAP Study Group. Dose dependent risk of malformations with antiepileptic drugs: An analysis of data from the EURAP epilepsy and pregnancy registry. *Lancet Neurol.* 2011;**10**(7):609–17.
3. Meador KJ, Baker GA, Browning N, et al. Fetal antiepileptic drug exposure and cognitive outcomes at age 6 years (NEAD study): A prospective observational study. *Lancet Neurol.* 2013;**12**(3):244–52.
4. Mosher WD, Jones J. Use of contraception in the United States: 1982–2008. *Vital Health Stat.* 2010; **23**(29):1–44.
5. Kavanaugh ML, Jerman J, Finer LB. Changes in use of long-acting reversible contraceptive methods among U.S. women, 2009–2012. *Obstet Gynecol.* 2015;**126**:917–27.
6. Practice Parameter. Management issues for women with epilepsy (summary statement): Report of the Quality Standards Subcommittee of the American Academy of Neurology. *Neurology.* 1998;**51**(4):944–8.
7. Herzog AG, Mandle HB, Cahill KE, et al. Contraceptive practices of women with epilepsy: Findings of the Epilepsy Birth Control Registry. *Epilepsia.* 2016;**57**(4):630–7.
8. Davis AR, Pack AM, Kritzer J, et al. Reproductive history, sexual behavior and use of contraception in women with epilepsy. *Contraception.* 2008;**77**(6):405–9.
9. Krauss GL, Brandt J, Campbell M, et al. Antiepileptic medication and oral contraceptive interactions: A national survey of neurologists and obstetricians. *Neurology.* 1996; **46**(6):1534–9.
10. Long L, Montouris G. Knowledge of women's issues and epilepsy (KOWIE-II): A survey of health care professionals. *Epilepsy Behav.* 2005;**6**(1):90–3.
11. Pack A, Davis AR, Kritzer J, et al. Antiepileptic drugs: Are women aware of interactions with oral contraceptives and potential teratogenicity? *Epilepsy Behav.* 2009;**14**(4):640–4.
12. Winner B, Peipert JF, Zhao Q, et al. Effectiveness of long-acting reversible contraception. *N Engl J Med.* 2012; **366**(21):1998–2007.
13. Ortiz ME, Croxatto HB. Copper-T intrauterine device and levonorgestrel intrauterine system: Biological bases of their mechanism of action. *Contraception.* 2007; **75**(6 Suppl):S16–S30.

14. ACOG Committee Opinion No. 735: Adolescents and long-acting reversible contraception: Implants and intrauterine devices. *Obstet Gynecol.* 2018;**131**(5):e130–e139.
15. Davis AR, Saadatmand HJ, Pack A. Women with epilepsy initiating a progestin IUD: A prospective pilot study of safety and acceptability. *Epilepsia.* 2016;**57**(11):1843–8.
16. Mohllajee AP, Curtis KM, Peterson HB. Does insertion and use of an intrauterine device increase the risk of pelvic inflammatory disease among women with sexually transmitted infection? A systematic review. *Contraception.* 2006;**73**(2):145–53.
17. Farley TM, Rosenberg MJ, Rowe PJ, et al. Intrauterine devices and pelvic inflammatory disease: An international perspective. *Lancet.* 1992;**339**(8796):785–8.
18. Vieira CS, Pack A, Roberts K, Davis AR. A pilot study of levonorgestrel concentrations and bleeding patterns in women with epilepsy using a levonorgestrel IUD and treated with antiepileptic drugs. *Contraception.* 2019;**99**(4):251–5.
19. Marions L, Lövkvist L, Taube A, et al. Use of the levonorgestrel releasing-intrauterine system in nulliparous women: A non-interventional study in Sweden. *Eur J Contracept Reprod Health Care.* 2011;**16**(2):126–34.
20. Madden T, McNicholas C, Zhao Q, et al. Association of age and parity with intrauterine device expulsion. *Obstet Gynecol.* 2014;**124**(4):718–26.
21. Johnson EL. Contraception for women with epilepsy. *Curr Obstet Gynecol Rep.* 2018;7:146–52.
22. Isley MM, Kaunitz AM. Update on hormonal contraception and bone density. *Rev Endocr Metab Disord.* 2011;**12**(2):93–106.
23. Centers for Disease Control and Prevention. US Medical Eligibility Criteria for Contraceptive Use, 2010. *MMWR Recomm Rep.* 2010;**59**(RR–4):1–86.
24. Kenyon IE. Unplanned pregnancy in an epileptic. *Br Med J.* 1972;**1**:686–7.
25. Gaffield ME, Culwell Kelly R, Lee CR. The use of hormonal contraception among women taking anticonvulsant therapy. *Contraception.* 2011; **83**:16–29.
26. Stoffel-Wagner B, Bauer J, Flügel D, et al. Serum sex hormones are altered in patients with chronic temporal lobe epilepsy receiving anticonvulsant medication. *Epilepsia.* 1998;**39**:1164–73.
27. Bounds W, Guillebaud J. Observational series on women using the contraceptive Mirena concurrently with anti-epileptic and other enzyme-inducing drugs. *J Fam Plann Reprod Health Care.* 2002;**28**:78–80.
28. Sabers A, Ohman I, Christensen J, et al. Oral contraceptives reduce lamotrigine plasma levels. *Neurology.* 2003;**61**(4):570–1.
29. Ohman I, Luef G, Tomson T. Effects of pregnancy and contraception on lamotrigine disposition: New insights through analysis of lamotrigine metabolites. *Seizure.* 2008;**17**:199–202.
30. Wegner I, Edelbroek PM, Bulk S, et al. Lamotrigine kinetics within the menstrual cycle, after menopause, and with oral contraceptives. *Neurology.* 2009;**73**(17):1388–93.
31. Herzog AG, Blum AS, Farina EL, et al. Valproate and lamotrigine level variation with menstrual cycle phase and oral contraceptive use. *Neurology.* 2009;**72**:911–14.
32. Herzog AG, Harden CL, Liporace J, et al. Frequency of catamenial seizure exacerbation in women with localization-related epilepsy. *Ann Neurol.* 2004;**56** (3):431–4.
33. Harden CL, Pennell PB. Neuroendocrine considerations in the treatment of men and women with epilepsy. *Lancet Neurol.* 2013; **12**(1):72–83.
34. Herzog AG. Differential impact of antiepileptic drugs on the effects of contraceptive methods on seizures: Interim findings of the Epilepsy Birth Control Registry. *Seizure.* 2015;**28**:71–5.

35. Herzog AG, Mandle HB, MacEachern DB. Differential risks of changes in seizure frequency with transitions between hormonal and non-hormonal contraception in women with epilepsy: A prospective cohort study. *Epilepsy Behav.* 2021;**120**:108011.
36. Mattson RH, Cramer J, Caldwell BV, et al. Treatment of seizures with medroxyprogesterone acetate: Preliminary report. *Neurology.* 1984;**34**:1255–8.
37. Herzog AG, Fowler KM, Smithson SD, et al. Progesterone vs. placebo therapy for women with epilepsy: A randomized clinical trial. *Neurology.* 2012;**78**(24):1959–66.
38. Fairgrieve SD, Jackson M, Jonas P, et al. Population based, prospective study of the care of women with epilepsy in pregnancy. *BMJ* (Clinical research ed). 2000;**321** (7262):674–5.
39. Bell GS, Nashef L, Kendall S, et al. Information recalled by women taking anti-epileptic drugs for epilepsy: A questionnaire study. *Epilepsy Res.* 2002;**52**(2):139–46.
40. May TW, Pfafflin M, Coban I, et al. Fears, knowledge, and need of counseling for women with epilepsy: Results of an outpatient study. *Der Nervenarzt.* 2009;**80** (2):174–83.
41. Vazquez B, Gibson P, Kustra R. Epilepsy and women's health issues: Unmet needs. Survey results from women with epilepsy. *Epilepsy Behav.* 2007;**10**(1):163–9.
42. Winterbottom JB, Smyth RM, Jacoby A, et al. Preconception counselling for women with epilepsy to reduce adverse pregnancy outcome. *Cochrane Database Syst Revi.* 2008;**3**:CD006645.
43. Crawford P. Best practice guidelines for the management of women with epilepsy. *Epilepsia.* 2005; **46**(Suppl 9): 117–24.
44. Aguglia U, Barboni G, Battino D, et al. Italian Consensus Conference on Epilepsy and Pregnancy, Labor and Puerperium. *Epilepsia.* 2009;**50**(Suppl 1):7–23.
45. Davis AR, Pack AM, Kritzer J, et al. Reproductive history, sexual behavior and use of contraception in women with epilepsy. *Contraception.* 2008;**77**(6):405–9.
46. Johnson EL, Burke AE, Wang A, Pennell PB. Unintended pregnancy, prenatal care, newborn outcomes, and breastfeeding in women with epilepsy. *Neurology.* 2018;**91**(11):1031–9.
47. Crawford P, Hudson S. Understanding the information needs of women with epilepsy at different lifestages: Results of the "Ideal World" survey. *Seizure.* 2003;**12**(7):502–7.
48. Helbig KL, Bernhardt BA, Conway LJ, et al. Genetic risk perception and reproductive decision making among people with epilepsy. *Epilepsia.* 2010;**51**(9):1874–7.
49. Winawer MR, Shinnar S. Genetic epidemiology of epilepsy or what do we tell families? *Epilepsia.* 2005;**46**(Suppl 10):24–30.
50. Peljto AL, Barker-Cummings C, Vasoli VM, et al. Familial risk of epilepsy: A population-based study. *Brain.* 2014;**137** (Pt 3):795–805.
51. Holmes LB, Harvey EA, Coull BA, et al. The teratogenicity of anticonvulsant drugs. *New Engl J Med.* 2001;**344**(15):1132–8.
52. Morrow J, Russell A, Guthrie E, et al. Malformation risks of antiepileptic drugs in pregnancy: A prospective study from the UK Epilepsy and Pregnancy Register. *J Neurol Neurosurg Psychiatry.* 2006;**77**(2):193–8.
53. Hernandez-Diaz S, Smith CR, Shen A, et al. Comparative safety of antiepileptic drugs during pregnancy. *Neurology.* 2012;**78**(21):1692–9.
54. Tomson T, Battino D, Bonizzoni E, et al. Comparative risk of major congenital malformations with eight different antiepileptic drugs: A prospective cohort study of the EURAP registry. *Lancet Neurol.* 2018;**17**(6):530–8.
55. Vajda FJE, Graham JE, Hitchcock AA, et al. Antiepileptic drugs and foetal malformation: Analysis of 20 years of data in a pregnancy register. *Seizure.* 2019;**65**:6–11.
56. Thomas SV, Jose M, Divakaran S, Sankara Sarma P. Malformation risk of antiepileptic

drug exposure during pregnancy in women with epilepsy: Results from a pregnancy registry in south India. *Epilepsia.* 2017;**58**(2):274–81.

57. Tomson T, Battino D. Teratogenic effects of antiepileptic drugs. *Lancet Neurol.* 2012;**11**(9):803–13.
58. FDA Drug Safety Communication: Risk of oral clefts in children born to mothers taking Topamax (topiramate). 2011. www.fda.gov/Drugs/DrugSafety/ucm245085.htm.
59. Shallcross R, Bromley RL, Irwin B, et al. Child development following in utero exposure: Levetiracetam vs. sodium valproate. *Neurology.* 2011;**76**(4):383–9. PubMed PMID: 21263139.
60. Banach R, Boskovic R, Einarson T, et al. Long-term developmental outcome of children of women with epilepsy, unexposed or exposed prenatally to antiepileptic drugs: A meta-analysis of cohort studies. *Drug Saf.* 2010;**33**(1):73–9.
61. Cohen MJ, Meador KJ, May R, et al. Fetal antiepileptic drug exposure and learning and memory functioning at 6 years of age: The NEAD prospective observational study. *Epilepsy Behav.* 2019;**92**:154–64.
62. Meador KJ, Baker GA, Browning N, et al. Effects of fetal antiepileptic drug exposure: Outcomes at age 4.5 years. *Neurology.* 2012;**78**(16):1207–14.
63. Meador KJ, Baker GA, Browning N, et al. Fetal antiepileptic drug exposure and cognitive outcomes at age 6 years (NEAD study): A prospective observational study. *Lancet Neurol.* 2013;**12**(3):244–52.
64. Meador K, Reynolds MW, Crean S, et al. Pregnancy outcomes in women with epilepsy: A systematic review and meta-analysis of published pregnancy registries and cohorts. *Epilepsy Res.* 2008;**81**(1):1–13.
65. Holmes LB, Mittendorf R, Shen A, et al. Fetal effects of anticonvulsant polytherapies: Different risks from different drug combinations. *Arch Neurol.* 2011;**68**(10):1275–81.
66. Blencowe H, Cousens S, Modell B, et al. Folic acid to reduce neonatal mortality from neural tube disorders. *J Epidemiol.* 2010;**39**(Suppl 1):i110–i21.
67. Medical Research Council Vitamin Study Research Group. Prevention of neural tube defects: Results of the Medical Research Council Vitamin Study.*Lancet.* 1991;**338**(8760):131–7.
68. Kaaja E, Kaaja R, Hiilesmaa V. Major malformations in offspring of women with epilepsy. *Neurology.* 2003;**60**(4):575–9.
69. Kjaer D, Horvath-Puho E, Christensen J, et al. Antiepileptic drug use, folic acid supplementation, and congenital abnormalities: A population-based case control study. *BJOG* 2008;**115**(1):98–103.
70. Pittschieler S, Brezinka C, Jahn B, et al. Spontaneous abortion and the prophylactic effect of folic acid supplementation in epileptic women undergoing antiepileptic therapy. *J Neurol.* 2008;**255**(12):1926–31.
71. Harden CL, Pennell PB, Koppel BS, et al. Practice parameter update: Management issues for women with epilepsy. Focus on pregnancy (an evidence-based review). Vitamin K, folic acid, blood levels, and breastfeeding. Report of the Quality Standards Subcommittee and Therapeutics and Technology Assessment Subcommittee of the American Academy of Neurology and American Epilepsy Society. *Neurology.* 2009; **73**(2):142–9.
72. Meador KJ, Pennell PB, May RC, et al. Effects of periconceptional folate on cognition in children of women with epilepsy: NEAD study. *Neurology.* 2020; **94**(7):729–40.
73. Bjørk M, et al. Association of folic acid supplementation during pregnancy with the risk of autistic traits in children exposed to antiepileptic drugs in utero. *JAMA Neurology.* 2018;**75**(2):160–8.
74. Wilson RD, Davies G, Desilets V, et al. The use of folic acid for the prevention of neural tube defects and other congenital anomalies. *J Obstet Gynaecol Can.* 2003;**25**(11):959–73.

75. Harden CL, Hopp J, Ting TY, et al. Practice parameter update: Management issues for women with epilepsy. Focus on pregnancy (an evidence-based review). Obstetrical complications and change in seizure frequency. Report of the Quality Standards Subcommittee and Therapeutics and Technology Assessment Subcommittee of the American Academy of Neurology and American Epilepsy Society. *Neurology.* 2009;**73**(2):126–32.

76. Pennell PB, French JA, May RC, et al. Changes in seizure frequency and antiepileptic therapy during pregnancy. *N Engl J Med.* 2020;**383**(26):2547–56.

77. Pennell PB, Peng L, Newport DJ, et al. Lamotrigine in pregnancy: Clearance, therapeutic drug monitoring, and seizure frequency. *Neurology.* 2008;**70**(22 Pt 2):2130–6.

78. Sabers A, Petrenaite V. Seizure frequency in pregnant women treated with lamotrigine monotherapy. *Epilepsia.* 2009;**50**(9):2163–6.

79. Kaplan PW, Norwitz ER, Ben-Menachem E, et al. Obstetric risks for women with epilepsy during pregnancy. *Epilepsy Behav.* 2007;**11**(3):283–91.

80. Adab N, Kini U, Vinten J, et al. The longer term outcome of children born to mothers with epilepsy. *J Neurol Neurosurg Psychiatry.* 2004;**75**(11):1575–83.

81. EURAP Study Group. Seizure control and treatment in pregnancy: Observations from the EURAP epilepsy pregnancy registry. *Neurology.* 2006;**66**(3):354–60.

82. Rauchenzauner M, Ehrensberger M, Prieschl M, et al. Generalized tonic-clonic seizures and antiepileptic drugs during pregnancy: A matter of importance for the baby? *J Neurol.* 2013;**260**(2):484–8.

83. Chen YH, Chiou HY, Lin HC, Lin HL. Affect of seizures during gestation on pregnancy outcomes in women with epilepsy. Arch Neurol. 2009;66(8):979–84. https://doi.org/10.1001/archneurol.2009.142. PMID: 19667219.

84. Birnbaum AK, Meador KJ, Karanam A, et al. Antiepileptic drug exposure in infants of breastfeeding mothers with epilepsy. *JAMA Neurol.* 2020;**77**(4):441–50.

85. Meador KJ, Baker GA, Browning N, et al. Breastfeeding in children of women taking antiepileptic drugs: Cognitive outcomes at age 6 years. *JAMA Pediatr.* 2014;**168**(8):729–36.

86. Klein A. The postpartum period in women with epilepsy. *Neurol Clin.* 2012;**30**(3):867–75.

87. Lossius MI, Hessen E, Mowinckel P, et al. Consequences of antiepileptic drug withdrawal: A randomized, double-blind study (Akershus Study). *Epilepsia.* 2008;**49**(3):455–63.

88. Decker BM, Thibault D, Davis KA, Willis AW. A nationwide analysis of maternal morbidity and acute postpartum readmissions in women with epilepsy. *Epilepsy Behav.* 2021;**117**:107874.

89. Espinera AR, Gavvala J, Bellinski I, Kennedy J, Macken MP, Narechania A, Templer J, VanHaerents S, Schuele SU, Gerard EE. Counseling by epileptologists affects contraceptive choices of women with epilepsy. Epilepsy Behav. 2016;**65**:1–6. https://doi.org/10.1016/j.yebeh.2016.08.021.

Chapter 11

Teratogenicity and Antiseizure Medications

Anna Serafini

Key Points

- Teratogenicity associated with antiseizure medications (ASMs) is variable and multifactorial.
- Observational data from international pregnancy registries, with large numbers, allow for a confident comparison of the teratogenicity of each specific ASM.
- The goal during pregnancy is to achieve an optimal, individualized balance between seizure control and the potential teratogenic risks of ASMs.
- Valproic acid (VPA) is the most teratogenic ASM, making it the least preferred for patients of reproductive potential.
- Antiseizure medications with the lowest teratogenic risk to date are lamotrigine and levetiracetam.
- The use of folic acid is recommended in women of childbearing potential, though the optimal dose is unknown.

Teratogenesis

Introduction

Teratology is the study of abnormal prenatal development that results from exposure to a "teratogen" that can produce structural and functional abnormalities in the conceptus [1]. A teratogenic agent is a chemical infectious agent, physical condition, or deficiency that, on fetal exposure, can alter fetal morphology or subsequent function [2].

Concerns related to the teratogenic effects of medications were highlighted during the thalidomide crisis in the 1960s, when women who took thalidomide while pregnant were giving birth to children with phocomelia. More concerns were raised after the teratogenic effects related to the use of diethylstilbestrol were discovered in 1971 [3]. These events led the US Food and Drug Administration (FDA) to establish regulations regarding the use of medications in pregnancy requiring proof of safety and efficacy of any drug before it becomes commercially available.

In 1979, the FDA developed a system determining the teratogenic risk of drugs based on data from animal and human studies. This classification aim is to provide therapeutic guidance for the clinician. The FDA established five lettered risk categories – A, B, C, D, and X – to indicate the potential of a drug to cause birth defects if used during pregnancy [4]. Category A is considered the safest category and category X is absolutely contraindicated in pregnancy. A specific agent is classified as teratogenic if the frequency of congenital malformations in women exposed to the agent is prospectively greater than the background frequency in the general population. However, pregnant women are often excluded from majority of clinical trials; therefore, data come mostly from animal studies. For this reason, drug use during pregnancy has limited high-quality safety data in the majority of cases. Antiseizure medications (ASMs) are all included in classes C and D. Older ASMs are categorized as category D, whereas newer ASMs are categorized as category C, except for topiramate, which was moved from category C to category D in 2010 due to observed increased risk of oral cleft.

However, throughout the years, this letter classification has posed challenges. Under this classification, different drugs were categorized within the same class even if the number of pregnancies enrolled for each drug highly varied. Having a drug with 3% risk with 30 pregnancies is not the same as having a drug with 3% risk with 2,000 pregnancies. This type of classification would not allow more individualized drug evaluation. Therefore, in 2015, the FDA replaced the letter classifications with new information to make them more meaningful to both patients and healthcare providers. This new system, also known as the Pregnancy and Lactation Labeling Rule (PLLR), allows better patient-specific counseling and informed decision-making for pregnant women seeking medication therapies. The drug labeling includes a section called "Pregnancy" that provides a narrative risk summary and detailed animal data, a background risk statement, and the estimated background risk for major birth defects and miscarriage [5].

Principles of Teratogenesis

The development of a fetus from conception to birth can be divided into three phases: preimplantation, embryonic, and fetal [6]. The effect of teratogens is different in each one of these phases. The preimplantation phase occurs 2–3 weeks after the start of the last menstrual period. During this phase, the fertilized egg (zygote) develops from one cell to a ball of many cells (the conceptus), which will move from the fallopian tubes to the uterus. The possible effect of teratogens in this phase often results in the loss of the conceptus (a miscarriage, often before the woman realizes she is pregnant).

Teratogens usually cause the most severe damage during the second or embryonic phase. This phase occurs 3–10 weeks after the start of the last menstrual period. The embryo is most susceptible to teratogenic agents during periods of rapid differentiation, in particular, between the third week and the eighth week after fertilization, which is the period of organogenesis [6]. During these crucial weeks, many women take medications before realizing they are pregnant. Each organ has a critical period during which its development may be disrupted. The type of congenital malformation produced depends upon which organ is most susceptible at the time of the teratogenic exposure (see Figure 11.1).

The third phase (fetal phase) starts after the ninth week and lasts until delivery. Development during this time is primarily maturation and growth. Exposure to drugs during this period is not associated with major congenital malformations, but they may alter the growth and function of normally formed organs and tissues. For example, the fetal brain can still be affected in this phase by some teratogens and exposure after the first trimester can cause cognitive and behavioral impairment.

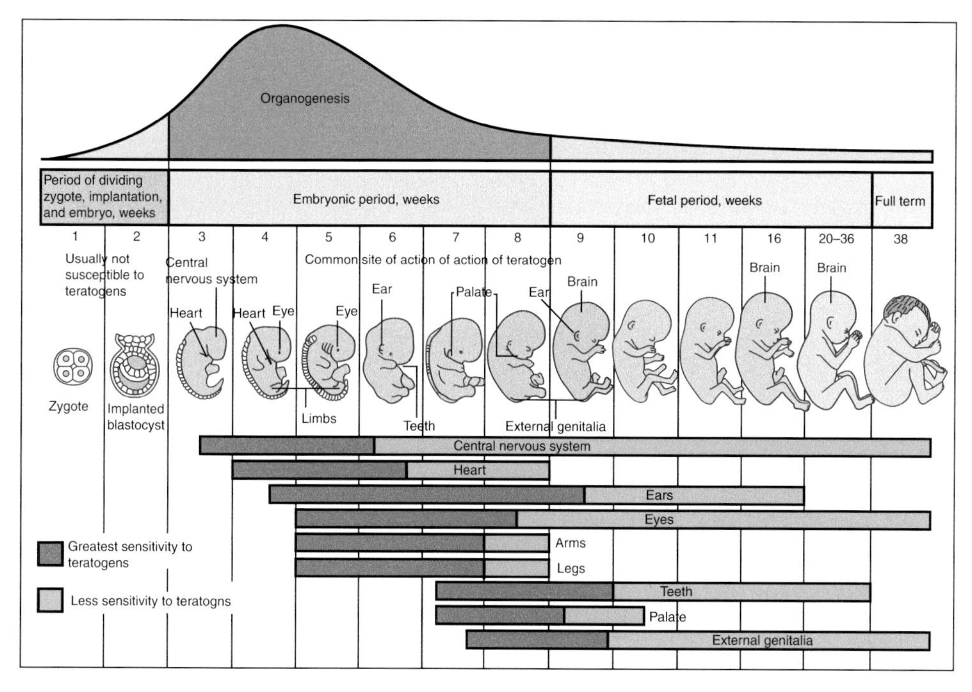

Figure 11.1 Sensitivity to teratogens during pregnancy

Congenital Malformations

Congenital malformations are defined as structural or functional anomalies that develop during intrauterine life and can be identified prenatally or at birth, or sometimes they may be detected only later in infancy. Congenital malformations may be classified based on clinical and etiologic as well as pathogenetic criteria. Malformations are classified as major or minor based on their clinical significance.

Minor malformations are usually defects not producing function impairment and not requiring medical assistance (birth prevalence < 4%). Examples include epicanthal folds, single transverse palmar crease, and fifth-finger clinodactyly. Minor malformations may be objective (e.g., preauricular tags) or more subjective (e.g., low-set ears) [7]. The presence of minor malformations may be indicative of an associated major malformation. For example, a single umbilical artery can be associated with congenital heart problems [8]. The greater the number of minor malformations, the greater the likelihood of an associated major malformation.

A major congenital malformation (MCM) is defined as a defect detected by imaging or clinical examination in the development of a body part or organ that would significantly impede the quality of life of the child or require surgical intervention or close monitoring and follow-up [7]. Typical MCMs can be external such as orofacial clefts, neural tube defects (NTDs), or limb deficiencies. These external MCMs are easily recognized on physical examination at or shortly after birth. On the other hand, internal MCMs (such as congenital heart defects, intestinal malrotation, or unilateral kidney agenesis) require specific tests to be detected. Among the general population, MCMs occur in 2–3% of infants [9].

Malformations may also be classified based on etiology. Primary malformations are morphogenetic defects arising from intrinsic errors of the developmental process with a genetic origin. Secondary malformations are the consequence of environmental factors that interfere with a normal developmental process [7]. Malformations attributed to teratogenic agents are considered secondary malformations. International pregnancy registries monitor for secondary malformations attributed to antiseizure drug exposure. Approximately 10–15% of congenital structural anomalies are the result of the adverse effect of environmental factors on prenatal development [2].

Overall, MCMs can cause significant health and developmental complications. They remain a major contributor to infant mortality and lifelong disabilities. According to a congenital anomalies survey conducted by the World Health Organization (WHO) in 193 countries in 2010, 270,000 of the 3.1 million newborn deaths were caused by congenital anomalies [10]. In the general population, 2% of newborns have an MCM. Less than 5% of them are caused by medications or toxins. This means that every pregnancy has a base risk independent of drug intake.

Teratogenesis and Epilepsy

Epidemiological Data and Pregnancy Registries

One and a half million women with epilepsy (WWE) are of childbearing age in the United States, and 3–5 births per 1,000 will be to WWE. However, when considering ASMs are used for other indications such as neuropathy, chronic pain, and other neurological and psychiatric disorders, the total number of children exposed in utero to ASMs is considerably greater [11]. Most WWE need to continue use of ASMs during pregnancy because uncontrolled seizures might harm the mother and fetus.

It is extremely important to keep a balance between seizure control and the potential teratogenic risks of ASMs. The original reports of ASMs teratogenicity date from the 1960s. In 1968, Meadow reported orofacial clefts and other abnormalities among babies of mothers who received primidone, phenytoin, or phenobarbital [12]. More than 50 years after this first report, more studies have confirmed higher birth defects rates among children of WWE [13, 14]. Malformations in the offspring of WWE typically follow a similar pattern to what is seen in the general population, with cardiac defects being the most common followed by facial clefts and hypospadias, but with some variation between different ASMs. Reassuringly, 96% of pregnancies in WWE result in a child without MCMs.

This increased risks of malformations in pregnant WWE can be the consequence of many factors: genetics, the type of maternal epilepsy, seizure frequency during pregnancy, and socioeconomic status. The most important risk factor however, remains the type of ASM used [15]. In the past 15–20 years, a number of pregnancy registries have been established all over the world. These registries aim to better understand the effects of each specific drug on pregnancy by enrolling prospectively large numbers of women taking ASMs.

Observational data comparing the teratogenicity of each specific ASM are currently available through these registries, which include independent, national, or international registries, population-based registries, and registries sponsored by pharmaceutical companies. The North American AED Pregnancy Registry (NAAPR) and the UK Pregnancy Registry (UKEPR) are two independent national registries. The NAAPR includes data on pregnant women from the United States and Canada and enrolls women taking ASMs during pregnancy (also for reasons outside of epilepsy) [16].

The UKEPR includes data on WWE with or without ASMs from the United Kingdom and Ireland [17]. The International Registry of Antiepileptic Drugs and Pregnancy (EURAP) includes data on pregnant women from more than 40 countries worldwide [18]. Like NAAPR, EURAP enrolls pregnant women taking ASMs for any clinical reason (not limited to epilepsy) but retrospectively excludes women not affected by epilepsy. The Australian Pregnancy Register (APR) and the Kerala Registry of Epilepsy and Pregnancy in India are two independent national registries that also contribute to EURAP [19, 20]. The GSK-LTG registry, focusing exclusively on lamotrigine (LTG), is sponsored by a pharmaceutical company [21]. Population-based registries have been established in Northern European countries: the Finnish Drug Prescription database [22], the Danish registry [23], the Swedish National Registry [24], and the Norwegian Medical Birth (MBRN) registry [25].

Although all registries have similar objectives and outcome measures, they all have differences in methodology; therefore, their results cannot be directly compared (see Table 11.1 for main differences among registries). They differ in methods of enrollment (self-referred vs. physician referred), moment of enrollment (first trimester vs. any moment during pregnancy), inclusion criteria (any women taking ASMs vs. only WWE taking ASMs), duration of follow-up (3 months after delivery vs. 1 year after delivery), and different definitions of malformations (all types vs. only major malformations).

Variation in malformations rates observed between registries is felt to be, at least in part, a result of these methodological differences. One of the most important differences is in regards to the duration of follow-up after birth. The EURAP registry, for example, has a longer follow-up (up to 1 year after birth), and of the 383 cases with MCMs reported, only 59 (15%) were detected in the first 2 months [18]. This explains why the frequency of MCMs is higher in EURAP than in other registries with shorter follow-up. Some malformations are not apparent immediately after birth and can be picked up only with an extended time window. In EURAP analysis, cardiac, hip, and renal malformations were the most commonly missed MCMs early after birth. Information regarding patients' epilepsy also is different between registries. The source for patients' epilepsy is acquired directly from the treating physician in EURAP, making these data more reliable. On the other hand, EURAP lacks direct access to patient-provided information for more detailed follow-up questions, which is possible with NAAPR.

A limitation of EURAP and UKEPR is the lack of a control with WWE not on ASMs or healthy women. Those registries rely mainly on internal comparisons between ASMs. In contrast, NAAPR utilizes internal as well as external unexposed control groups. The external control group for NAAPR comes from the Active Malformations Surveillance Program at Brigham and Women's Hospital in Boston, where the malformation rate was 1.62% after excluding infants with genetic disorders and chromosomal abnormalities.

It is important to also take into consideration how the method of enrollment might affect the results. Study participants referred by healthcare providers tend to be women with more severe epilepsy. On the other hand, self-referred patients are likely more motivated and probably better informed. Lastly, some registries only collected information on major congenital malformations, excluding minor malformations. Others included minor malformations as well, increasing the overall number of malformations and making comparisons extremely hard to do.

Table 11.1 Characteristics of different pregnancy registries

	NAAPR [16]	UKEPR [17]	EURAP [18]	APR [19]	GSK [21]	Kerala [20]	Finland [22]	Medical birth registry of Norway (MBRN) [25]	Danish registry [23]	Swedish [24]
Pregnancies (n)	5,667 monotherapy	6,130 total (5412 monotherapy)	7,355 monotherapy	2,148 total (1,593 monotherapy)	1,558 monotherapy	1,436 (1021 monotherapy)	3,067 total (1,231 monotherapy)	2,559 total (2,309 monotherapy)	1,532 total	1,398 total (1,256 monotherapy)
Year established	1997	1996 (Ireland joined 2007)	1999	1999	1992	1998	1985	1999	1996	1994
Setting	United States Canada	United Kingdom Ireland	International (42 countries between Europe, Asia, Oceania, Australia, and South America)	Australia (contributes to EURAP)	International	Kerala-India (contributes to EURAP)	Population based	Population based	Population based	Population based
Method of enrollment	Self-referred	Self-referred and physician-referred	Physician-referred	Self-referred	Physician-referred	Self-referred and physician-referred	National medical birth registry	National registry	National medical birth registry	National Registry
Moment of enrollment	Any moment during pregnancy	First trimester (<16 weeks gestation); outcome unknown	First trimester (<16 weeks from conception); outcome unknown	Any moment during pregnancy	Any moment during pregnancy	Within first trimester; outcome unknown	n/a – national registry	n/a – national registry	n/a – national registry	n/a – national registry
Study design	Prospective/ retrospective	Prospective	Prospective/ retrospective	Prospective/ retrospective	Prospective/ retrospective	Prospective	Retrospective	Retrospective	Retrospective	Retrospective
Eligibility criteria	Treatment with ASMs for any reason (not only epilepsy)	Pregnant WWE with or without ASMs	Treatment with ASMs (not only epilepsy)	Treatment with ASMs for any reason (not only epilepsy); WWE not treated with ASMs	Pregnant women on LTG	Pregnant WWE with or without ASMs	Pregnant women on ASMs	Pregnant women on ASMs	Pregnant women on ASMs	Pregnant women on ASMs

Classification of outcomes	MCM (minor malformations excluded)	Minor and MCMs according to EUROCAT criteria	MCMs according to EUROCAT criteria	Birth defects as defined by Victorian birth register	MCM as defined by CDC Metropolitan Atlanta Congenital Defects Program (MACDP)	MCM	Malformations as defined by ICD-9 system (minor malformations excluded)	Malformations as defined by ICD-10 system	Malformations classified according to EUROCAT criteria (minor malformations excluded)	Malformations as defined by ICD-9 and Swedish Register of Congenital Malformations
Outcome assessment	Telephone interview	Questionnaire to primary physician	Physician report	Interviews and hospital records	Physician report	Physician report	Finnish Malformation Register	Hospital records and national registry	Hospital records and national registry	Hospital records and national registry
Latest follow-up after birth	3 months after birth	3 months after birth	12 months after birth	12 months after birth	Shortly after birth	12 months after birth		Within 12 months from birth	Cases identified through national patient registry within 12 months from birth	/
Control population	External group; internal comparisons between different ASMs	Internal comparisons between different ASMs	Internal comparisons between different ASMs	AEDs not exposed pregnancies	1) general population cohorts 2) cohorts of WWE exposed to ASMs monotherapy identified from the literature	Internal control: WWE not on ASMs; external control group: 319 women without epilepsy not using ASMs	Offspring of women with no epilepsy diagnosis and no AED use	Unexposed children born to mothers without epilepsy	Malformations rates in infants from unexposed pregnancies	Malformation rate of all infants in the population

Even though the majority of data come from these pregnancy registries, there are also some meta-analyses that have evaluated the different teratogenic effects of ASMs [26–28]. A limitation of meta-analyses is the heterogeneity of data across studies in terms of populations, ascertainment methods, and endpoints. Veroniki's meta-analysis for example, included studies with different outcome criteria and some studies listing abnormalities that many would not consider MCMs, and excluded data from large prospective registries.

One last consideration is the possible teratogenic risk of epilepsy alone. Data coming from registries so far have not shown an increased risk due to the disease itself. Similar rates of MCM were seen between children of WWE who were not taking ASMs and a healthy control group: the MCM rate was 6.1% in the offspring of WWE who were treated with ASMs versus 2.8% among children of women with untreated epilepsy versus 2.2% in the healthy control group [29].

Malformation Risks for Each Antiseizure Medication

Phenobarbital

Phenobarbital (PB) is one of the oldest first-generation ASMs. It is rarely used as a first-line treatment in adults due to side effects, but it is still broadly used in the developing world due to its low cost. Considering all data gathered across pregnancy registries, there are a little over 800 pregnancies exposed to PB (an even higher number of pregnancies when considering meta-analysis as well). Pregnancy registries demonstrated that PB increases the risk of MCMs compared with either unexposed women without epilepsy or unexposed WWE. The MCM rates range between 0% and 14% across pregnancy registries (see Table 11.2).

The highest percentage (14%) is reported by the Swedish registry, but it must be observed that the cohort is extremely small with only 7 patients on PB. When looking at the biggest cohorts (NAAPR and EURAP have around 200–300 patients each), the MCM rates stay around 6–7%. The EURAP registry shows MCM rates that are dose dependent: 2.7% (0.3–9.5) for doses less than 80 mg/daily, 6.2% (3.0–11.1) for doses of 80–130 mg/daily, and rates of 11.7% (4.8–22.6) for doses greater than 120 mg/day.

Compared with a LTG dose of less than 325 mg/day, the odds of MCMs were significantly higher for PB at doses of greater than 80 mg/day: OR of 5.81 (2.40–14.08) for doses greater than 130 mg/day, and OR 2.46 (1.16–5.23) for doses of 80–130 mg/day [18]. When looking at the different types of MCMs seen with PB, cardiac abnormalities are the most common [30]. This was confirmed in two meta-analyses as well [26, 27]. In conclusion, the malformation risk is increased with PB when compared to the general population. However, it must be noted that the number of pregnancies on PB recorded across registries is still low.

Carbamazepine

The overall prevalence of malformations with the use of monotherapy carbamazepine (CBZ) ranges between 2.6% and 5.9% (see Table 11.2). These data come from different pregnancy registries with almost 8,000 pregnancies of women on CBZ. Similar percentages are observed in different meta-analyses [26, 27]. The range reflects the study methodologies of each registry. As mentioned before, the different timing of assessment between registries can give different malformations rates. Malformations most likely to be picked up between 2 and 12 months were cardiac, hip, and renal malformations, which are the ones usually seen with CBZ use. This explains why rates of malformations with CBZ exposures are highest in

Table 11.2 The rate of major congenital malformations reported for monotherapy with antiseizure medications by major pregnancy registries and population-based studies.

	Prospective pregnancy registries						Population-based studies			
	NAAPR [16]	**APR [19]**	**EURAP [18]**	**KREP [93]**	**GSK Lamotrigine [21]**	**UKEPR [17, 41, 52]**	**Danish [23]**	**Finland [2005]**	**Swedish [24]**	**Medical birth registry of Norway (MBRN) [25]**
	5,667 monotherapy	2,148 total (1,593 monotherapy)	7,355 monotherapy	1,988 (1,343 monotherapy)	1,558 monotherapy	6,130 total (5,369 monotherapy)	1,532 total	3,067 Total (1,231 monotherapy)	1,398 total (1,256 monotherapy)	2,559 total (2,309 monotherapy)
CBZ	3.0% (31/1,033)	5.9% (24/409)	5.5% (107/1957)	4.7% (44/490)		2.6% (43/1657)		2.7% (32/805)	2.7% (46/1430)	2.9% (20/685)
LTG	2.0% (31/ 1,562)	4.9% (20/406)	2.9% (74/2514)	2.00% (1/50)	2.2% (35/1558)	2.3% (49/2098)	3.7% (38/1019)		2.9% (32/1100)	3.4% (28/833)
LEV	2.4% (11/450)	3.6% (5/139)	2.8% (17/599)	4.71% (5/106)		0.70% (2/304)	0% (0/58)		0% (0/61)	1.7% (2/118)
OXC	2.2% (4/182)	5.3% (1/19)	3.0% (10/333)	7.00% (5/71)			2.8 (11/393)	1.0% (1/99)	3.7% (1/27)	1.8% (1/57)
PB	5.5% (11/199)	0% (0/2)	6.5% (19/294)	5.80% (8/137)					14% (1/7)	7.4% (2/27)
PHT	2.9% (12/416)	2.3% (1/44)	6.4% (8/125)	5.88% (7/119)		3.7% (3/82)		2.6% (7/263)	6.7% (11/103)	
TPM	4.2% (15/359)	1.9% (1/53)	3.9% (6/152)	0.00% (0/9)		4.8% 3/62	4.6% (5/108)		7.7% (4/52)	4.2% (2/48)
VPA	9.3% (30/323)	14.8% (43/290)	10.3% (142/1381)	7.91% (27/341)		6.7% (82/1220)		10.7% (28/263)	4.7% (29/619)	6.3% (21/333)
ZNS	0% (0/98)		0% (0/9)			13.04% (3/23)				
CLZ	3.1% (2/64)	0% (0/26)		0.00% (0/4)					6.2% (3/48)	1.8% (2/113)
CBZ		0% (0/2)		21.4% (3/14)						
GBP	0.7% (1/145)					3.2% (1/31)	1.7% (1/59)		0% (0/18)	

the Australian and EURAP registries, which follow enrolled infants up to 1 year of age. When looking at the number of cases for each specific type of malformation observed with CBZ, the most common ones were NTD (0.3%), cardiac malformations (0.8%), hypospadias (0.4%), and oral clefts (0.36%) [30]. Overall, the malformations observed with CBZ also include genitourinary tract defects, skeletal malformations including clubfoot and polydactyly, and respiratory and gastrointestinal malformations. A Cochrane meta-analysis of 31 observational studies reported a risk ratio of MCM of 2.01 (95% CI, 1.20–3.36) for the offspring of women using CBZ when compared with the offspring of women without epilepsy. Compared with controls, odds ratios (ORs) for MCMs were increased with CBZ (1.37; 95% CI, 1.10–1.71) [27].

Different studies have demonstrated a dose-dependent effect. In EURAP, conception doses were divided into two groups: those taking less than 700 mg/day and those taking more than 700 mg/day. The rates of MCMs at 1 year were 4.5% (3.5–5.8) for the dose group taking less than 700 mg/day were, and 7.2% (5.4–9.4) for those taking more than 700 mg/day [18]. Compared with LTG doses of less than 325 mg/day, the odds of MCMs were significantly higher for all doses of CBZ. A high dose of CBZ (>700 mg/day) was associated with increased odds compared with levetiracetam (LEV) and oxcarbazepine [18]. In UKEPR, the MCM rate seen with exposure to doses of more than 1,000 mg/day was lower (5.2%), but the OR observed was similar to EURAP's (OR 2.7) [17]. In conclusion, considering all registries and meta-analysis, the number of pregnancies on CBZ is high. The average malformation rates are around 4–5% at doses of less than 700 mg/day. These rates are higher than the overall risk of malformation seen in the general population (2–3%).

Lamotrigine

Lamotrigine is the ASM that has been studied the most across pregnancy registries and meta-analyses, with almost more than 9,000 pregnancies exposed to LTG. The range of MCMs with LTG monotherapy use is 1.9–4.9%. It is important to note that the three registries with the most data on LTG exposure (almost 6,000 pregnancies between the three registries) all showed similar low MCM rates: 2.9% in EURAP, 2.0% in NAAPR, and 2.3% in UKEPR [16–18]. Higher rates were reported by the APR (4.9%), but there was a much smaller cohort of LTG-exposed pregnancies (only 406 pregnancies) [31]. The risk of MCMs with LTG seems to be dose dependent. The EURAP study group demonstrated an increased risk with increased dose at the time of conception. An MCM risk of 4.3% (28/644) was seen for doses of LTG greater than 325 mg/day compared with 2.5% (46/1,870) for doses of LTG less than 325 mg/day (OR 1.68 [95% CI, 1.01–2.80]) [18].

The UKEPR shows a similar dose-dependent trend, but with a smaller difference of a 1.3% increase between low doses (>400 mg/day) and high doses (<200 mg/day). This difference, however, was not statistically significant [17]. A population-based cohort study using data from Danish health registers found no difference in MCM risk in a preplanned analysis that evaluated the risks associated with first-trimester mean daily doses of LTG of less than 250 mg/day (n = 766) or greater than 250 mg/day (n = 253) [23]. The most commonly observed MCMs in LTG-exposed fetuses are cardiac congenital malformations (21 cases over 3,291 pregnancies [0.6%]), hypospadias (12 cases over 3,291 pregnancies [0.36%]), NTDs (4 cases over 3,291 pregnancies [0.1%]), and cleft palate and cleft lip (5 cases over 3,291 pregnancies [0.15%]) [30]. Recent studies evaluating only LTG monotherapies did not confirm previous results on higher incidences of oral clefts with LTG. Those older studies probably reflected a contamination of the polytherapy data. In conclusion, LTG is one of the preferred ASMs for WWE of childbearing age. It is a broad-spectrum ASM that can be used for both focal and generalized epilepsy. The overall MCM rate across the three biggest pregnancy registries is comparable to the risk of malformations for the general population (2–3%).

Valproic Acid

Valproic acid (VPA) is a broad-spectrum ASM frequently prescribed for epilepsy as well as for bipolar disorder and migraine headache. It is considered one of the drugs of choice for generalized epilepsies. All pregnancy registries and meta-analyses have shown how VPA is associated with the highest rates of malformations among all ASMs. Rates of malformations range between 6.3% and 14.8% (see Table 11.2). A dose-dependent risk was reported by some pregnancy registries; EURAP reported a MCM rate of 6.4% with doses of less than 650 mg/day, 11.3% with doses of 650–1,450 mg/day, and 24.2% with doses of more than 1,450 mg/day [18]. A similar dose-dependent effect was observed in UKEPR, which reported a statistically significant higher risk with doses greater than 1,000 mg/day: 5.0% risk for VPA doses less than 600 mg, 6.1% for VPA doses 600–1,000 mg, and 10.4% for VPA doses greater than 1,000 mg [17]. Compared with LTG doses of less than 325 mg/day, the odds of MCMs were significantly higher with all doses of VPA. The low-dose category of VPA (≤650 mg/day) is associated with increased odds compared with LEV [18].

Valproic acid is consistently associated with a higher risk of NTDs (50 cases over 2,721 pregnancies [1.8%]), cardiac congenital malformations (47 cases over 2,721 pregnancies [1.7%]), hypospadias (38 cases over 2,721 pregnancies [1.3%]), and cleft palate and cleft lip (25 cases over 2,721 pregnancies [0.9%]) [30]. The UKEPR results showed that the risk of NTDs, facial clefts, and genitourinary and skeletal malformations were significantly increased for VPA compared with CBZ or LTG, but no significant difference was found for cardiac malformations between CBZ and VPA [17].

The European Surveillance of Congenital Anomalies database showed how the use of VPA monotherapy was associated with significantly increased risks for 6 of the 14 malformations under consideration. In the past, a polymalformative syndrome was described in association with the use of VPA. This syndrome consists of cardiac malformations, neural tube closure defect, hypospadias and renal malformations, cleft palate or cleft lip, craniostenosis, limb malformations, and characteristic facial dysmorphia. Due to growing evidence of increased teratogenic risks with VPA, the European guidelines recommend avoiding the use of VPA in pregnancy unless alternative treatments are not available. Additionally, most women of reproductive potential should not be prescribed VPA unless they are taking contraception. Due to those recommendations, the use of VPA for WWE has declined. A recent study evaluated the reduction of VPA-associated risk in Europe from 2005 to 2014: the incidence significantly decreased from 0.22 to 0.03 per 10,000 births in 2005/6 compared to 2013/14 [32].

Phenytoin

Phenytoin (PHT) is a first-generation, narrow-spectrum ASM of low cost, often used for focal epilepsies. Rates of MCMs associated with PHT are 2.4–6.7% across registries (see Table 11.2), but individual cohorts are small. The largest cohort studied in NAAPR published an MCM rate of 2.9% among 416 PHT-exposed pregnancies [16]. This MCM rate is not significantly different than the one observed with CBZ and with a risk ratio of 1.5

(95% CI, 0.7–2.9) when compared with LTG [16]. Only limited studies have analyzed the dose-dependent risk with PHT [16, 33–35]. Overall, their data do not consistently show an association between dose and risks of MCMs. Phenytoin is mostly associated with increased risks of cardiac malformations (4 cases over 1,002 pregnancies [0.39%]) and hypospadias (5 cases over 1,002 pregnancies [0.49%]) [30]. Phenytoin can induce carnitine deficiency in the fetus, which may lead to cardiomyopathies and ventricular septum defects [36].

In 1975, Hanson and Smith described a specific fetal hydantoin syndrome associated with in utero PHT exposure. The characteristic features of fetal hydantoin syndrome include microcephaly, craniofacial anomalies, hypertelorism, flattened nasal root, ptosis, wide mouth, cleft palate or cleft lip, cardiac defects, urogenital malformations, and hypoplastic distal phalanx and nails. They later reported that this was present in 11% of 35 exposed infants and that 31% of exposed infants had some aspects of the syndrome [37]. In 1988, Gaily and colleagues reported no evidence of the hydantoin syndrome in 82 women exposed in utero to PHT. Some patients had hypertelorism and hypoplasia of the distal phalanges, but none had the full hydantoin syndrome. Fetal hydantoin syndrome can be seen in approximately 5–10% of infants with in utero exposure to PHT, whereas AN incomplete clinical syndrome can be seen in about one-third of them [18].

Levetiracetam

Levetiracetam (LEV), due to its simple pharmacokinetics and limited side effects, is one of the most prescribed ASMs for both focal and generalized epilepsies. The overall malformation risk for LEV ranges between 0% and 4.7% across different pregnancy registries with more than 1,000 pregnancies (see Table 11.2). The largest cohort of patients comes from EURAP with 599 pregnant patients on LEV. This registry reported a very low rate of malformations of 2.8%. No association between the dose of LEV and MCM rate was found [18].

Different rates of malformations were published in 2019, in an LEV-only registry initiated by a pharmaceutical company. This registry was based on pregnancies with exposure to the name-brand version of LEV between 2004 and 2012. The assessment of malformations was based on the Metropolitan Atlanta Congenital Defects Program (MACDP), a modified version of criteria in the Centers for Disease Control and Prevention (CDC). The registry reported a malformation rate of 10.4% (95% CI, 7.7–13.6). The study reported that 46 of 444 live births with in utero LEV exposure (monotherapy or polytherapy) had malformations. Among 309 live births with monotherapy exposure were 29 malformations (9.4%: 95% CI, 6.4–13.2). Representatives from EURAP and NAAPR later reviewed the criteria used for the assessment of the malformations. Different rates of malformations were found after they applied the same criteria used in the EURAP and NAAPR registries. Based on the EURAP criteria, of the 444 live births exposed to LEV in monotherapy or polytherapy, only 4.9% would have been classified as having an MCM (compared to 10.4% considered MCM by the MACDP criteria). Using the NAAPR criteria, the rate of confirmed MCMs among all exposures was 1.5% [39]. The LEV registry had no external unexposed control group, so it is difficult to make direct comparisons to baseline malformation rates.

In conclusion, the risks associated with the use of LEV are not increased compared to the general population, suggesting that LEV could be a safe drug for WWE. It has become one of the drugs of choice for WWE of childbearing age, especially for generalized epilepsies, given the limited use of VPA. However, cohorts of pregnant patients using LEV are still small, requiring more data to confirm the safe profile of this medication in pregnancy.

Oxcarbazepine

Oxcarbazepine (OXC) is a narrow-spectrum ASM, derivative of CBZ. There are a little more than 1,000 OXC-exposed pregnancies and overall rates of MCM are low at 0–5.3% (see Table 11.2). It must be noted that the pregnancy registries with higher numbers (200–300) of pregnancies showed rates of 1.6–3%, values similar to MCM rates in the general population. A 2018 study by Tomson and colleagues, which is the largest of the individual studies, compared the risk seen with OXC (dose ≥ 75 mg/day to 4,500 mg/day) to that seen with other individual ASMs, and these data do not suggest that the risk differs significantly from that seen with LTG (≤325 mg/day), LEV (250–4,000 mg/day), or CBZ (≤700 mg/day) [18]. The study showed how high doses of CBZ (>700 mg/day) are associated with increased odds compared with OXC. Given the limited number of pregnant patients on OXC, further data will be required to adequately counsel women who use OXC in pregnancy.

Topiramate

Topiramate (TPM) is a broad-spectrum ASM used for epilepsy but also for other conditions such as migraine. Data are available on almost 1,000 TPM-exposed pregnancies. The risk of malformations is 1.9–7.0% (see Table 11.2). The lower risk of 1.9% comes from a very small cohort of only 53 pregnancies. Overall, these data support an increased risk of malformations in offspring of pregnant WWE who took TPM compared with controls (unexposed women with or without epilepsy).

A population-based study evaluated the presence of oral clefts specifically with TPM. This study included a cohort of 1,360,101 pregnant women with a live-born infant from 3 months before conception through 1 month after delivery. Oral clefts were defined as the presence of a recorded diagnosis in claims during the first 90 days after birth. The risk of oral clefts at birth was 4.1 per 1,000 in the 2,425 infants born to women exposed to TPM compared with 1.1 per 1,000 in the unexposed group. This same study showed a dose-dependent effect. The risk ratio for oral clefts associated with TPM doses less than or equal to 100 mg was 1.64 (95% CI, 0.53–5.07) and for TPM doses greater than 100 mg, it was 5.16 (95% CI, 1.94–13.73) [40]. However, results must be interpreted with caution as the cohort of pregnant WWE treated with a lower dose was much smaller.

The UKEPR evaluated all cases of TPM monotherapy exposure (70 pregnancies) and reported that three infants had MCMs. For these three patients, the average total daily dose was 400 mg of TPM compared to 238 mg in those without an MCM [41]. In addition to oral cleft being the most frequent malformation observed with TPM, hypospadias and cardiac malformations were reported, but no NTDs [16].

Zonisamide

Zonisamide is a broad-spectrum ASM used for generalized epilepsy. Data about this medication come from a total of only 142 pregnancies worldwide. Different rates have been reported by different studies, and UKEPR recently released information about risk of MCMs with zonisamide in monotherapy and polytherapy. Only 26 patients using zonisamide on monotherapy were enrolled between 1996 and 2020 (and 86 exposed to polytherapy). Among the 26 monotherapy exposures were three spontaneous and two induced abortions. This group of 26 patients reported three MCMs: two of those were severe malformations (anencephaly and an omphalocele with exstrophy and anal-spinal defects in another) that occurred in the two induced abortions. The third malformation was an inguinal hernia. The MCM rate calculated among live births and induced abortions was 13% (3/23). In the polytherapy group, the MCM rate was 6.9% [42].

The NAAPR did not find a high rate of MCMs in pregnancies exposed to zonisamide monotherapy. In their cohort of 98 patients on zonisamide, no MCMs were reported [16, 42]. A Maternal Outcomes and Neurodevelopmental Effects of Antiepileptic Drugs (MONEAD) study reported one MCM in 13 pregnancies, EURAP reported zero in 3 pregnancies, and APR reported one MCM in 5 exposures [18, 44, 45]. These cohorts are still small; more pregnancies will be needed to have a better understanding of the teratogenic risk related to zonisamide.

Other Antiseizure Medications

For other ASMs such as lacosamide, eslicarbazepine, retigabine/ezogabine, and perampanel, very little data is available on their use during pregnancy. A cohort population-based study evaluated the presence of malformations with pregabalin. Of 477 infants exposed to pregabalin during the first trimester, 28 (5.9%) had malformations compared to 3.3% in nonexposed infants [46]. Animal models (rodents) have shown an association between lacosamide and embyrolethality as well as behavioral abnormalities [47]. An abstract from a commercial global pharmacovigilance database reported one malformation in 16 monotherapy exposures [48]. Unpublished data available online from the NAAPR report 65 pregnancies exposed to lacosamide monotherapy with no identified malformations [49].

Very small cohorts of patients exposed to benzodiazepines are reported. Rates of MCMs with clonazepam exposure in small cohorts is 0–6.8%. The largest cohort from the medical birth registry of Norway reported a rate of 1.8% in 113 pregnancies exposed to clonazepam monotherapy [25]. Given these limited data, the use of these new ASMs in pregnancy remains uncertain due to unknown risks of malformations. Therefore, these medications should be avoided in pregnant WWE.

Monotherapy versus Polytherapy

Previous studies suggested that MCMs were occurring more frequently with ASM polytherapy than with monotherapy [50]. However, more recent results coming from three prospective registries demonstrated how the type of ASMs included in the polytherapy regimen is more important than whether the therapy is monotherapy or polytherapy [51, 52]. All registries showed similar findings with an increased risk of malformations with polytherapies that involve either VPA or TPA.

The Australian registry showed similar results with higher MCM rates in polytherapy pregnancies: MCMs occurred in 44 of the 508 polytherapy pregnancies (8.7%) versus 87 of the 1,302 monotherapy pregnancies (6.7%). This difference, however, was not significant (OR = 2.25; 95% CI, 0.90, 5.62). Excluding all pregnancies involving VPA, the malformed fetus rates became 8.18% (27 in 330) for polytherapy pregnancies and 4.77% (87 in 1,007) for monotherapy pregnancies (OR = 1.78; 95% CI, 1.09, 2.90). Excluding only TPM-exposed pregnancies, the malformation rates were 7% (29 in 415) for polytherapy pregnancies and 6.87% (86 in 1,252) for monotherapy pregnancies (OR = 1.02; 95% CI, 0.66, 1.58). Of note, the mean valproate dose was 859 ± 635 mg per day in the polytherapy pregnancies and 904 ± 574 mg per day in the monotherapy ones. For TPM, the mean dose was 246 ± 138 mg/day in polytherapy and 196 ± 118 mg per day for monotherapy pregnancies [53].

The UKEPR also showed an increased risk of MCMs in infants exposed to ASM polytherapy compared with monotherapy. The MCM rates were higher with polytherapy use at 6% (95% CI, 4.5–8.0) compared with 3.7% (95% CI, 3.4–5.0) in monotherapy, but MCM rates were highest when polytherapy regimens contained VPA [52]. Treatment including VPA with TPM either as part of a dual therapy regimen (n = 12, MCM rate 36.4%; 95% CI, 15.2–64.6) or as part of a regimen of three or more ASMs (n = 23, MCM rate 23.8%; 95% CI, 10.6–45.1) was associated with the highest rates of MCMs [41].

Data from Norway seem to indicate a similar trend for minimal increase in the rates of MCMs for polytherapy with "newer" ASMs, except TPM, which, similar to VPA, seemed to elevate the MCM rate [25].

In 2011, NAAPR data revealed that not all ASMs polytherapy combinations are alike. The MCM rates were 9.1% for LTG plus VPA (OR = 5.0; 95% CI, 1.5–14.0) but only 2.9% for LTG with any other ASM (OR = 1.5; 95% CI, 0.7–3.0); likewise, the risks were 15.4% for CBZ plus VPA (OR = 6.2; 95% CI, 2.0–16.5) and 2.5% for CBZ plus any other ASM (OR = 0.8; 95% CI, 0.3–1.9) [53]. In conclusion, polytherapy per se does not seem to be increasing the MCM risk but more specifically the inclusion of VPA or TPA as part of the polytherapy is associated with the observed increased risks of malformations.

Teratogenesis in Repeated Pregnancies

Few data exist about outcomes of subsequent pregnancies within the same pregnant WWE taking ASM. In 2001, Duncan reported two cases of WWE taking moderate doses of VPA who repeatedly bore children with NTDs, despite folate supplementation [94]. Authors hypothesized that these women were more susceptible to the effects of VPA because of failure of upregulation of the human form of folate-binding protein (FR α and FR β), MTHFR, or some of the other candidate genes thought to play a role in neural tube development.

Data about repeated pregnancies come from the Australian registry, which reported data on 15 women who had two or more pregnancies that resulted in fetuses with malformations. Women taking any ASM who had given birth to a malformed baby in their first enrolled pregnancy and who continued taking the same drug were at increased risk of having a malformed offspring in their next pregnancy (35.7% vs. 3.1%). These results seemed to be mostly related to the use of VPA. They indicated that, if a woman taking VPA in one pregnancy gave birth to a malformed fetus, her absolute risk of having a malformed fetus in her next pregnancy if she continued to take the drug was greater than 50% (57.2% vs. 7.0%; OR 17.8), as compared with women continuing to take the drug whose index pregnancies produced non-malformed fetuses.

There was also a trend of an increased risk of a malformed fetus in women who had a malformed fetus in previous pregnancies in which they took an ASM other than VPA, although this trend was not as strong and did not attain statistical significance [54]. These results suggest a possible inherent individual vulnerability of some women to the pro-teratogenic effects of ASMs, in particular VPA. This raises the possibility that specific genetic characteristics in women or their partners render such women more likely to have fetuses with malformations.

A genetic role in teratogenesis has been suggested by other studies as well. In the EURAP registry, a personal history of an MCM in one parent was associated with a fourfold increased risk of having a child with ASM-associated MCMs (OR = 4.4; 95% CI, 2.06–9.23, p = 0.0001)

[55]. Among ASM-exposed children, de novo copy number variants (CNVs) and de novo single-nucleotide variants/indels (SNVs/indels) were not seen more frequently in children with birth defects compared to those without [56]. Authors suggest that these findings argue against ASM-associated mutagenesis. Further research is needed to understand how teratogenesis due to ASMs occurs. In particular, it would be incredibly helpful to understand if a genetic susceptibility could identify which mother–infant pairs are at greatest risk.

Cognitive Outcome

It is now well established that the first trimester is the crucial period during which malformations due to ASMs exposure occur. However, in the past 10–20 years, more studies started evaluating the effects of ASMs on cognitive development and how this might be the consequence of drug exposures that occur throughout the entire pregnancy, even beyond the first trimester.

Most human studies have been retrospective or prospective observational studies of pregnant WWE. All studies have shown a strong association between VPA and developmental delay. A Cochrane Review reported a significant reduction in IQ in VPA-exposed children compared to children of mothers treated with CBZ, children of mothers with untreated epilepsy, and children of mothers without epilepsy [57]. It is very important to take into consideration the maternal IQ as an important predictor of the child IQ. The major studies that have incorporated the maternal IQ in their analyses are: the Neurodevelopmental Effects of Antiepileptic Drugs (NEAD) study [58, 59], the Liverpool and Manchester Neurodevelopmental Group (LMNG) study, and an Australian cohort [60].

The US- and UK-based NEAD study has been the most comprehensive prospective multicenter observational study of exposure and neurodevelopmental effects, assessing outcomes such as IQ and behavior in children up to 6 years post-exposure [61]. The NEAD study enrolled women on ASM monotherapy (CBZ, LTG, PHT, or VPA) between October 1999 and February 2004, across 25 epilepsy centers in the United Kingdom and the United States. The primary outcome was the child's IQ at 6 years of age adjusted for maternal IQ. At 3- and 6-year follow-ups, fetal exposure to VPA was associated with an IQ reduced by 7–10 points compared with exposure to CBZ, LTG, and PHT [61]. Exposure to VPA was also associated with worse verbal and memory abilities compared with exposure to other drugs and reduced nonverbal and executive functions compared with LTG exposure. Those cognitive deficits due to VPA were dose-related but no dose-related effects were observed with the other drugs [59, 61]. The LMNG study demonstrated a dose-dependent relationship. Even though exposure to lower doses of VPA (<800 mg daily) was associated with mildly reduced IQ, the difference was not statistically significant. However, lower doses were still associated with impaired verbal abilities and a sixfold increase in need for educational intervention. Higher doses of daily VPA (>800 mg daily) were associated with a 9.7-point-lower adjusted IQ and an eightfold increased need for educational intervention [62]. Of note, a subset of the patients in the LMNG study participated in the NEAD study as well.

A study that assessed children between the ages of 5 and 9 showed similar results. Increasing the dose of VPA was associated with poorer full-scale IQ (CI 216.3–25.0, p, 0.001), verbal abilities (CI 216.8–25.5, p, 0.001), nonverbal abilities (CI 217.3–24.9, p, 0.001), and expressive language ability (CI 23.4–21.6, p, 0.001) [63].

A recent population-based study from the Danish National Prescription registry included all children born between January 1, 1996, and December 31, 2011. The aim was to evaluate the risk of intellectual disability and delayed development in childhood. Among mothers with epilepsy, offspring exposed prenatally to valproate had increased risk of intellectual disability (aHR, 1.95; 95% CI, 1.21–3.14) and intellectual disability with delayed childhood milestones (aHR, 3.07; 95% CI, 2.24–4.20) compared with offspring without prenatal exposure [64].

Regarding other ASMs, very few data are available on their possible effect on cognitive development. A study from Denmark from 1995 raised the concern that PB exposure during early development can have long-term deleterious effects on cognitive performance, especially on verbal intelligence scores [65]. These findings led to recommendations to avoid PB if possible during pregnancy [15].

Carbamazepine does not seem to affect neurocognitive development [66, 67]. IQ appears to be comparable in school-aged children to controls, as well as children exposed to LTG. With regard to specific skills, the NEAD study raised the possibility of dose relationship with poorer verbal and motor skills [61]. Recently, the Danish population-based study showed that compared with offspring without prenatal exposure to ASMs, children with prenatal exposure to maternal monotherapy use of CBZ were at increased risk of intellectual disability (aHR, 3.84; 95% CI, 2.32–6.38), clonazepam (aHR, 2.41; 95% CI, 1.09–5.35), and OXC (aHR, 3.70; 95% CI, 2.11–6.51), but not LTG (aHR, 1.33; 95% CI, 0.71–2.48) [64].

Fewer data are available regarding other ASMs. Other studies have also shown that children exposed to LGT are comparable to controls in terms of global neurodevelopment and adaptive behavior. The NEAD study showed how right-handedness was less frequent than expected in LTG-exposed children, raising the concern that verbal abilities were worse than nonverbal abilities in LTG-exposed children [59]. Baker and colleagues found that children exposed to LTG in utero did not have significantly lower IQ or specific verbal, nonverbal, or spatial disabilities in comparison to control children [62]. No dose effect on cognition has been demonstrated for LTG.

Few studies have assessed the effects of LEV on cognitive development. The LMNG study showed that following in utero exposure to LEV, the developmental scores at 3 years were similar to controls but better than those of VPA-exposed children [58, 59]. Similar results came from UKEPR, where no associations were found between prenatal exposure to LEV and reductions in children's cognitive abilities. Additionally, adverse outcomes were not associated with increasing the dose [70]. The UK study assessing children at school age also showed how increased doses of LEV were not associated with poorer outcomes in comparison to control children and were documented to have superior outcomes to the children exposed to higher doses of valproate [63]. Animal studies have also suggested LEV does not cause the cellular changes seen with exposure to other ASMs.

One study investigated the abilities of nine school-aged children prenatally exposed to TPM in utero. This study reported lower IQ scores across several domains as well as poorer motor and visual spatial skills in the children exposed to TPM in comparison to control children [71]. A later study on 27 children exposed to TPM did not observe any association between TPM use and reduced cognitive abilities, even with higher doses of TPM. These results, however, should be evaluated with caution given the small sample of patients.

Behavioral Outcome

In addition to its effect on cognitive development, ASM exposure has been associated with adverse effects on behavioral outcomes. A retrospective study assessed 242 children aged between 6 and 16 years born to WWE [72]. Exposure to VPA in utero was associated with high levels of parental stress induced by the child's maladaptive behavior. Children also showed lower scores on tasks relating to daily living and socialization skills than children exposed to other ASMs. A diagnosis of autism spectrum disorder (ASD) was made in 4 (6%) of 64 children exposed to VPA monotherapy in pregnancy. None of 76 children exposed in utero to CBZ and 1 of 44 exposed to LTG monotherapy had ASD [73]. The association between exposure to VPA and ASD was later confirmed in a population-based Danish register study, showing that even doses as low as 750 mg/day increase the risk of ASD significantly. The cohort of patients (N = 913,302) was followed up from birth until the day of the ADHD diagnosis, death, emigration, or December 31, 2015, whichever came first. This study showed a 48% increased risk of attention deficit hyperactivity disorder (ADHD) compared with children with no VPA exposure [74].

The NEAD study showed how children of mothers who took VPA during their pregnancies were at a significantly greater risk of a diagnosis of ADHD [59]. Taking into account all developmental problems, it has been estimated that 30–40% of preschool children exposed to VPA in utero may be affected [75].

A recent prospective observation study (2015–18) examined the behavioral functioning of children exposed to CBZ, LTG, LEV, and VPA. The Child Behavior Checklist and the Social Emotional Questionnaire were used to assess behavioral problems. The study included a total of 81 children. Behavioral problems were found in 32% of VPA-exposed children, 14% of CBZ-exposed children, 16% of LTG-exposed children, and 14% of LEV-exposed children. Children exposed to VPA had significantly more social problems than those exposed to LTG or LEV and more attention problems than those exposed to LEV. Children exposed to LTG had more attention deficit but were less anxious than LEV-exposed children [76]. Other studies did not find any significant increase in ASD in children exposed in utero to CBZ [77, 78].

The Role of Folic Acid

Folate, or vitamin B9, is thought of as one of the 13 essential vitamins. It cannot be synthesized de novo by the body and must be obtained either from diet or from supplementation. Folic acid (FA), on the other hand, is a synthetic dietary supplement present in artificially enriched foods and pharmaceutical vitamins. Neither folate nor FA are metabolically active. To become metabolically active, FA must first be converted to dihydrofolate (DHF) and then tetrahydrofolate (THF) through enzymatic reduction, a process catalyzed by the enzyme DHF reductase (DHFR). Afterward, THF can be converted to the biologically active L-methylfolate by the enzyme methylenetetrahydrofolate reductase (MTHFR).

The active metabolite of FA plays an important role in cellular metabolic activities, such as functioning as a cofactor in one-carbon metabolism for DNA and RNA synthesis as well as nucleotide and amino acid biosynthesis in the body. Demands for folate increase during pregnancy as it is required for THE growth and development of the fetus. Folate deficiency has been associated with abnormal growth and development in experimental animal and human studies, and it has been hypothesized as one of the possible mechanisms involved in teratogenesis [79]. Randomized controlled trials, systematic reviews, and meta-analyses have shown how FA supplementation reduces teratogenic risks [80]. In particular, FA decreases the risk of birth of infants with NTDs, obstructive urinary tract anomalies, limb deficiencies, orofacial clefts, and congenital hypertrophic pyloric stenosis. The role of periconceptional FA in the prevention of NTDs has been investigated since the 1980s. A randomized controlled trial in Hungary was one of the first to show a reduction in recurrent NTDs with FA supplementation [81]. Due to the known risks associated with folate deficiency, many countries have introduced mandatory fortification of cereals and grains with FA, which has been associated with a risk reduction of 20–60% [82]. Additionally, many countries started developing policies on the supplementation of FA in pregnancy: a prescription of a 0.4 mg FA tablet daily to all women planning pregnancy and 4 mg of FA to those with a previous pregnancy affected by NTDs.

In 2009, the American Academy of Neurology posited that preconception FA supplementation in WWE may be considered to reduce the risk of MCMs (Level C) [15]. Due to ASM treatment, WWE are at greater risk for low folate serum levels than the general population: both enzyme inducers ASM and VPA can interfere with folate metabolism [83, 84]. Serum and red blood cell folate are reduced in up to 90% of patients receiving PHT, CBZ, or barbiturates [85]. Antiseizure medications that do not induce cytochrome P450 enzymes are not associated with low levels of FA. Evidence from experimental models of epilepsy in rats showed that valproate lowered brain folate levels and partially blocked the reuptake of folinic acid [86]. Because of this, WWE are often recognized as a high-risk group and the recommended FA supplementation in this group of patients is of high doses (up to 4 mg/day).

The reduction of MCMs in WWE who take an FA supplement has not been demonstrated conclusively. In the Australian registry, the rate of MCM was 5.08% in 1,495 pregnancies treated with preconception folate and 4.94% in 628 untreated pregnancies (relative risk 1.02; 95% CI, 0.69, 1.55) [19]. The UKEPR reported rates of MCMs in offspring of women on ASMs with appropriate folate intake that were at least as high as those in women on ASMs without appropriate folate intake. The total MCM rate for women taking FA during the first trimester was 3.6% (95% CI, 3.1–4.2) compared with 2.7% (95% CI, 1.5–4.8) for those not taking FA ($p = 0.39$) [87]. In the MONEAD study, there was no effect of periconceptional folate on MCMs; however, the use of folate in pregnant WWE was high at 86% [44]. Similarly, there was no effect of periconceptional folate on MCMs in the NEAD study [61]. these findings should not discourage WWE from taking folic acid. Most likely those results are biased by the fact that women at greater risk are more likely to take folate.

Studies evaluating the effect of FA on cognitive and behavioral development showed good results. A large cohort study from Norway has suggested reduced rates of autism with periconceptional FA supplementation [88]. The NEAD study also demonstrated the protective effects of FA against reduced measures of cognitive development. At 6-year follow-up, periconceptional FA exposure was associated with a higher IQ compared with no FA exposure for each of the four ASMs studied, including VPA. For all 311 children in the study, periconceptional FA was associated with an average of 5 points higher in their IQ [61]. In the large prospective Norwegian mother and child cohort study, periconceptional FA exposure prior to and during the first trimester was associated with a fourfold reduction in the risk of delayed language skills at 18 months in the children of mothers exposed to many different ASMs, including VPA [89]. In similar Norwegian mother and child cohorts [88, 90] and in other studies [91, 92], periconceptional FA also reduced the risk of autistic traits in children of ASM-treated mothers and of mothers without epilepsy or exposure to ASMs.

In conclusion, recommendations from the American Academy of Neurology and the American Epilepsy Society in 2009 stated that the data are insufficient to show that folate is effective in reducing MCMs in pregnant WWE, but noted that risk of MCMs in the offspring of WWE is possibly decreased by FA supplementation based on two adequate Class III studies. Guidelines recommend up to 4 mg of FA daily prior to and during at least the first trimester of any pregnancy in WWE on VPA or other ASMs. Additionally, since it is estimated that half of pregnancies are not planned, FA supplementation should be recommended at the time of prescription of any ASM in women of childbearing age.

References

1. Finnell RH. Teratology: General considerations and principles. *J Allergy Clin Immunol.* 1999;**103**(2 Pt 2):S337–42.
2. Gilbert-Barness E. Teratogenic causes of malformations. *Ann Clin Lab Sci.* 2010;**40**(2):99–114.
3. Veurink M, Koster M, de Jong–van den Berg LTW. The history of DES, lessons to be learned. *Pharm World Sci.* 2005;**27**(3):139–43.
4. Archives N, Administration R. Federal Register: 44 Fed. Reg. 37191 (June 26, 1979). Vol. **44**. 1979. 37191–0.
5. Pernia S, DeMaagd G. The new pregnancy and lactation labeling rule. *PT.* 2016;**41**(11):713–15.
6. Carlson B. *Human embryology and developmental biology.* 5th ed. Philadelphia: Elsevier; 2014.
7. Corsello G, Giuffrè M. Congenital malformations. *J Matern Neonatal Med.* 2012;**25**(Suppl. 1):25–9.
8. Leppig KA, Werler MM, Cann CI, Cook CA, Holmes LB. Predictive value of minor anomalies. I. Association with major malformations. *J Pediatr.* 1987;**110**(4):531–7.
9. Update on overall prevalence of major birth defects: Atlanta, Georgia, 1978–2005. *MMWR Morb Mortal Wkly Rep.* 2008;**57**(1):1–5.
10. Smulian JC, Beres-Sochka L, DePrince K, et al. Birth defects surveillance. *N J Med.* 2002;**99**(12):25–31.
11. Viinikainen K, Heinonen S, Eriksson K, Kälviäinen R. Community-based, prospective, controlled study of obstetric and neonatal outcome of 179 pregnancies in women with epilepsy. *Epilepsia.* 2006;**47**(1):186–92.
12. Meadow SR. Anticonvulsant drugs and congenital abnormalities. *Lancet.* 1968;**2**(7581):1296.
13. Meador K, Reynolds MW, Crean S, Fahrbach K, Probst C. Pregnancy outcomes in women with epilepsy: A systematic review and meta-analysis of published pregnancy registries and cohorts. *Epilepsy Research.* 2008;**81**(1):1–13.
14. Tomson T, Battino D, Perucca E. Teratogenicity of antiepileptic drugs. *Curr Opin Neurol.* 2019;**32**(2):246–52.
15. Harden CL, Pennell PB, Koppel BS, et al. Practice parameter update: Management issues for women with epilepsy. Focus on pregnancy (an evidence-based review): Vitamin K, folic acid, blood levels, and breastfeeding. 2009. www.neurology.org.
16. Hernández-Díaz S, Smith CR, Shen A, et al. Comparative safety of antiepileptic drugs during pregnancy. *Neurology.* 2012;**78**(21):1692–9.
17. Campbell E, Kennedy F, Russell A, et al. Malformation risks of antiepileptic drug monotherapies in pregnancy: Updated results from the UK and Ireland epilepsy and pregnancy registers. *J Neurol Neurosurg Psychiatry.* 2014;**85**(9):1029–34.
18. Tomson T, Battino D, Bonizzoni E, et al. Comparative risk of major congenital malformations with eight different antiepileptic drugs: A prospective cohort study of the EURAP registry. *Lancet Neurol.* 2018;**17**(6):530–8.

19. Vajda FJE, Graham JE, Hitchcock AA, et al. Antiepileptic drugs and foetal malformation: Analysis of 20 years of data in a pregnancy register. *Seizure*. 2019;**65** (December 2018):6–11. https://doi.org/10.1016/j.seizure.2018.12.006.
20. Thomas SV, Jose M, Divakaran S, Sankara Sarma P. Malformation risk of antiepileptic drug exposure during pregnancy in women with epilepsy: Results from a pregnancy registry in south India. *Epilepsia*. 2017;**58**(2):274–81.
21. Cunnington MC, Weil JG, Messenheimer JA, et al. Final results from 18 years of the International Lamotrigine Pregnancy Registry. *Neurology*. 2011;**76**(21):1817–23.
22. Artama M, Auvinen A, Raudaskoski T, Isojärvi I, Isojärvi J. Antiepileptic drug use of women with epilepsy and congenital malformations in offspring. *Neurology*. 2005;**64**(11):1874–8.
23. Mølgaard-Nielsen D, Hviid A. Newer-generation antiepileptic drugs and the risk of major birth defects. *Obstet Gynecol Surv*. 2011;**66**(9):543–4.
24. Wide K, Winbladh B, Källén B. Major malformations in infants exposed to antiepileptic drugs in utero, with emphasis on carbamazepine and valproic acid: A nation-wide, population-based register study. *Acta Paediatr Int J Paediatr*. 2004;**93**(2):174–6.
25. Veiby G, Daltveit AK, Engelsen BA, Gilhus NE. Fetal growth restriction and birth defects with newer and older antiepileptic drugs during pregnancy. *J Neurol*. 2014;**261**(3):579–88.
26. Veroniki AA, Rios P, Cogo E, et al. Comparative safety of antiepileptic drugs for neurological development in children exposed during pregnancy and breast feeding: A systematic review and network meta-analysis. *BMJ Open*. 2017;7(7): e017248. 1–11.
27. Weston J, Bromley R, Jackson CF, et al. Monotherapy treatment of epilepsy in pregnancy: Congenital malformation outcomes in the child. *Cochrane Database Syst Rev*. 2016;**11**(11):CD010224.
28. Viale L, Allotey J, Cheong-See F, et al. Epilepsy in pregnancy and reproductive outcomes: A systematic review and meta-analysis. www.thelancet.com. http://dx.doi.org/10.1016.
29. Tomson T, Marson A, Boon P, et al. Valproate in the treatment of epilepsy in girls and women of childbearing potential. *Epilepsia*. 2015;**56**(7):1006–19.
30. Tomson T, Battino D. Teratogenic effects of antiepileptic drugs. *Lancet Neurol*. 2012;**11**(9):803–13.
31. Vajda FJE, O'Brien TJ, Graham J, Lander CM, Eadie MJ. Prediction of the hazard of foetal malformation in pregnant women with epilepsy. *Epilepsy Research*. 2014;**108**:1013–17.
32. Morris JK, Garne E, Loane M, et al. Prevalence of valproate syndrome in Europe from 2005 to 2014: A registry based multi-centre study. *Eur J Med Genet*. 2018;**61**(9):479–82.
33. Nulman I, Scolnik D, Chitayat D, Farkas LD, Koren G. Findings in children exposed in utero to phenytoin and carbamazepine monotherapy: Independent effects of epilepsy and medications. *Am J Med Genet*. 1997;**68**(1):18–24.
34. Samrén EB, Van Duijn CM, Koch S, et al. Maternal use of antiepileptic drugs and the risk of major congenital malformations: A joint European prospective study of human teratogenesis associated with maternal epilepsy. *Epilepsia*. 1997;**38**(9):981–90.
35. Kaaja E, Kaaja R, Hiilesmaa V. Major malformations in offspring of women with epilepsy. *Neurology*. 2003;**60**(4):575–9.
36. Nicolai J, Vles JSH, Aldenkamp AP. Neurodevelopmental delay in children exposed to antiepileptic drugs in utero: A critical review directed at structural study-bias. *J Neurol Sci*. 2008;**271**(1–2):1–14.
37. Hanson JW, Smith DW. The fetal hydantoin syndrome. *J Pediatr*. 1975;**87**(2):285–90.
38. Correa-Villaseñor A, Cragan J, Kucik J, et al. The Metropolitan Atlanta Congenital

Defects Program: 35 years of birth defects surveillance at the Centers for Disease Control and Prevention. *Birth Defects Res Part A – Clin Mol Teratol.* 2003;**67**(9):617–24.

39. Scheuerle AE, Holmes LB, Albano JD, et al. Levetiracetam pregnancy registry: Final results and a review of the impact of registry methodology and definitions on the prevalence of major congenital malformations. *Birth Defects Res.* 2019;**111**(13):872–87.

40. Hernandez-Diaz S, Huybrechts KF, Desai RJ, et al. Topiramate use early in pregnancy and the risk of oral clefts A pregnancy cohort study. *Neurology.* 2018;**90**(4):E342–51.

41. Hunt S, Russell MA, Smithson WH, et al. Levetiracetam in pregnancy: Preliminary experience from the UK Epilepsy and Pregnancy Register. *Neurology.* 67(10):1876–9.

42. McCluskey G, Kinney MO, Russell A, et al. Zonisamide safety in pregnancy: Data from the UK and Ireland epilepsy and pregnancy register. *Seizure.* 2021;**91**:311–15.

43. Hernández-Díaz S, Mittendorf R, Smith CR, et al. Association between topiramate and zonisamide use during pregnancy and low birth weight. *Obstet Gynecol.* 2014;**123**(1):21–8.

44. Meador KJ, Pennell PB, May RC, et al. Fetal loss and malformations in the MONEAD study of pregnant women with epilepsy. *Neurology.* 2020;**94**(14):E1502–11.

45. Vajda FJE, Perucca P, O'Brien TJ, Lander CM, Eadie MJ. Teratogenic effects of zonisamide. *Seizure.* 2021;**91**(July):490.

46. Patorno E, Bateman BT, Huybrechts KF, et al. Pregabalin use early in pregnancy and the risk of major congenital malformations. *Neurology.* 2017;**88**(21):2020–5.

47. López-Escobar B, Fernández-Torres R, Vargas-López V, et al. Lacosamide intake during pregnancy increases the incidence of foetal malformations and symptoms associated with schizophrenia in the offspring of mice. *Sci Rep.* 2020;**10**(1):1–14.

48. Golembesky A, Cooney M, Craig J, et al. Outcomes following exposure to the antiepileptic drug lacosamide during pregnancy: Results from a global safety database (P5.231). *Neurology.* 2017;**88**(16 Supplement):P5.231.

49. The North American Antiepileptic Drug Pregnancy Registry. Updated data available online. 2020.

50. Harden CL, Meador KJ, Pennell PB, et al. Management issues for women with epilepsy-Focus on pregnancy (an evidence-based review): II. Teratogenesis and perinatal outcomes: Report of the Quality Standards Subcommittee and Therapeutics and Technology Subcommittee of the American Academy of Neurol. *Epilepsia.* 2009;**50**(5):1237–46.

51. Holmes LB, Mittendorf R, Shen A, Smith CR, Hernandez-Diaz S. Fetal effects of anticonvulsant polytherapies: Different risks from different drug combinations. *Arch Neurol.* 2011;**68**(10):1275–81.

52. Morrow J, Russell A, Guthrie E, et al. Malformation risks of antiepileptic drugs in pregnancy: A prospective study from the UK Epilepsy and Pregnancy Register. *J Neurol Neurosurg Psychiatry.* 2006;**77**(2):193–8.

53. Vajda FJE, O'Brien TJ, Graham JE, et al. Antiepileptic drug polytherapy in pregnant women with epilepsy. *Acta Neurol Scand.* 2018;**138**(2):115–21.

54. Vajda FJE, O'Brien TJ, Lander CM, et al. Teratogenesis in repeated pregnancies in antiepileptic drug-treated women. *Epilepsia.* 2013;**54**(1):181–6.

55. Tomson T, Battino D, Bonizzoni E, et al. Dose-dependent risk of malformations with antiepileptic drugs: An analysis of data from the EURAP epilepsy and pregnancy registry. *Lancet Neurol.* 2011;**10**(7):609–17.

56. Perucca P, Anderson A, Jazayeri D, et al. Antiepileptic drug teratogenicity and de novo genetic variation load. *Ann Neurol.* 2020;**87**(6):897–906.

57. Bromley R, Weston J, Adab N, et al. Treatment for epilepsy in pregnancy: Neurodevelopmental outcomes in the

child. *Cochrane Database of Systematic Reviews*. 2014;**10**:CD010236.

58. Meador KJ, Baker GA, Browning N, et al. Cognitive function at 3 years of age after fetal exposure to antiepileptic drugs. *N Engl J Med*. 2009;**360**(16):1597–1605.
59. Cohen MJ, Meador KJ, Browning N, et al. Fetal antiepileptic drug exposure: Adaptive and emotional/behavioral functioning at age 6 years. *Epilepsy Behav*. 2013;**29**(2):308–15. http://dx.doi.org/10.1016/j.yebeh.2013.08.001.
60. Nadebaum C, Anderson V, Vajda F, Reutens D, Wood A. Neurobehavioral consequences of prenatal antiepileptic drug exposure. *Dev Neuropsychol*. 2012;**37**(1):1–29. www.ncbi.nlm.nih.gov/pubmed/22292829.
61. Meador KJ, Baker GA, Browning N, et al. Fetal antiepileptic drug exposure and cognitive outcomes at age 6 years (NEAD study): A prospective observational study. *Lancet Neurol*. 2013;**12**(3):244–52. http://dx.doi.org/10.1016/S1474-4422(12)70323-X.
62. Baker GA, Bromley RL, Briggs M, et al. IQ at 6 years after in utero exposure to antiepileptic drugs: A controlled cohort study. *Neurology*. 2015;**84**(4):382–90.
63. Bromley RL, Calderbank R, Cheyne CP, et al. Cognition in school-age children exposed to levetiracetam, topiramate, or sodium valproate. *Neurology*. 2016;**87**(18):1943–53.
64. Daugaard CA, Pedersen L, Sun Y, Dreier JW, Christensen J. Association of prenatal exposure to valproate and other antiepileptic drugs with intellectual disability and delayed childhood milestones. *JAMA Netw Open*. 2020;**3**(11): e2025570.
65. Reinisch JM, Sanders SA, Mortensen EL, Rubin DB. In utero exposure to phenobarbital and intelligence deficits in adult men. *JAMA*. 1995;**274**(19):1518–25.
66. Wide K, Henning E, Tomson T, Winbladh B. Psychomotor development in preschool children exposed to antiepileptic drugs in utero. *Acta Paediatr*. 2002;**91**(4):409–14.
67. Bromley RL, Mawer G, Love J, et al. Early cognitive development in children born to women with epilepsy: A prospective report. *Epilepsia*. 2010;**51**(10):2058–65.
68. Shallcross R, Bromley RL, Cheyne CP, et al. In utero exposure to levetiracetam vs. valproate: Development and language at 3 years of age. *Neurology*. 2014;**82**(3):213–21.
69. Shallcross R, Bromley BRL, Irwin B, et al. Child development following in utero exposure: Levetiracetam vs sodium valproate. 2011. www.epilepsyandpregnancy.co.uk.
70. Bromley RL, Baker GA. Fetal antiepileptic drug exposure and cognitive outcomes. *Seizure*. 2017;**44**:225–31.
71. Rihtman T, Parush S, Ornoy A. Preliminary findings of the developmental effects of in utero exposure to topiramate. *Reprod Toxicol*. 2012;**34**(3):308–11.
72. Vinten J, Bromley RL, Taylor J, et al. The behavioral consequences of exposure to antiepileptic drugs in utero. *Epilepsy Behav*. 2009;**14**(1):197–201.
73. Bromley RL, Mawer G, Clayton-Smith J, Baker GA. Autism spectrum disorders following in utero exposure to antiepileptic drugs. *Neurology*. 2008;**71**(23):1923–4.
74. Christensen J, Grønborg TK, Merete M, et al. Prenatal valproate exposure and risk of autism spectrum disorders and childhood autism. *JAMA*. 2013;**309**(16):1696–1703.
75. Wieck A, Jones S. Dangers of valproate in pregnancy. *BMJ* (Clinical research ed.). 2018;**361**:k1609.
76. Huber-Mollema Y, Oort FJ, Lindhout D, Rodenburg R. Behavioral problems in children of mothers with epilepsy prenatally exposed to valproate, carbamazepine, lamotrigine, or levetiracetam monotherapy. *Epilepsia*. 2019;**60**(6):1069–82.
77. Bromley RL, Mawer GE, Briggs M, et al. *NIH Public Access*. 2014;**84**(6):637–43.
78. Veiby G, Daltveit AK, Schjolberg S, et al. Exposure to antiepileptic drugs in utero and child development. *NIH*. 2013;**54**(8):1462–72.

79. Ritter AC, Wagner AK, Fabio A, et al. Incidence and risk factors of posttraumatic seizures following traumatic brain injury: A traumatic brain injury model systems study. *Epilepsia.* 2016;**57**(12):1968–77.

80. Shannon GD, Alberg C, Nacul L, Pashayan N. Preconception health care and congenital disorders: Mathematical modelling of the impact of a preconception care programme on congenital disorders. *BJOG.* 2013;**120**(5):555–66.

81. Czeizel AE, Dudás I, Métneki J. Pregnancy outcomes in a randomised controlled trial of periconceptional multivitamin supplementation: Final report. *Arch Gynecol Obstet.* 1994;**255**(3):131–9.

82. Mills JL, Molloy AM, Reynolds EH. Do the benefits of folic acid fortification outweigh the risk of masking vitamin B(12) deficiency? *BMJ.* 2018;**360**:k724.

83. Dansky LV, Rosenblatt DS, Andermann E. Mechanisms of teratogenesis: Folic acid and antiepileptic therapy. *Neurology.* 1992;**42**(4 Suppl 5):32–42.

84. Spiegelstein O, Merriweather MY, Wicker NJ, Finnell RH. Valproate-induced neural tube defects in folate-binding protein-2 (Folbp2) knockout mice. *Birth Defects Res A Clin Mol Teratol.* 2003;**67**(12):974–8.

85. Ogawa Y, Kaneko S, Otani K, Fukushima Y. Serum folic acid levels in epileptic mothers and their relationship to congenital malformations. *Epilepsy Res.* 1991;**8**(1):75–8.

86. Reynolds EH, Green R. Valproate and folate: Congenital and developmental risks. *Epilepsy Behav.* 2020;**108**:107068. https://doi.org/10.1016/j.yebeh.2020.107068.

87. Morrow JI, Hunt SJ, Russell AJ, et al. Folic acid use and major congenital malformations in offspring of women with epilepsy: A prospective study from the UK Epilepsy and Pregnancy Register. *J Neurol Neurosurg Psychiatry.* 2009;**80**(5):506–11.

88. Surén P, Roth C, Bresnahan M, et al. Association between maternal use of folic acid supplements and risk of autism spectrum disorders in children. *JAMA.* 2013;**309**(6):570–7. https://doi.org/10.1001/jama.2012.155925.

89. Husebye ESN, Gilhus NE, Riedel B, et al. Verbal abilities in children of mothers with epilepsy: Association to maternal folate status. *Neurology.* 2018;**91**(9):e811–21.

90. Bjørk M, Riedel B, Spigset O, et al. Association of folic acid supplementation during pregnancy with the risk of autistic traits in children exposed to antiepileptic drugs in utero. *JAMA Neurol.* 2018;**75**(2):160–8.

91. Roth C, Magnus P, Schjølberg S, et al. Folic acid supplements in pregnancy and severe language delay in children. *JAMA.* 2011;**306**(14):1566–73. https://doi.org/10.1001/jama.2011.1433.

92. Schmidt RJ, Iosif A-M, Guerrero Angel E, Ozonoff S. Association of maternal prenatal vitamin use with risk for autism spectrum disorder recurrence in young siblings. *JAMA Psychiatry.* 2019;**76**(4):391–8. https://doi.org/10.1001/jamapsychiatry.2018.3901.

93. Thomas SV, Jeemon P, Pillai R, et al. Malformation risk of new anti-epileptic drugs in women with epilepsy: Observational data from the Kerala Registry of Epilepsy and Pregnancy (KREP). *Seizure.* 2021;**93**:127–32. https://doi.org/10.1016/j.seizure.2021.10.015.

94. Duncan S, Mercho S, Lopes-Cendes I, et al. Repeated neural tube defects and valproate monotherapy suggest a pharmacogenetic abnormality. Epilepsia. 2001;**42**:750–3.

Chapter 12

Seizure Management in Pregnancy

Ginette Moores

Key Points

- Most women with epilepsy have a normal pregnancy and delivery. Women with epilepsy warrant special attention by both neurologic and obstetrical teams given the increased risk of complications, including seizure destabilization during pregnancy and delivery.
- Preconception counseling is essential for all women with epilepsy of childbearing age.
- Generalized tonic-clonic and focal unaware seizures are most likely associated with maternal and fetal obstetrical risks.
- Monitoring antiseizure medication (ASM) levels and appropriately adjusting doses during pregnancy is critical to seizure control as ASM pharmacokinetics are altered by pregnancy.
- Measuring preconception serum drug level(s) help identify the serum level associated with preconception seizure control.
- Successful management of epilepsy in pregnancy balances the risk of congenital malformations against the considerable fetal and maternal risk levied by seizures.

Course of Seizures during Pregnancy

Though the majority of women will have either stable or improved seizure control, a small proportion of women may experience seizure deterioration [1]. Seizure deterioration in pregnancy is driven by a number of factors. These include nonadherence with an antiseizure medication (ASM) regimen, altered pharmacokinetics of ASMs, hormonal changes, and difficulty retaining medication due to hyperemesis gravidarum. Additional stressors, anxiety, and sleep deprivation may contribute.

The landmark study by Schmidt published in 1982 is well cited for estimating the course of epilepsy in pregnancy. This meta-analysis of articles published until 1980 included 2,165 pregnancies. Researchers found that seizure frequency increased in 24% of women, decreased in 23% of women, and remained unchanged in 53% of women [2]. Since then, multiple observational studies have demonstrated similar results [3–5]. No conclusion could be drawn from these data, as to whether the changes in seizure frequency were due to pregnancy itself or the natural history of epilepsy as it had no control group.

Recently, Pennell and colleagues published the first prospective observational multicenter cohort comparing seizure frequency in women with epilepsy during pregnancy and peripartum to seizure frequency in nonpregnant controls [6]. They found no significant difference in seizure incidence during pregnancy as compared to epilepsy controls. Overall,

39.2% of pregnant women and 36.8% of the control group had no change in seizure frequency; 28.8% of pregnant women and 29.5% of the control group experienced increased seizure frequency during the observed period. Thirty-two percent of pregnant women and 33.7% of the control group had decrease in seizure frequency. However, ASM dose adjustments occurred much more frequently (74% of pregnant women had a dose increase and 31% of the control group had a dose increase) in the pregnant women when compared to controls, reflecting gestation-related pharmacokinetic changes and compensatory dose adjustments. This is likely why no difference was observed [6].

Women in this study were more likely to be highly educated (72%) and white (87%), cared for exclusively at highly specialized epilepsy centers. Based on this study, when closely managed by a knowledgeable healthcare practitioner, pregnancy itself does not appear to increase the risk of seizures in women with epilepsy. However, these results may not be broadly applicable to different demographic populations as well as those receiving care in less specialized centers where access to therapeutic drug monitoring (TDM) may not be available.

Preconception seizures are the most important predictor of seizures in pregnancy. Seizure occurrence in the month prior to pregnancy increases the risk of seizures during pregnancy 15-fold [5]. Good seizure control in the 9 months before conception is associated with an 84–92% chance of remaining seizure free in pregnancy [7]. In other studies, a period of 1 year was the most significant factor associated with ongoing seizure remission in pregnancy. Importantly, being more than 2 years without a seizure prior to pregnancy offered negligible advantage over being 1 year seizure free in achieving seizure freedom in pregnancy [8].

Most studies have found that women with focal epilepsy are less likely to be seizure free during pregnancy as compared to those with generalized epilepsies (OR 2.97, 95% CI 1.0–8.81) [3, 5, 8, 9]. Those with frontal lobe epilepsy seem to be at a higher risk [10, 11]. However, this is confounded as women with focal epilepsy are more likely to have active epilepsy and be medically refractory prior to becoming pregnant [8]. Women with catamenial epilepsy have demonstrated better seizure control and more likely to be seizure free during pregnancy compared to women without catamenial epilepsy (OR 2.6, 95% CI 1.9–3.2).

Additionally, more than half of women with catamenial epilepsy experienced a decrease in seizure frequency during pregnancy, which was significantly higher than non-catamenial epilepsy (OR 2.5, 95% CI 1.7–3.1) [12, 13]. This may be attributable to pregnancy-associated changes in hormones (i.e., increased progesterone levels and absence of cyclical changes in circulating hormones). Therefore, other than catamenial epilepsy, the type of epilepsy disorder on its own might not be a significant factor in determining seizures during pregnancy.

Other factors that may inform the likelihood of seizures in pregnancy include preconception drug therapy. Seizures are more likely to occur in women who are not on ASM at the time of conception [8]. Similarly, ASM noncompliance, which occurs in up to 20% of cases, is associated with seizures [9]. Polytherapy (more than one ASM) has also been associated with an increased risk for seizures (OR 2.98, 95% CI 2.3–3.9) [5], but is highly confounded by the fact that polytherapy is used in women with more refractory seizure disorders who are less likely to be seizure free prior to pregnancy. This highlights the importance of ongoing ASM management of women with epilepsy both before and throughout pregnancy to optimize seizure control.

Pharmacokinetics Affecting Antiseizure Medication Efficiency

Seizure control during pregnancy is challenging due to marked changes in pharmacokinetics that can alter ASM efficacy. Pregnancy increases plasma volume, circulating sex hormones, and decreases albumin concentration. Clearance is substantially affected by increased fluid volume and sex hormones. Renal function and glomerular filtration rate (GFR) increase, which leads to increased excretion of renally excreted drugs. Glucuronidation is induced by sex hormones thereby leading to increased metabolism of drugs such as lamotrigine, which are then cleared by hepatic enzymes [7, 14]. Decreased albumin levels enhance these changes by increasing the free fraction of protein-bound medications available for excretion [15].

Increased knowledge about ASM changes in pregnancy can serve to better inform management [15]. A large prospective study looked to characterize pregnancy-related clearance changes for levetiracetam, oxcarbazepine, topiramate, phenytoin, and valproate. The magnitude and time of change varied between ASM, influenced by mechanism of drug clearance. Levetiracetam was maximally cleared in the first trimester, whereas peak oxcarbazepine and topiramate clearance occurred in the second trimester [15]. Lamotrigine clearance begins as early as the fifth gestational week and continues to increase through the first, second, and third trimesters [15, 16]. This highlights the importance of beginning therapeutic drug level monitoring early in pregnancy when significant changes can be seen.

Lamotrigine metabolism has been well documented during pregnancy. Consistently, studies have demonstrated that lamotrigine clearance, which is dependent on glucuronidation, increases throughout pregnancy with an average 264% increase by delivery [17]. Large variation in drug clearance can be seen between individuals, making ASM dose adjustments in the absence of serum drug levels challenging. Polepally and colleagues performed frequent serum monitoring to create pharmacokinetic modeling of lamotrigine clearance throughout pregnancy [18]. There was a linear increase in lamotrigine clearance with gestational age with rapid return to baseline in the postpartum period. They found two distinct subpopulations of women. While the majority of women (77%) had a 219% increased rate of lamotrigine clearance, a smaller subgroup (23%) had a minimal increase in clearance (21%) that was 10-fold less than most [18].

Interestingly, one study found that two different genetic polymorphisms as well as the sex of the fetus influenced changes in lamotrigine clearance seen during pregnancy and that the observed pharmacokinetic changes differed between the variants [19]. Greater understanding into pharmacogenetic differences will serve for improved understanding of lamotrigine clearance in pregnancy and serve to optimize medical management.

Levetiracetam, which is largely excreted renally, has an average 207% increased clearance with 40–62% decrease in serum concentration compared to prepregnancy baseline. Oxcarbazepine is metabolized through glucuronidation prior to excretion through the kidneys. It can similarly experience significantly increased excretion in pregnancy. One study demonstrated that seizure frequency doubled in about half of pregnant women taking oxcarbazepine, with correlation between seizure deterioration and decrease in plasma concentration of oxcarbazepine's active metabolite [7].

A more recent study comparing dose-normalized concentrations (DNC) between pregnant women and nonpregnant controls across different trimesters in pregnancy demonstrated reductions in the DNC of both oxcarbazepine (32.6%) and unbound oxcarbazepine (30.6%) in pregnancy [16]. Incremental increases in drug dosage for lamotrigine, levetiracetam, and oxcarbazepine may be needed to maintain therapeutic drug levels of these medications.

Studies have shown that during pregnancy, total concentrations decline by an average of 50% for phenobarbital. Topiramate clearance is increased during pregnancy with a gradual decline in the concentration-to-dose ratio in the third trimester being 34–78% less than baseline values [17]. In a more recent study by Pennell and colleagues, a decrease in third-trimester topiramate DNC was observed; however, this change was not statistically significant (29.83 μg/L/mg to 13.77 μg/L/mg; $p = 0.18$) [16]. This was limited by a small number of pregnant women taking topiramate during this study and suggests a need for further evaluation.

By contrast, free carbamazepine and carbamazepine 10,11-epoxide DNC are not substantially altered by pregnancy. Total carbamazepine DNC decreased by 17.3% in pregnancy. However, this has not consistently been observed in other studies [17]. Free carbamazepine levels are felt to be more predictive of seizure worsening. Pregabalin and vigabatrin are both eliminated renally and therefore changes in serum concentrations of these drugs are expected to change as GFR changes [7, 17].

Valproic acid total serum levels decrease in the second and third trimesters without a significant change in free drug levels [20]. During pregnancy, decreasing binding to albumin may cause measurements of lower total drug levels, while the unbound and pharmacologically active plasma concentration changes minimally, if at all. This effect has also been observed in phenytoin and tiagabine, all of which are highly protein-bound. Therefore, it is important that women on these medications use free drug levels instead of total drug levels to avoid inappropriate dose adjustments.

Limited information is available regarding gestational-induced pharmacokinetic changes for newer ASMs, including pregabalin, clobazam, lacosamide, perampanel, brivaracetam, eslicarbazepine, rufinamide, and zonisamide. Lacosamide clearance is complex, metabolized by CYP2C19 and excreted by the kidneys. While CYP2C19 activity is decreased during pregnancy, GFR increases, and they may balance each other out. A recent case report modeled lacosamide pharmacokinetics during pregnancy in a woman with temporal lobe epilepsy on polytherapy with lacosamide, carbamazepine, and clobazam. They found that the lacosamide serum concentration and the concentration-to-dose ratio declined during pregnancy, before returning to preconception levels postpartum [21]. Similarly, in the study by Pennell and colleagues, three women were taking lacosamide in the first trimester of pregnancy. They observed a significant decline in lacosamide DNC (39.9%) during pregnancy compared to the postpartum period [16]. Zonisamide DNC were also observed to decline during pregnancy by almost 30% among the small sample [16].

Current knowledge about the pharmacokinetics of ASMs in pregnancy is summarized in Table 12.1. More data are required to fully assess the safety of newer ASMs.

Consequences of Seizures during Pregnancy

Compared to those without the condition, women with epilepsy are 5–10 times more likely to die during pregnancy and during the hospitalization for their delivery [22–24]. Despite the significant increase in the relative risk, the absolute risk remains low, observed in one study to be 80 deaths per 100,000 pregnancies during in-hospital delivery compared to 6 deaths per 100,000 pregnancies among women without epilepsy [24]. When causes of death were analyzed, seizure-related trauma or sudden unexpected death in epilepsy (SUDEP)

Table 12.1 Antiseizure medication treatment in pregnancy

Drug	Metabolism	Expected change in pregnancy	Protein-binding	Recommendation for therapeutic drug monitoring
Brivaracetam	Renal	Data lacking	Negligible	Unknown
Carbamazepine	Hepatic	Declines < 25%	75%	Optional
Ethosuximide	Hepatic	Data lacking	Negligible	Unknown
Lamotrigine	Hepatic	Variable, 77% of population 69% decline; 23% of population have 17% decline	55%	Yes
Levetiracetam	Renal	Declines 40–62%	Negligible	Yes
Lacosamide	Renal with hepatic metabolism	Data lacking	Negligible	Unknown
Gabapentin	Renal	Negligible	0%	Optional
Oxcarbazepine	Hepatic	Declines 30–40%	40% for active metabolite (10-monohydroxy derivative)	Yes
Perampanel	Hepatic	Data lacking	Highly protein-bound, >90%	Unknown
Phenobarbital	Hepatic	Declines 50–55%	50%	Yes
Phenytoin	Hepatic	Free level declines 16–40% minimally; total level declines 60–70%	Highly protein-bound, >90%	Yes, monitor free concentration
Pregabalin	Renal	Data lacking	0%	Unknown
Tiagabine	Hepatic	Data lacking	Highly protein-bound, >90%	Unknown
Topiramate	Renal predominance	Declines 30–40%	15%	Yes
Valproic Acid	Hepatic	Free drug changes minimally; total level declines < 40%	Highly protein-bound, >90%	Optional but monitor free concentration if done
Vigabatrin	Renal	Data lacking	0%	Unknown
Zonisamide	Hepatic	Declines 25–50%	60%	Yes

accounted for the majority of cases [22, 25]. A retrospective review of all maternal deaths in Japan from 2010 to 2019 found 6 deaths related to SUDEP. These deaths were evenly distributed in the second trimester, third trimester, and postpartum period. All women were on ASM monotherapy (4/6) or not on any ASM therapy (2/6) with relatively well-controlled seizures. This highlights the absence of typical SUDEP risk factors and the need for greater understanding of SUDEP in pregnancy [25].

Seizures with impaired awareness put the mother at risk for falls or other traumatic injuries. Premature labor or placental abruption can be the consequence of this trauma, occurring in 1–5% of minor and 20–50% of major blunt injuries [26]. Additionally, generalized tonic-clonic seizures affect electrolytes, blood pressure, and oxygenation, all of which can negatively impact the fetus.

A systematic review and meta-analysis of studies from 1990 to 2015 calculated the risk of maternal and fetal outcomes among women with epilepsy. Thirty-eight studies comprising 2,809,984 pregnancies were compiled for analysis. Of these studies, most (25/38) were retrospective with data obtained from population-based cohorts (21/38). Women with epilepsy had increased risk of spontaneous miscarriage (OR 1.54, 95% CI 1.02–2.32), antepartum hemorrhage (OR 1.49, 95% CI 1.01–2.20), postpartum hemorrhage (OR 1.29, 95% CI 1.13–1.49), hypertensive disorders (OR 1.37, 95% CI 1.21–1.55), induction of labor (OR 1.67, 95% CI 1.31–2.11), caesarean section (OR 1.40, 95% CI 1.23–1.58), and preterm birth (OR 1.16, 95% CI 1.01–1.34).

Additionally, women with epilepsy on ASMs had a small increased risk of postpartum hemorrhage (OR 1.33, 95% CI 1.16–1.54) and induction of labor (OR 1.30, 95% CI 1.05–1.85) compared to women with epilepsy not taking ASMs. Women with epilepsy were also more likely to deliver a baby with fetal growth restriction (OR 1.26, 95% CI 1.20–1.33). This risk is significantly increased with exposure to ASM polytherapy (OR 3.51, 95% CI 1.23–10.01). Notably, no increased risk of fetal or perinatal death was observed [27].

Studies examining major congenital malformations that did not also assess reproductive outcomes were excluded from these analyses and therefore these estimates are potentially higher. Additionally, many studies involved older ASMs such as carbamazepine, topiramate, lamotrigine, valproate, and phenytoin and may not be applicable to newer ASMs such as levetiracetam, oxcarbazepine, and brivaracetam.

Occurrence of one or more generalized tonic-clonic seizures during pregnancy has been associated with increased risk of preterm birth and small-for-gestational-age infants in two studies [28, 29]. One study demonstrated an association between five or more generalized tonic-clonic seizures in pregnancy and unfavorable neurodevelopment in infants [30]. In a study by Adab and colleagues, five or more generalized tonic-clonic seizures in pregnancy resulted in approximately 10-point decrease in average verbal IQ scores compared to women without seizures in pregnancy. This effect was seen independently of valproic acid use [31].

Data regarding the effects of individual seizures on the fetus are limited. Two case reports demonstrated fetal heart rate deceleration during maternal focal seizures with impaired awareness. Fetal heart rate returned to normal several minutes after the seizure. In one of the cases, the patient was in labor and there was associated prolonged uterine contraction during the seizure. However, in both cases, babies were delivered without complications identified [12].

An additional two cases of generalized tonic-clonic seizures during pregnancy were reported with associated fetal bradycardia-tachycardia and decreased fetal heart rate.

A single case of intracranial hemorrhage with in utero fetal demise following maternal seizure, of unclear semiology, has been reported. Several mechanisms, including baseline increased risk of fetal intracranial bleed related to history of epilepsy, coagulation defect as a result of ASM, abdominal trauma during seizure, and fetal anoxia during seizure leading to arterial hypertension, were proposed by the authors to explain the association between seizure and fetal intraventricular hemorrhage [32]. Besides these direct health consequences, seizures during pregnancy also have a negative impact on daily life. Seizures are associated with anxiety and stress. The loss of a driver's license affects employment, social interactions, interpersonal relationships, and quality of life [33].

A common criticism of most of these studies is that they failed to discern if these increased risks are attributable to a diagnosis of epilepsy, seizures themselves, or treatment. What we can infer, however, is the overall impact of seizures and the use of ASM during pregnancy is both complex and can influence both maternal and fetal outcomes.

Preconception Management

Preconception Planning

Preconception counseling is essential for all women with epilepsy of childbearing age. A recent retrospective cohort study based in the United States found that among women with epilepsy, 65% of pregnancies are unplanned [17]. Given that organogenesis occurs at 3–8 weeks' gestation, the bulk of risk for major congenital malformations (MCMs) happens during the first trimester before many women are aware they are pregnant. Therefore, preconception counseling is important to decrease adverse outcomes. This should occur at disease diagnosis and at the initiation of ASMs. This includes a discussion of contraception, maternal and fetal risks in pregnancy, selection and management of ASM, and folate supplementation. Preconception care is discussed in detail in Chapter 10.

Antiseizure Medication

Successful management of epilepsy in pregnancy balances the risk of congenital malformation against the considerable fetal and maternal risk levied by seizures. There has been an increase in ASM options within the past two decades. Newer ASMs offer a favorable risk-to-benefit ratio; however, data in pregnancy are not always available. Although pregnant women with epilepsy were excluded from drug trials, several pregnancy registries have been established to gather potential risk and safety data regarding medication use during pregnancy.

Epilepsy itself has not proven teratogenic, but ASMs have a clear, dose-dependent relationship to birth defects. Antiseizure medications are not equal when considering MCM risks. Lamotrigine, levetiracetam, and oxcarbazepine are associated with the lowest risk (2–3%). In contrast, valproate has the highest observed risk of MCM (5–15%) [34]. Antiseizure medications with potential teratogenicity should be replaced with acceptable alternatives prior to conception when possible. Switching ASMs is usually avoided in an established pregnancy as it poses a potential risk of seizure recurrence. Ideally, the management of seizure disorder in pregnancy begins prior to conception with the patient on the lowest effective dose of a single ASM, preferably one with the lowest risk of teratogenesis.

Folic Acid

In women without epilepsy, the benefits of preconception folic acid are well established to reduce the risk of neural tube defect (NTD) by up to 93%. Several ASMs are known to alter folate metabolism, which is one mechanism by which they are thought to be teratogenic. Optimal periconceptual folate dosage and duration of folic acid supplementation intrapartum in women with epilepsy remains unclear. However, some experts suggest that 1 mg of folate be given to all women of childbearing age taking ASMs, with higher doses up to 4–5 mg daily considered for women at high risk of MCMs (e.g., valproic acid, high doses of medications, or polytherapy). See Chapter 10 for a more detailed discussion on preconception counseling of WWE.

Antiseizure Medication Management during Pregnancy

Antiseizure Medication Withdrawal and Switches

For any individual with epilepsy, there is always the unknown efficacy and tolerability of any newly initiated ASM. Switching medications typically involves a transition period with bridging of two medications. In the case of pregnancy, this exposes the fetus to polytherapy, which is associated with an increased risk of teratogenicity.

The European and International Registry of Antiepileptic Drugs and Pregnancy (EURAP) group assessed seizure control among pregnancies in which valproic acid was withdrawn or switched to another medication in the first trimester. Generalized tonic-clonic seizures occurred twice as often among women in whom valproic acid was withdrawn or switched as compared to those who were maintained on their prepregnancy therapy [35]. A similar study with Australian Pregnancy Registry data examined women on valproic acid whose dose was reduced, unchanged, or discontinued prior to pregnancy. While the fetal malformation rate was lower when the valproic acid dose was reduced prior to pregnancy, there was a 50% increased risk of seizures during pregnancy if the valproic acid dose was changed during pregnancy [36].

Ideally, medication optimization has occurred during the preconception period. However, with unplanned pregnancy, physicians may consider withdrawal or switching from the current ASM(s) during pregnancy. This strategy is unlikely to reduce the risk of teratogenicity, which typically occurs before a pregnancy is recognized, but poses significant risk to loss of seizure control. In a study by Asranna and colleagues, Kerala Registry of Epilepsy and Pregnancy Registry data were used to compare MCM rates between those who had ASM changes during the second and third trimesters. Dose reduction or discontinuation occurred in 6.5% of pregnancies (93/1,454) [37]. There was no difference in MCM frequency or developmental quotient at 1 year among those whose ASMs were reduced or stopped as compared to those in whom ASM dose was unchanged or escalated [37]. Therefore, caution should be taken for any ASM switch or withdrawal during pregnancy.

An exception to this exists for women on lamotrigine therapy who discontinue a combined oral contraceptive for pregnancy planning. Ethinyl estradiol contained within combined hormonal contraceptives is known to decrease lamotrigine levels through glucuronidation. Therefore, upon discontinuation of these contraceptives for pregnancy, lamotrigine levels will increase, and dose reduction should be considered to avoid toxicity.

In the cases of valproic acid or phenytoin, which are associated with adverse cognitive outcomes, is it unknown whether withdrawal of medication during pregnancy is associated with improved neurodevelopmental outcomes.

Therapeutic Drug Monitoring

In general, there is variability in the extent to which pregnancy affects serum drug concentrations in each individual woman. International League against Epilepsy guidelines recommend TDM during pregnancy, but do not provide recommendations on the frequency and timing of such monitoring [17, 38].

A systematic review and meta-analysis compared different monitoring strategies for pregnant women on lamotrigine. Six studies, none of which were randomized controlled trials, were included. They demonstrated that seizure deterioration was less frequent among those with TDM (rate 0.3; 95% CI 0.21–0.41) compared to those who were monitored by clinical features (i.e., seizures) alone (rate 0.73; 95% CI 0.56–0.86) [39].

While an AntiEpileptic drug Monitoring in PREgnancy (EMPiRE) study found no difference in seizure numbers or time to first seizure between women randomized to TDM or clinical judgment alone, non-inferiority was not proven as this study did not reach target recruitment for sample size estimation and not all women included in this study had prepregnancy serum trough levels [40]. Also, inclusion of individuals up to 24 weeks' gestational age may have missed significant changes in drug levels, which are known to occur early in pregnancy [15]. In light of this and more recently published data on pregnancy outcomes with TDM, a role remains for TDM in pregnancy as correction of a declining serum level may prevent a seizure [6].

It is generally recommended to establish a prepregnancy baseline serum drug level to identify the level that provides optimal seizure control. If a preconception serum level is not available, it should be drawn as early as possible in the first trimester. Once a woman is pregnant, her preconception serum level can serve as a reference to guide dosing of ASM.

The serum level should be monitored at least once per trimester during pregnancy, with monthly monitoring in certain circumstances. Medications likely to experience marked changes such as levetiracetam, lamotrigine, and oxcarbazepine require more frequent – usually monthly – monitoring. Consideration may be given to monitoring of medications where there is a lack of understanding of pharmacokinetic changes in pregnancy but serum drug levels are available (e.g., clobazam, clonazepam, lacosamide). More frequent monitoring may also be considered for individuals who are sensitive to medication adjustments and drug level fluctuations, irrespective of the ASM they are taking. Additional drug levels should be done if clinically indicated (e.g., change in seizure frequency, medication side effects, or rapidly changing drug levels) [7]. A greater than 35% decline in the baseline serum drug level is associated with increased risk for seizures. Therefore, dose adjustments may be necessary throughout pregnancy, ideally targeting maintenance of a serum drug level greater than 65% that of preconception.

The physiologic changes of pregnancy rapidly resolve over the first 2–3 weeks postpartum. Importantly, if ASM levels are increased during pregnancy, they need to be tapered shortly after delivery to avoid postpartum toxicity. Postpartum sleep deprivation may lower the seizure threshold and therefore the ASM dose may be kept at a slightly higher level than the preconception baseline for the initial months postpartum. This tapering plan should be established in the late third trimester so the woman is prepared once she delivers to avoid toxic side effects.

Seizures during Labor and Delivery

Labor and delivery are a common time for breakthrough seizures during pregnancy, second only to the beginning of pregnancy. Sleep deprivation, especially during a prolonged labor, pain, hyperventilation, emotional stress, reduced ASM levels, or missed doses of ASM may contribute. An early epidural is usually recommended so a woman can sleep during labor, thereby reducing pain and sleep deprivation.

The risk of seizures during labor in women with epilepsy was found to be 3.5% in the EURAP study, with one case of status epilepticus during delivery. While seizures during labor and delivery are most likely to occur in women who had seizures during pregnancy (OR 4.8; CI 2.3–10), 14 of the 60 women (23%) had been seizure free throughout pregnancy [41].

More recent data from the EURAP pregnancy registry found that seizures occurred in 1.4–2.3% of deliveries. This was influenced by ASM therapy, with higher rates among women taking carbamazepine or lamotrigine and the lowest rates among those exposed to valproate [3]. This is likely somewhat explained by the major pharmacokinetic effect of pregnancy on lamotrigine clearance.

Another retrospective study of 99 pregnancies among women with epilepsy in the United States found that seizures during labor and delivery occurred in 12.5% of women with generalized epilepsy but none in women with focal epilepsy. Almost half of women in this study had a subtherapeutic serum drug level at the time of delivery. No women with therapeutic drug levels had seizures during labor and delivery, suggesting that maintenance of therapeutic drug levels during the third trimester is important to prevent seizures during labor and delivery, especially among women with generalized epilepsy [42].

The Kerala Registry of Epilepsy and Pregnancy found that seizure relapse was highest during the first 3 days peripartum; however, this study was limited to women who were not on ASMs or were on low doses of ASMs [5]. Breakthrough seizures can additionally be related to missed doses of ASMs during labor, sleep deprivation, pain, fatigue, or dehydration. Women with epilepsy should be encouraged to bring their own ASMs to delivery and medications should be administered at the usual times during labor.

Women with epilepsy are known to have an increased risk of preeclampsia (1.37; CI 1.21–1.55) [27]. When considering seizure workup and management during labor and delivery, it is important to distinguish between seizures related to epilepsy and those occurring due to eclampsia (Table 12.2).

Seizures Secondary to Epilepsy

Seizures secondary to epilepsy have characteristics of a patient's established seizure type. It would be unusual to develop a de novo seizure type during pregnancy. If this does occur, consider other causes of new-onset seizures in pregnancy (see Table 12.3). In the context of seizure recurrence in patients with established epilepsy, it is important to stabilize the patient once a seizure is recognized. This involves protection of airway, patient positioning in the left lateral decubitus, monitoring of the patient's vitals, and continuous fetal monitoring. Basic tests should be done to assess for common provoking factors (e.g., electrolytes, glucose, toxicity screen), serum drug levels, and screening for preeclampsia.

No studies have directly assessed the optimal management of seizures in labor. Rather, guidelines are based on expert opinion as well as principles guiding the management of seizure outside of pregnancy. Intravenous lorazepam is typically the preferred medication for acute seizure management, but diazepam may be an alternative. If seizures remain uncontrolled,

Table 12.2 Seizures from eclampsia versus epilepsy

	Eclampsia	Epilepsy
History of epilepsy	Yes or no	Yes
Timing of seizures	After 20 weeks' gestational age or postpartum (often in third trimester or within first 2 weeks postpartum)	Any time during pregnancy or postpartum
Seizure semiology	Generalized tonic-clonic seizures	Focal onset seizures (more likely to have seizure worsening) or generalized seizures (myoclonic, absence or generalized tonic-clonic)
Associated features	Headache, visual disturbance, right upper quadrant or epigastric pain, or pulmonary edema	Often none
Vitals	BP > 140/90	Often normal but can be elevated immediately after a seizure
Physical examination	Altered level of consciousness, hyperreflexia, or edema	Often normal
Laboratory investigations	Possible proteinuria, low platelets, low fibrinogen, elevated liver enzymes, elevated creatine, elevated lactate dehydrogenase, lactic acidosis	Can have lactic acidosis depending on seizure type

consider administration of a loading dose of intravenous phenytoin or levetiracetam followed by normal treatment of status epilepticus as outside of pregnancy [43]. It is important to be aware that benzodiazepines and barbiturates can cause neonatal sedation and potentially a neonatal withdrawal syndrome. Therefore, continuous fetal monitoring should occur whenever such medications are administered. Delivery is not required for the treatment of epileptic seizures but may be necessary for obstetrical indications such as persistent fetal heart rate deceleration [43].

Seizures Secondary to Eclampsia

Eclampsia is the manifestation of new seizures or altered level of consciousness in a woman with preeclampsia. This is a multisystem disorder that affects both mother and fetus and is characterized by hypertension, proteinuria, and other systemic disturbances in the second half of pregnancy or postpartum. Clinically, women with eclampsia often have preceding headache, visual disturbance, right upper quadrant or epigastric pain, and ankle clonus [43]. Eclampsia typically manifests with generalized tonic-clonic seizures.

Management of eclampsia begins with assessment of blood pressure. Hypertension should be immediately addressed with hypertensive agents. Intravenous magnesium sulfate remains the treatment of choice for seizures in this setting [44]. If seizures persist despite magnesium, benzodiazepines should be used as a second-line therapy. Delivery of the baby is indicated at any gestational age. Management of seizures during labor and delivery is summarized in Figure 12.1. If doubt exists as to whether seizures in the second half of pregnancy are due to epilepsy or eclampsia, women should be treated with magnesium sulfate until a definitive diagnosis can be made.

Table 12.3 Differential diagnosis of new-onset seizures in pregnancy

Potential causes of new-onset seizures in pregnancy
Epilepsy • Undiagnosed preexisting epilepsy • New-onset epilepsy during pregnancy
Structural • Intracranial hemorrhage • Cerebral venous sinus thrombosis • Ischemic stroke • Ruptured aneurysm or vascular malformation • Reversible cerebral vasoconstriction syndrome • Posterior reversible encephalopathy syndrome • Brain tumor • Hydrocephalus
Eclampsia Trauma Infectious • Meningitis • Encephalitis • Brain abscess
Metabolic • Hypoglycemia • Hypernatremia • Hyponatremia • Hyperosmolar nonketotic hyperglycemia • Hypocalcemia • Hypomagnesemia • Uremia • Liver failure • Acute hepatitis • Renal failure
Genetic • Congenital brain defects • Acute intermittent porphyria • Sturge Weber syndrome
Autoimmune disorders • Antiphospholipid syndrome • Systemic lupus erythematous • Thrombotic thrombocytopenic purpura
Drug or alcohol overdose or withdrawal Psychogenic non-epileptic events

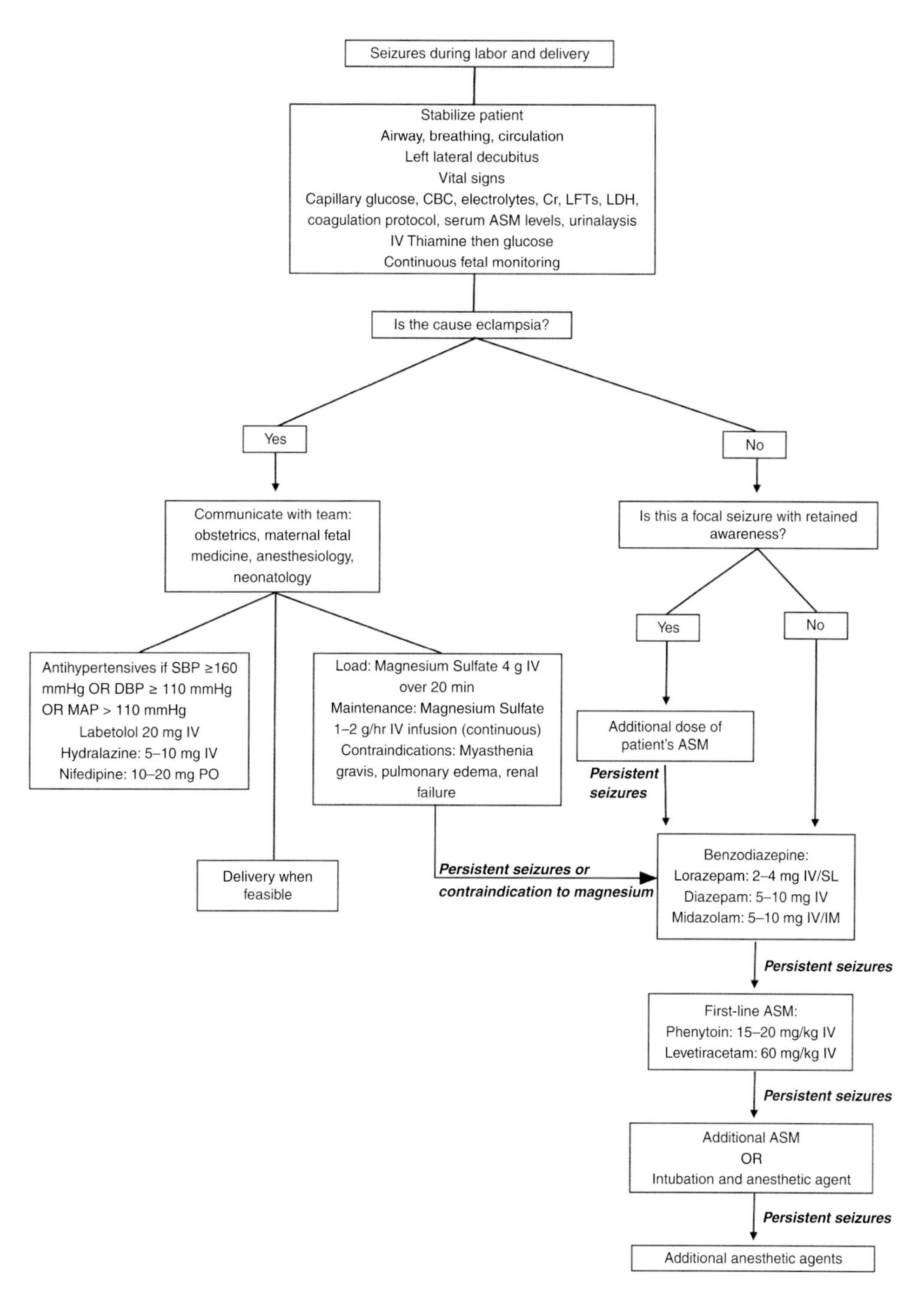

Figure 12.1 Management of seizures during labor and delivery

Status Epilepticus

Status epilepticus is rare during pregnancy, but it is of concern as it is associated with increased fetal and maternal mortality [7]. It is unique in that it can occur at any stage of pregnancy from the first trimester through delivery. In the EURAP registry, 21 cases of status epilepticus were documented among 1,956 pregnant women (incidence 0.6%). Only 10 of the 21 cases were convulsive status epilepticus. Status epilepticus occurred evenly over the three trimesters. No maternal mortality was observed; however, one case of status epilepticus in the third trimester resulted in perinatal death. Additionally, three offspring born to women who had status epilepticus were diagnosed with MCMs [3]. Pregnancy-associated status epilepticus accounted for 2.1% of all cases of status epilepticus in a recent cohort [45].

A more recent systematic review reported 29 cases of status epilepticus in seven articles. The most common etiology for status epilepticus in pregnancy was acute symptomatic causes, most commonly due to eclampsia (5 cases), posterior reversible encephalopathy syndrome not secondary to eclampsia (6 cases), and cerebral venous thrombosis. Only 3 cases, accounting for 10%, occurred in women with preexisting epilepsy in whom there was ASM noncompliance. Poor outcomes occurred in 21% of pregnant women with status epilepticus, including two maternal deaths. Twenty-four out of 29 cases resulted in delivery of live-born offspring. There were three cases of medical termination of pregnancy and one case of spontaneous abortion and one case of intrauterine fetal death [46].

In a longitudinal cohort of pregnant women with medically refractory epilepsy in Brazil, the prevalence of status epilepticus was 8.5%. Status epilepticus occurred evenly throughout the three trimesters. There was no maternal or fetal mortality; however, women who had status epilepticus had increased rates of obstetrical complications, caesarian sections, and premature deliveries [47]. The approach to seizure management including status epilepticus is summarized in Figure 12.1.

Conclusion

Preconception counseling is important to establish the lowest effective dose of the least teratogenic medication. Women can be reassured that when followed closely in a specialized clinic, pregnancy alone does not increase the risk of seizures. Optimization of seizure control during pregnancy is still recommended to prevent adverse outcomes. Baseline ASM trough and free drug levels should be measured and monitored throughout pregnancy with dose adjustment to maintain prepregnancy levels. This is particularly important for levetiracetam, lamotrigine, and oxcarbazepine, which are known to undergo significantly increased clearance. Medication adherence is important throughout pregnancy and delivery. Postpartum, ASM dosages should be reduced to or slightly above prepregnancy levels to avoid drug toxicity.

References

1. Schmidt D, Canger R, Avanzini G, et al. Change of seizure frequency in pregnant epileptic women. *J Neurol Neurosurg Psychiatry*. 1983;**46**(8):751–5.
2. Bag S, Behari M, Ahuja GK, Karmarkar MG. Pregnancy and epilepsy. *Journal of Neurology*. 1989;**236**:311–13.
3. Battino D, Tomson T, Bonizzoni E, et al. Seizure control and treatment changes in pregnancy: Observations from the EURAP epilepsy pregnancy registry. *Epilepsia*. 2013;**54**:1621–7.
4. La Neve A, Boero G, Francavilla T, et al. Prospective, case-control study on the effect of

pregnancy on seizure frequency in women with epilepsy. *Neurol Sci*. 2014;**36**:79–83.

5. Thomas SV, Syam U, Devi JS. Predictors of seizures during pregnancy in women with epilepsy. *Epilepsia*. 2012;**53**:e85–e88.
6. Pennell PB, French JA, May RC, et al. Changes in seizure frequency and antiepileptic therapy during pregnancy. *New England Journal of Medicine*. 2020;**383**(26):2547–56.
7. Burakgazi E, Pollard J, Harden C. The effect of pregnancy on seizure control and antiepileptic drugs in women with epilepsy. *Reviews in Neurological Diseases*. 2011;**8**:16–22.
8. Vajda FJE, O'Brien TJ, Graham JE, et al. Predicting epileptic seizure control during pregnancy. *Epilepsy & Behavior*. 2018;**78**:91–5.
9. Shahla M, Hijran B, Sharif M. The course of epilepsy and seizure control in pregnant women. *Acta Neurol Belg*. 2018;**118**(3):459–64.
10. Mostacci B, Troisi S, Bisulli F, et al. Seizure worsening in pregnancy in women with sleep-related hypermotor epilepsy (SHE): A historical cohort study. *Seizure*. 2021;**91**:258–62.
11. Voinescu PE, Ehlert AN, Bay CP, Allien S, Pennell PB. Variations in seizure frequency during pregnancy and postpartum by epilepsy type. *Neurology*. 2022;**98**:e802–e807.
12. Sveberg L, Svalheim S, Taubøll E. The impact of seizures on pregnancy and delivery. *Seizure*. 2015;**28**:35–8.
13. Cagnetti C, Lattanzi S, Foschi N, Provinciali L, Silvestrini M. Seizure course during pregnancy in catamenial epilepsy. *Neurology*. 2014;**83**(4):339–44.
14. Eadie MJ. Treating epilepsy in pregnant women. *Expert Opinion on Pharmacotherapy*. 2014;**15**:841–50.
15. Voinescu P, Park S, Chen L, et al. Antiepileptic drug clearances during pregnancy and clinical implications for women with epilepsy. *Neurology*. 2018;**91**: e1228–e1236.
16. Pennell PB, Karanam A, Meador KJ, et al. Antiseizure medication concentrations during pregnancy: Results from the Maternal Outcomes and Neurodevelopmental Effects of Antiepileptic Drugs (MONEAD) study. *JAMA Neurol*. 2022;**79**(4):370–9.
17. Tomson T, Battino D, Bromley R, et al. Management of epilepsy in pregnancy: A report from the International League against Epilepsy Task Force on Women and Pregnancy. *Epileptic Disorders*. 2019;**21**(6) 497–517.
18. Polepally AR, Pennell PB, Brundage RC, et al. Model-based lamotrigine clearance changes during pregnancy: Clinical implication. *Ann Clin Transl Neurol*. 2014;**1**(2):99–106.
19. Petrenaite V, Sabers A, Hansen-Schwartz J. Seizure deterioration in women treated with oxcarbazepine during pregnancy. *Epilepsy Research*. 2009;**84**(2):245–9.
20. Johannessen Landmark C, Farmen AH, Burns ML, et al. Pharmacokinetic variability of valproate during pregnancy: Implications for the use of therapeutic drug monitoring. *Epilepsy Res*. 2018;**141**:31–7.
21. Fukushima Y, Yamamoto Y, Yamazaki E, et al. Change in the pharmacokinetics of lacosamide before, during, and after pregnancy. *Seizure*. 2021;**88**:12–14.
22. Edey S, Moran N, Nashef L. SUDEP and epilepsy-related mortality in pregnancy. *Epilepsia*. 2014;**55**(7):e72–4.
23. Christensen J, Vestergaard C, Hammer Bech B. Maternal death in women with epilepsy: Smaller scope studies. *Neurology*. 2018;**91**(18):e1716–e1720.
24. MacDonald SC, Bateman BT, McElrath TF, Hernández-Díaz S. Mortality and morbidity during delivery hospitalization among pregnant women with epilepsy in the United States. *JAMA Neurol*. 2015;**72**(9):981–8.
25. Tanaka H, Katsuragi S, Hasegawa J, et al. Maternal death related to sudden unexpected death in epilepsy: A nationwide survey in Japan. *Brain Sci*. 2021;**11**(8):995.
26. Pennell P. Pregnancy, epilepsy, and women's issues. *Continuum*. 2013;**19**:697–714.

27. Viale L, Allotey J, Cheong-See F, et al. Epilepsy in pregnancy and reproductive outcomes: A systematic review and meta-analysis. *Lancet*. 2015;**386**:1845–52.
28. Chen Y, Chiou H, Lin H, Lin H. Affect of seizures during gestation on pregnancy outcomes in women with epilepsy. *Archives of Neurology*. 2009;**66**:979–84.
29. Rauchenzauner M, Rauchenzauner M, Ehrensberger M, et al. Generalized tonic-clonic seizures and antiepileptic drugs during pregnancy: A matter of importance for the baby? *J Neurol*. 2013;**260**:484–8.
30. Cummings C, Stewart M, Stevenson M, Morrow J, Nelson J. Neurodevelopment of children exposed in utero to lamotrigine, sodium valproate and carbamazepine. *Archives of Disease in Childhood*. 2011;**96**:643–7.
31. Adab N, Kini U, Vinten J, et al. The longer term outcome of children born to mothers with epilepsy. *Journal of Neurology, Neurosurgery & Psychiatry*. 2004;**75**:1575–83.
32. Minkoff H, Schaffer RM, Delke I, Grunebaum AN. Diagnosis of intracranial hemorrhage in utero after a maternal seizure. *Obstet Gynecol*. 1985; **65**: 22S–4S.
33. Loring DW, Meador KJ, Lee GP. Determinants of quality of life in epilepsy. *Epilepsy & Behavior*. 2004;**5**(6):976–80.
34. Tomson T, Battino D, Craig J, et al. Comparative risk of major congenital malformations with eight different antiepileptic drugs: A prospective cohort study of the EURAP registry. *Lancet Neurology*. 2018;**17**:530–8.
35. Tomson T, Battino D, Bonizzoni E, et al. Withdrawal of valproic acid treatment during pregnancy and seizure outcome: Observations from EURAP. *Epilepsia*. 2016;**57**(8):e173–e177.
36. Vajda FJE, O'Brien TJ, Graham JE, et al. Pregnancy after valproate withdrawal: Fetal malformations and seizure control. *Epilepsia*. 2020;**61**(5):944–50.
37. Asranna A, Jose M, Philip RM, Sarma PS, Thomas SV. Do anti-epileptic drug modifications after first trimester of pregnancy influence fetal malformation or cognitive outcome? *Epilepsy Research*. 2018;**146**:121–5.
38. Harden CL, Pennell PB, Kaplan PW, et al. Practice parameter update: Management issues for women with epilepsy. Focus on pregnancy (an evidence-based review). Vitamin K, folic acid, blood levels, and breastfeeding. Report of the Quality Standards Subcommittee and Therapeutics and Technology Assessment Subcommittee of the American Academy of Neurology and American Epilepsy Society. *Neurology*. 2009;**73**(2):142–9.
39. Pirie DAJ, Wattar BHA, Pirie AM, et al. Effects of monitoring strategies on seizures in pregnant women on lamotrigine: A meta-analysis. *European Journal of Obstetrics & Gynecology and Reproductive Biology*. 2013;**172**:26–31.
40. Thangaratinam S, Marlin N, Newton S, et al. AntiEpileptic drug monitoring in PREgnancy (EMPiRE): A double-blind randomised trial on effectiveness and acceptability of monitoring strategies. *Health Technol Assess*. 2018;**22**(23):1–152.
41. EURAP Study Group. Seizure control and treatment in pregnancy: Observations from the EURAP epilepsy pregnancy registry. *Neurology*. 2006;**66**(3):354–60.
42. Katz JM, Devinsky O. Primary generalized epilepsy: A risk factor for seizures in labor and delivery? *Seizure*. 2003;**12**(4):217–19.
43. Bollig KJ, Jackson DL. Seizures in pregnancy. *Obstetrics and Gynecology Clinics of North America*. 2018;**45**(2):349–67.
44. Eclampsia Trial Collaborative Group. Which anticonvulsant for women with eclampsia? Evidence from the collaborative eclampsia trial. *Lancet*. 1995;**345**:1455–63.
45. Lu Y, Hsu C, Tsai W, et al. Status epilepticus associated with pregnancy: A cohort study. *Epilepsy & Behavior*. 2016;**59**:92–7.
46. Rajiv KR, Radhakrishnan A. Status epilepticus in pregnancy: Can we frame a uniform treatment protocol? *Epilepsy & Behavior*. 2019;**101**:106376.
47. Kusznir Vitturi B, Barreto Cabral F, Mella Cukiert C. Outcomes of pregnant women with refractory epilepsy. *Seizure*. 2019;**69**:251–7.

Chapter 13

Obstetric and Fetal Monitoring in Women with Epilepsy

John W. Snelgrove and Mathew Sermer

Key Points

- Most women with epilepsy (WWE) will have no change in seizure frequency during pregnancy.
- The risk of seizure during labor and delivery is low (2–3%).
- Women with epilepsy are more likely than women without epilepsy (WWoE) to experience spontaneous abortion or preterm birth and to have small-for-gestational-age (SGA) infants. Women with epilepsy are also at higher risk of the hypertensive disorders of pregnancy, postpartum hemorrhage, peripartum depression, and maternal death – although the latter remains rare. Poor seizure control preceding pregnancy, unplanned pregnancy, and polytherapy are associated with higher risks.
- The reported associations between epilepsy and adverse pregnancy outcomes may be affected to some extent by differences in baseline maternal characteristics and other confounders.
- Valproic acid (VPA) has the highest risk of fetal major congenital malformations (MCMs) and should be avoided in reproductive-aged WWE, if possible. Monotherapy with an appropriate antiseizure medication (ASM) at the lowest-effective dose to achieve seizure freedom is the goal. The ASM levels should be monitored in pregnancy and postpartum, as dose adjustments may be necessary.
- Daily folic acid supplementation is ideally initiated 2–3 months prior to conception and continued through pregnancy and the postpartum period or until breastfeeding completion.
- The best modality to detect neural tube defects (NTDs) and MCMs is second-trimester fetal anatomical sonography.
- Women with epilepsy should have coordinated antenatal care involving an obstetrician and a neurologist with experience in managing epilepsy. Delivery should occur in an obstetric unit with proper expertise and resources for the care of WWE.
- Epilepsy is not an indication for a caesarean delivery. Caesarean delivery should be performed for the usual obstetrical indications, or in the setting of intractable generalized seizures during labor.

Effects of Pregnancy on Epilepsy

Most pregnant people with epilepsy will have maintained seizure control during their pregnancy. The risk of increased seizure activity that is directly attributable to pregnancy is minimal. Older literature comparing seizure frequency in pregnant WWE to the seizure frequency preceding their pregnancy reported seizure freedom 50–75% of the time. These findings were corroborated by a larger dataset from the European & International Registry of Antiepileptic Drugs and Pregnancy (EURAP) [1]. A 2013 update reported pregnancy outcomes, antiseizure medication (ASM) use, and seizure type and frequency for 3,806 prospectively followed pregnancies among 3,451 WWE. Two-thirds (66.6%) of WWE remained seizure free throughout their pregnancy, while 15.8% experienced an increase in seizure activity. Women with epilepsy with idiopathic generalized epilepsies were significantly more likely to remain seizure free (73.6%) than those with localized-related epilepsies (59.5%; $p < 0.001$) [1]. More recent studies have compared seizure activity in pregnant WWE to that in nonpregnant WWE controls, permitting evaluation of the pregnancy-associated effects on epilepsy course and seizure risk. The Maternal Outcomes and Neurodevelopmental Effects of Antiepileptic Drugs (MONEAD) multicenter, prospective cohort study reported seizure outcomes among pregnant and postpartum WWE compared with nonpregnant WWE controls who were similar with respect to age, sociodemographic characteristics, epilepsy diagnosis, baseline seizure frequency, and ASM type and dose [2]. To estimate changes in seizure activity during pregnancy, the authors compared seizure frequency over 18 months divided between two epochs, from conception up to 6 weeks postpartum (total, 10.5 months), and then from 6 weeks postpartum to 9 months postpartum. The nonpregnant WWE control group was similarly assessed over the same follow-up time period, using time of enrollment to define the start of epoch 1, and 10.5 months following enrollment to define the start of epoch 2. Increased seizure frequency during pregnancy and the first 6 weeks postpartum occurred in 23% of pregnant WWE and in 25% of nonpregnant WWE controls during the corresponding epoch, and the discrepancy in these proportions was not statistically significant (adjusted odds ratio (aOR) 0.93, 95% CI 0.54–1.60) [2]. This study was important in demonstrating that overall seizure activity was no different for pregnant WWE compared to similar nonpregnant WWE over the same time period. Seizures during pregnancy were approximately equal in frequency during the second and third trimesters, and postpartum (15%, 15%, and 12%, respectively) and were less likely in the first trimester (7%) [2].

The MONEAD study also found that ASM dose or type was changed at least once in significantly more pregnant WWE (74%), compared with nonpregnant WWE (31%; OR 6.36, 95% CI 3.82–10.59) [2]. This finding is not surprising, given that pharmacodynamic changes in pregnancy warrant careful monitoring and titration of ASM doses. Drug levels in pregnancy are affected by multiple factors and may be reduced in relation to nausea and vomiting, decreased gastrointestinal motility and absorption, increased circulating blood volume, and increased drug metabolism. Lower compliance with ASM therapy over concerns about teratogenicity and other negative effects may also complicate dosing and drug bioavailability. Large observational studies have evaluated changes in ASM prescribing and adherence trends over time. These studies suggest that while there is an overall increase in the number of pregnancies with corresponding ASM use, the use of specific ASMs associated with higher teratogenicity potential has decreased. For example, population-linked registry data from Australia and five Nordic countries, combined with US drug claims data, showed a reduction in valproic acid (VPA) use from 2006 to 2016 – although notable prescribing pattern differences exist between countries [3]. In the United States over a similar time frame, Ajinkya and colleagues [4] reported an increase in levetiracetam (LEV) use among almost 400,000 WWE of reproductive age with data from the Medical Expenditure Panel Survey Household Component. Combined, these representative population-based studies suggest that changes in ASM prescription patterns among WWE reflect the evolving availability of drug safety data, an increased understanding of teratogenic risks among certain ASMs, and the benefits of monotherapy during pregnancy. The teratogenic effects of ASMs are addressed further in Chapter 11, and ASM dosing and monitoring for seizure control management during pregnancy are discussed in Chapter 12.

Fetal and Neonatal Outcomes Associated with Epilepsy

In addition to the risks of major congenital malformations (MCMs) described in Chapter 11, increased fetal risks exist for pregnant WWE, including fetal growth restriction, intrauterine fetal death, and preterm birth. This suggests that epilepsy as a maternal medical condition may pose a risk to fetal development and maturation to some extent. However, it is challenging to disentangle these effects as many studies compare pregnancies of WWE to those of women without epilepsy (WWoE) and are therefore unable to evaluate whether risks are mainly driven by the epilepsy condition itself, or by seizure control and frequency, ASM use, or other possible confounders. For example, pregnant WWE are more likely to have pregestational diabetes, hypertension, mental illness, and substance use disorders, and have lower educational attainment, all of which are associated with adverse perinatal outcomes [5].

A 2015 meta-analysis including more than 2.8 million pregnancies evaluated adverse maternal and fetal outcomes among WWE compared to WWoE and found small but significant risk increases for spontaneous abortion (pooled OR 1.54, 95% CI 1.02–2.32), preterm birth at less than 37 weeks of gestation (pooled OR 1.16, 95% CI 1.01–1.34), and fetal growth restriction (pooled OR 1.26, 95% CI 1.20–1.33), although not for stillbirth, perinatal death, or neonatal intensive care unit (NICU) admission [6]. A 2017 population-based Swedish study by Razaz and colleagues examined more than 1.4 million singleton births, including 5,373 births among 3,586 WWE [5]. This study compared birth outcomes between WWE and WWoE pregnancies, but also between WWE pregnancies with and without ASM exposure. The authors found that almost all fetal adverse outcomes were more likely in WWE pregnancies than in WWoE pregnancies, including preterm birth (7.7% vs. 4.7%, aOR 1.49, 95% CI 1.34–1.66), stillbirth (0.6% vs. 0.3%, aOR 1.55, 95% CI 1.05–2.30), and small-for-gestational-age (SGA) fetal size (8.4% vs. 6.3%, aOR 1.25, 95% CI 1.13–1.30) [5]. Neonatal adverse outcomes were also more prevalent among WWE, including asphyxia-related complications (meconium aspiration, hypoxic ischemic encephalopathy, neonatal seizure), respiratory distress syndrome, hypoglycemia, and low APGAR scores [5]. An important caveat for this study was that WWE were more likely than WWoE to have pregestational diabetes, hypertension, mental illness, and substance use – all of which are significant risk factors for each of the fetal outcomes reported. Use of ASMs among WWE was not associated with these potential confounders. When comparing WWE pregnancies with ASM use to WWE pregnancies without ASM use, the authors found no significant differences in fetal or neonatal outcomes. This corroborates a study by Viale and colleagues, apart from a minimal increase in NICU admissions found in their meta-analysis (pooled OR 1.42, 95% CI 1.13–1.78) [6]. In contrast, an analysis using North American Antiepileptic Drug Pregnancy Registry data showed higher rates of preterm birth, SGA, and lower birth weight among women on ASMs in pregnancy, regardless of whether the medication was to used treat epilepsy or another neuropsychiatric condition [7]. Tomson and colleagues used EURAP data to compare different ASM types and found no differences in spontaneous abortion and stillbirth outcomes between the six most frequently used monotherapies in the registry – carbamazepine, lamotrigine (LTG), VPA, LEV, phenobarbital, and oxcarbazepine [8]. However, the authors did find a significantly higher risk of overall fetal death with polytherapy (12.1%) compared to monotherapy (8.2%), with an adjusted risk ratio (aRR) of 1.38 (95% CI 1.14–1.66). The majority of fetal deaths occurred under 24 weeks of gestation, and stillbirths (fetal death occurring at ≥ 24 weeks of gestation) were below 1% across all ASM monotherapy types and the polytherapy category [8].

There is limited research on the direct fetal effects of seizure activity during pregnancy. Focal seizure activity that does not evolve to bilateral tonic-clonic seizures are thought to have minimal impact on fetal and overall maternal well-being. However, earlier studies have demonstrated transient fetal heart rate decelerations and fetal bradycardia lasting several minutes following a complex partial seizure [9, 10]. These case studies support the hypothesis that seizures with impaired awareness may transiently interfere with placental oxygen transport to the fetus. Complications associated with impaired awareness and fall-related maternal and fetal injury are also possible. Generalized tonic-clonic seizures have the added risk of direct fetal trauma during convulsive seizure activity, and the effects of imbalances in maternal blood pressure, oxygenation, and serum electrolytes can adversely impact the fetus. Few studies have demonstrated these fetal effects, and much of our understanding is inferred either from animal models or from studies on eclamptic seizures [11]. Two cases of prolonged fetal bradycardia followed by tachycardia immediately after maternal generalized tonic-clonic seizure were reported by Teramo and colleagues in 1979 [12]. Minkoff and colleagues described a fetal intracranial hemorrhage following maternal seizure in a case report from 1985, with the injury attributed to direct fetal trauma experienced during the seizure [13]. More recently, the effects of seizures during pregnancy have been evaluated with respect to fetal growth and maturity. Seizures are likely independently associated with adverse outcomes after accounting for ASM use and other maternal characteristics. For example, having one or more generalized tonic-clonic seizure during pregnancy was associated with low birth weight in male neonates, and with preterm birth for both sexes (OR 5.35, 95 % CI 1.37–20.93) compared to no seizure activity in pregnancy among WWE on similar ASMs [14].

A final concern among many pregnant WWE and their partners is the risk of epilepsy in their child. Maternal epilepsy is associated with a higher lifetime risk of epilepsy in their offspring (3–9%) compared to paternal epilepsy (1–3%), and the risk is greater if a sibling or both parents are affected [15]. Advances in genetic testing, including the advent of next-generation sequencing, has resulted in a proliferation of candidate genetic causes for epilepsies that were formerly considered idiopathic. More robust evidence from population-based family aggregation studies and twin concordance studies points to complex patterns of familial inheritance [16, 17]. It is now widely accepted that genetics play a much larger role in epilepsy than previously appreciated.

To summarize, WWE are more likely than WWoE to experience pregnancies complicated by preterm birth, fetal growth restriction/SGA, and spontaneous abortion. Some studies suggest a small but significant increase in stillbirth risk, although others do not. Adverse neonatal outcomes are also more prevalent among WWE pregnancies. An important limitation of the available evidence is the potential for confounding by underlying medical comorbidities such as preexisting diabetes, hypertension, mental illness, and substance use. The use of ASMs may be associated with some adverse fetal/neonatal outcomes, including preterm birth, SGA, low birth weight, and NICU admission, although the evidence is inconsistent across studies. Compared to monotherapy, ASM polytherapy is associated with increased rates of fetal death at less than 24 weeks of gestation.

Maternal Outcomes Associated with Epilepsy

Epilepsy is associated with increased risks of adverse maternal outcomes and with mode of delivery. In a 2015 meta-analysis by Viale and colleagues, increased pregnancy risks among WWE compared to WWoE were seen for antepartum hemorrhage (pooled OR 1.49, 95% CI 1.01–2.20), postpartum hemorrhage (pooled OR 1.29, 95% CI 1.13–1.49), and the hypertensive disorders of pregnancy (pooled OR 1.37, 95% CI 1.21–1.55) [6]. When evaluating only WWE pregnancies, those exposed to ASMs were more likely to experience postpartum hemorrhage than those not exposed (pooled OR 1.33, 95% CI 1.16–1.54); however, other adverse maternal outcomes were not increased. The association between ASM use and postpartum hemorrhage has been called into question more recently. The underlying etiology proposed for increased bleeding is that some ASMs are inducers of cytochrome P450 (e.g., carbamazepine, phenobarbital, phenytoin, oxcarbazepine, topiramate), which in turn could alter vitamin K activity. To evaluate this, Panchaud and colleagues performed a population-based cohort study of more than 11,500 publicly insured pregnant women in the US Medicaid Analytic eXtract dataset and compared maternal and neonatal hemorrhage complications between ASMs that induce P450 activity and those that do not, using propensity-score techniques to adjust for ASM indication and other potential confounders. They found no difference in postpartum hemorrhage among those taking a P450-inducing ASM (2.6%) and those taking other ASMs (3.6%; aRR 0.77, 95% CI 0.58–1.00), and no difference in neonatal hemorrhage complications [18]. Although epilepsy is associated with higher rates of the hypertensive disorders of pregnancy, comparisons between WWE and WWoE are likely affected to some extent by differences in underlying medical conditions and other variables [5, 19, 20]. Few studies address the specific effects of individual ASMs on hypertension in pregnancy. The use of VPA may be associated with non-severe preeclampsia compared to no ASM use in WWoE (aOR 2.9, 95% CI 1.3–6.4), while LEV and LTG were not associated in one Norwegian population-based cohort study [20].

Epilepsy is associated with a 5–10-fold higher risk of maternal death in studies from the United States, the United Kingdom, and Denmark [21–23]. However, this remains a rare outcome and studies that can measure absolute maternal mortality rates report 80–100 per 100,000 WWE pregnancies compared to 6–11 per 100,000 WWoE pregnancies [21, 23]. The majority of maternal deaths associated with epilepsy are seizure-related, mostly involving sudden unexpected death in epilepsy (SUDEP) [21–23].

Increased attention is now paid to the risk of maternal mental illness and the role of chronic conditions in exacerbating peripartum depression and anxiety. Women with epilepsy have higher rates of depression than the general population, and this is reflected in pregnancy as well, with up to 29% of WWE experiencing postpartum depression compared to 11% of WWoE [24, 25]. The risk of postpartum depression may be further increased for multiparous WWE and those on ASM polytherapy [25].

Studies evaluating maternal outcomes also typically investigate associations between epilepsy and delivery mode and other obstetrical interventions. Women with epilepsy are more likely to have an induction of labor and to be delivered by caesarean delivery [6]. Both emergency, unplanned caesarean delivery during labor [26] and planned elective caesarean delivery [19] are more common among WWE. Breech presentation is one indication for caesarean delivery and was found to be twice as likely among WWE pregnancies in one prospective cohort study [26]. Other reasons for higher caesarean delivery rates in this population may relate to fetal indications or to other obstetric indications, but rarely to intractable seizure activity necessitating urgent delivery [27].

To summarize, WWE have higher rates of adverse outcomes during pregnancy and postpartum, including the hypertensive disorders of pregnancy, postpartum hemorrhage, peripartum depression, and maternal death – although the latter remains a rare event. As with the associations between epilepsy and fetal outcomes, comparisons between WWE and WWoE for maternal outcomes are likely confounded to some extent by underlying medical conditions and other factors. Women with epilepsy are more likely to deliver by caesarean delivery, although uncommonly for indications directly related to seizure activity at the time of birth.

Antenatal Management

Preconception and Early Pregnancy

Preconception counseling for WWE is an important opportunity to identify additional risk factors, optimize ASM medication, and provide information for patients and their family (see Chapter 10). With the increasing awareness of the role genetics play in many forms of epilepsy, consideration should be given to a medical genetics consultation based on features of the patient's clinical and family history. Epilepsy associated with maternal congenital anomalies, neurodevelopmental disabilities, autism spectrum disorder, or a family history of epilepsy may warrant referral to a geneticist in advance of pregnancy [16]. Women with epilepsy of reproductive age should be counseled regarding folate deficiency and associated MCMs. Canadian pregnancy guidelines support folic acid supplementation from preconception through 12 weeks of gestation at a dose of 1.0 mg daily, and thereafter with doses of 0.4–1.0 mg daily for WWE taking ASMs [28]. If a WWE or their partner has a personal history of a neural tube defects (NTDs) or other congenital anomaly associated with folate deficiency, the recommended dose is increased to 4.0–5.0 mg daily from preconception through 12 weeks of gestation. National guidelines from the United Kingdom recommend a folic acid dose of 5.0 mg daily for all WWE from preconception through the first trimester, regardless of ASM use [29]. Given emerging data on neurodevelopmental benefits, it is likely that folic acid supplementation is beneficial throughout pregnancy, although more studies are needed to establish the optimal dose.

Routine aneuploidy screening for the most common significant fetal aneuploidies (trisomies 13, 18, 21) should be offered to pregnant WWE according to local standards of care. This ideally includes nuchal translucency ultrasound at between 11 and 13 weeks and biochemical or circulating cell-free fetal DNA screening for aneuploidy.

Fetal Anatomical Assessment

The best modality to assess for NTDs is a second-trimester anatomical sonography with detailed fetal spine and intracranial imaging [30]. This is performed between 18 and 22 weeks of gestation. The use of maternal serum alpha-fetoprotein is described as an alternative option in lieu of sonography for specific instances where geography or maternal factors such as elevated body mass index (e.g. BMI > 35 kg/m^2) prevent timely referral to detailed anatomical sonography. First-trimester fetal anatomical sonography – often performed in conjunction with nuchal translucency measurement – is increasingly offered by tertiary obstetrics centers for pregnancies at moderate-to-high risk of NTDs and other MCMs. In the context of epilepsy, this may be considered based on a patient's personal or previous pregnancy history, use of an ASM with higher teratogenicity, or other medical factors. Early anatomical sonography performed between 11 and 16 weeks at an experienced center can detect up to 86% of MCMs, although it must always be followed by routine second-trimester sonography to complete the assessment of fetal anatomy [31]. In cases where early anatomy sonography detects a significant MCM, patients should be referred for maternal-fetal medicine counseling to discuss pregnancy options, including termination of pregnancy.

Ongoing Pregnancy Care

Pregnant WWE should have regular antenatal care involving a multidisciplinary team that includes an obstetrician and a neurologist with experience in epilepsy. Referral to a maternal-fetal medicine specialist should be considered for pregnancies with high-risk features, including seizures during pregnancy, suboptimal or worsening seizure control, unplanned pregnancy, exposure to ASMs with higher risk of teratogenicity (VPA), or ASM polytherapy. Seizure control in the year before pregnancy is the best predictor of seizure control during pregnancy, and WWE who have experienced seizures should be monitored more closely. Pregnant WWE should be counseled regarding MCMs and other pregnancy risks associated with ASMs, but also about the risks of discontinuing medication, as nonadherence is a major cause of breakthrough seizures, which can have deleterious fetal effects. The lowest effective ASM dose – preferably monotherapy if possible – should be used, and the choice of medication should take into account potential teratogenicity. The use of LEV or LTG is associated with the lowest risk of MCMs and is preferred where appropriate [27]. The use of VPA should be avoided unless necessary to maintain seizure control. For WWE on VPA who are already pregnant, withdrawal or changing to a different ASM is reasonable under close observation, if seizure control can be maintained [32]. Drug-level monitoring should be considered for each case and based on ASM type. Notably, LTG and LEV have significantly reduced serum concentrations during pregnancy that may require dose adjustment [27]. Serial growth ultrasounds in the third trimester are necessary to detect SGA fetuses and to assist with delivery planning [29]. Table 13.1 presents the suggested maternal and fetal monitoring for WWE in pregnancy.

Intrapartum and Postpartum Management

The majority of pregnant WWE will experience an uncomplicated labor and birth. The risk of a seizure during labor and delivery for WWE is approximately 2–3% (EURAP) [1]. In the event of an intrapartum seizure, swift treatment with a fast-acting benzodiazepine is indicated – for example, lorazepam (0.1 mg/kg IV), usually given as a 4 mg bolus followed by a second 4 mg dose after 10–20 minutes, or diazepam (5–10 mg IV) administered slowly. If no IV access is available, rectal diazepam (10–15 mg followed by a second 10–15 mg dose after 15 minutes) or buccal midazolam (10 mg) are suitable alternative options [29]. Any seizure lasting longer than 5 minutes should raise concern for status epilepticus, prompting immediate treatment and expedited delivery. Delivery timing and mode are tailored to each individual case; however, epilepsy itself is not an indication for induction of labor or caesarean delivery in the absence of additional concerns or other obstetrical indications [27, 29]. Epidural analgesia should be offered as a safe, effective pain management strategy for WWE in labor. By alleviating the stressor of pain, the use of an epidural minimizes the risk of seizures in labor and provides added safety in situations where urgent caesarean delivery is required [29]. Delayed pushing in the second stage of labor should be considered, if appropriate, to allow passive descent of the fetus. Assisted vaginal birth with vacuum or forceps may be considered to expedite delivery if concerns arise about the maternal or fetal status. Continuous fetal heart rate monitoring in

Table 13.1 Suggested maternal and fetal components of pregnancy monitoring for women with epilepsy

Time period	Monitoring and management
Preconception	• Optimize ASM medication: Goal is seizure freedom with monotherapy at lowest effective dose, if possible • Baseline ASM levels • Start folic acid supplementation • Genetics referral if indicated • Preconception counseling (Chapter 10)
First trimester (0–12 weeks)	• Establish coordinated care plan, obstetrics and neurology • Routine aneuploidy screening, nuchal translucency ultrasound (11–13 weeks) • Early anatomy ultrasound if high-risk features (11–16 weeks) • Monitor ASM drug levels
Second trimester (13–27 weeks)	• Anatomy ultrasound (18–22 weeks) – special attention to spine, intracranial structures, cardiac and facial anatomy • Monitor ASM drug levels
Third trimester (28–42 weeks)	• Serial fetal growth ultrasounds (every 2–4 weeks) • Monitor ASM drug levels • Delivery planning
Intrapartum	• Maintain adequate hydration, minimize sleep deprivation • Consider epidural analgesia to minimize labor pain • Continuous fetal heart rate monitoring if indicated • Avoid missing ASM doses • Caesarean delivery for usual OB indications, or if status epilepticus (rare)
Postpartum	• Maintain adequate pain control, sleep • Postpartum ASM levels and dose titration (Chapter 16) • Postpartum depression screening (Chapter 2) • Support breastfeeding (Chapter 18) • Postpartum safety and counseling (Chapter 16) • Contraception counseling (Chapters 5 and 10)

labor is individualized based on an assessment of perinatal risk factors, patient characteristics, and labor interventions. In addition to the standard indications, continuous fetal monitoring is warranted in WWE with any seizure activity during the pregnancy or labor [29, 33]. Care must be taken to avoid missed ASM doses during labor and the postpartum period. The ASM dose should be reevaluated postpartum if it was increased during pregnancy to avoid supra-therapeutic levels and toxicity. Sleep deprivation, dehydration, pain, and other stressors need to be minimized as these are triggers for seizure deterioration. Finally, WWE should be informed about the symptoms of peripartum depression and provided with supports and urgent medical care contact options [29].

References

1. Battino D, Tomson T, Bonizzoni E, et al. Seizure control and treatment changes in pregnancy: Observations from the EURAP epilepsy pregnancy registry. *Epilepsia*. 2013;**54**(9):1621–7.
2. Pennell PB, French JA, May RC, et al. Changes in seizure frequency and antiepileptic therapy during pregnancy. *New England Journal of Medicine*. 2020;**383**(26):2547–56.
3. Cohen JM, Cesta CE, Furu K, et al. Prevalence trends and individual patterns of antiepileptic drug use in pregnancy 2006–2016: A study in the five Nordic countries, United States, and Australia. *Pharmacoepidemiology & Drug Safety*. 2020;**29**(8):913–22.
4. Ajinkya S, Fox J, Lekoubou A. Contemporary trends in antiepileptic drug treatment among women of childbearing age with epilepsy in the United States: 2004–2015. *Journal of the Neurological Sciences*. 2021;**427**:117500.
5. Razaz N, Tomson T, Wikstrom AK, Cnattingius S. Association between pregnancy and perinatal outcomes among women with epilepsy. *JAMA Neurology*. 2017;**74**(8):983–91.
6. Viale L, Allotey J, Cheong-See F, et al. Epilepsy in pregnancy and reproductive outcomes: A systematic review and meta-analysis. *Lancet*. 2015;**386**(10006):1845–52.
7. Hernandez-Diaz S, McElrath TF, Pennell PB, et al. Fetal growth and premature delivery in pregnant women on antiepileptic drugs. *Annals of Neurology*. 2017;**82**(3):457–65.
8. Tomson T, Battino D, Bonizzoni E, et al. Antiepileptic drugs and intrauterine death: A prospective observational study from EURAP. *Neurology*. 2015;**85**(7):580–8.
9. Nei M, Daly S, Liporace J. A maternal complex partial seizure in labor can affect fetal heart rate. *Neurology*. 1998;**51**(3):904–6.
10. Sahoo S, Klein P. Maternal complex partial seizure associated with fetal distress. *Arch Neurol*. 2005;**62**(8):1304–5.
11. Sveberg L, Svalheim S, Taubøll E. The impact of seizures on pregnancy and delivery. *Seizure*. 2015;**28**:35–8.
12. Teramo K, Hiilesmaa V, Bardy A, Saarikoski S. Fetal heart rate during a maternal grand mal epileptic seizure. *J Perinat Med*. 1979;**7**(1):3–6.
13. Minkoff H, Schaffer RM, Delke I, Grunebaum AN. Diagnosis of intracranial hemorrhage in utero after a maternal seizure. *Obstetrics and Gynecology*. 1985;**65**(3 Suppl):22S–4S.
14. Rauchenzauner M, Ehrensberger M, Prieschl M, et al. Generalized tonic-clonic seizures and antiepileptic drugs during pregnancy: A matter of importance for the baby? *Journal of Neurology*. 2013;**260**(2):484–8.
15. Winawer MR, Shinnar S. Genetic epidemiology of epilepsy or what do we tell families? *Epilepsia*. 2005;**46** Suppl 10:24–30.
16. el-Achkar CM, Olson HE, Poduri A, Pearl PL. The genetics of the epilepsies. *Current Neurology & Neuroscience Reports*. 2015;**15**(7):39.

17. Perucca P, Bahlo M, Berkovic SF. The genetics of epilepsy. *Annu Rev Genomics Hum Genet*. 2020;**21**:205–30.

18. Panchaud A, Cohen JM, Patorno E, et al. Anticonvulsants and the risk of perinatal bleeding complications: A pregnancy cohort study. *Neurology*. 2018;**91**(6):e533–e42.

19. Danielsson KC, Gilhus NE, Borthen I, Lie RT, Morken NH. Maternal complications in pregnancy and childbirth for women with epilepsy: Time trends in a nationwide cohort. *PLoS One*. 2019;**14**(11): e0225334.

20. Danielsson KC, Borthen I, Morken NH, Gilhus NE. Hypertensive pregnancy complications in women with epilepsy and antiepileptic drugs: A population-based cohort study of first pregnancies in Norway. *BMJ Open*. 2018;**8**(4):e020998.

21. MacDonald SC, Bateman BT, McElrath TF, Hernandez-Diaz S. Mortality and morbidity during delivery hospitalization among pregnant women with epilepsy in the United States. *JAMA Neurology*. 2015;**72**(9):981–8.

22. Christensen J, Vestergaard C, Hammer Bech B. Maternal death in women with epilepsy: Smaller scope studies. *Neurology*. 2018;**91**(18):e1716–20.

23. Edey S, Moran N, Nashef L. SUDEP and epilepsy-related mortality in pregnancy. *Epilepsia*. 2014;**55**(7):e72–4.

24. Turner K, Piazzini A, Franza A, et al. Postpartum depression in women with epilepsy versus women without epilepsy. *Epilepsy Behav*. 2006;**9**(2):293–7.

25. Galanti M, Newport DJ, Pennell PB, et al. Postpartum depression in women with epilepsy: Influence of antiepileptic drugs in a prospective study. *Epilepsy Behav*. 2009;**16**(3):426–30.

26. Farmen AH, Grundt JH, Nakling JO, et al. Increased rate of acute caesarean sections in women with epilepsy: Results from the Oppland Perinatal Database in Norway. *European Journal of Neurology*. 2019;**26**(4):617–23.

27. Tomson T, Battino D, Bromley R, et al. Management of epilepsy in pregnancy: A report from the International League Against Epilepsy Task Force on Women and Pregnancy. *Epileptic Disorders*. 2019;**21**(6):497–517.

28. Wilson RD, Wilson RD, Audibert F, et al. Pre-conception folic acid and multivitamin supplementation for the primary and secondary prevention of neural tube defects and other folic acid–sensitive congenital anomalies. *Journal of Obstetrics and Gynaecology Canada*. 2015;**37**(6):534–49.

29. Royal College of Obstetricians and Gynaecologists. *Epilepsy in pregnancy: Green-top guideline No. 68*. London: Royal College of Obstetricians and Gynaecologists; 2016.

30. Wilson RD, Van Mieghem T, Langlois S, Church P. Guideline No. 410: Prevention, screening, diagnosis, and pregnancy management for fetal neural tube defects. *Journal of Obstetrics and Gynaecology Canada*. 2021;**43**(1):124–39.

31. Nevo O, Brown R, Glanc P, Lim K. No. 352: Technical update. The role of early comprehensive fetal anatomy ultrasound examination. *Journal of Obstetrics and Gynaecology Canada*. 2017;**39**(12):1203–11.

32. The Epilepsy Implementation Task Force (EITF) and Epilepsy Research Program of the Ontario Brain Institute. *Provincial clinical guidelines for the management of epilepsy in adults and children*. Toronto, ON: The Epilepsy Implementation Task Force (EITF) and Epilepsy Research Program of the Ontario Brain Institute; 2020.

33. Dore S, Ehman W. No. 396: Fetal health surveillance. Intrapartum consensus guideline. *Journal of Obstetrics and Gynaecology Canada*. 2020;**42**(3):316–48.

Chapter 14

Neuroimaging in Pregnancy and Epilepsy

Paula Alcaide Leon and Kalliopi A. Petropoulou

Key Points

- Multidisciplinary decision-making in triaging imaging modality is recommended, as protocols can be optimized or deferred to minimize potential harm to the fetus.
- Computed tomography (CT) of the head does expose the fetus to scattered radiation, though the radiation dose is relatively low.
- Iodinated contrast for CT carries a negligible risk of newborn hypothyroidism and should not be withheld in pregnant or potentially pregnant patients when it is needed for diagnostic purposes.
- Gadolinium contrast for magnetic resonance imaging (MRI) should be administered to pregnant or potentially pregnant patients only if their usage is considered critical for diagnosis.
- Imaging helps differentiate causes of seizures in pregnancy, including eclampsia, cerebral venous thrombosis, postpartum angiopathy, and tumors.

Introduction

Pregnant women who present with seizure may or may not have a prior history of seizure or epilepsy. The imaging approach would vary depending on the medical history and presentation. The imaging protocols should be tailored to address the clinical question and for that, adequate and accurate history should be provided. For example, a pregnant woman with eclampsia should be approached from an imaging standpoint differently from a patient with known epilepsy prior to her pregnancy. The main focus of this chapter is discussion of pregnancy-related conditions associated with epilepsy and seizure, among other neurologic symptoms, along with their appropriate imaging.

Neuroimaging in Pregnancy

Computed tomography (CT) and magnetic resonance imaging (MRI) are the two main modalities available for evaluation of the brain. Patients with epilepsy are evaluated almost exclusively with MRI. However, CT may be the only modality available in a case of acute onset of seizure, when the patient's condition does not allow the lengthy imaging often required for MRI, or MRI is not available.

Computed tomography can accurately show acute intracranial hemorrhage, brain edema, mass effect, hydrocephalus, and many times, dural sinus thrombosis. Modern scanners allow the completion of imaging within seconds, which may be quite desirable for a patient with altered level of consciousness and otherwise limited available history. The multiplanar capability and superior soft tissue resolution renders MRI the modality of choice for evaluation of the brain parenchyma.

Pregnancy represents a challenge when it comes to choosing the appropriate imaging modality since potential risks to the fetus have to be taken into consideration. Pregnancy as well as breastfeeding may raise questions as to the appropriateness of the intravenous, iodinated, or gadolinium-based contrast administration. It is imperative that existing guidelines are followed any time a pregnant woman undergoes either CT or MRI.

Safety Considerations for the Unborn Child

Computed Tomography Imaging and Radiation Exposure

It has long been recognized that ionizing radiation can induce detrimental biological effects in organs and tissues by producing free radicals and damaging important molecules such as DNA. The amount of biological damage depends on the total energy deposited (dose) and the type of radiation. X-rays produce less biological damage than alpha particles for the same amount of energy (dose) deposited in the tissue. Data on the detrimental effects of radiation come from studies on atomic bomb survivors, radiation workers, and radiation therapy. The effects are categorized as deterministic and stochastic (random).

Determinist effects of radiation are short-term, adverse tissue reactions resulting from a dose that is significantly high enough to damage living tissues (dose > 0.5Gy). They are generally related to cell death and characterized by a threshold dose. Typical manifestations include skin erythema, cataract, hair loss, and induction of sterility. Exposure of the fetus to radiation dose greater than 0.5Gy may result in malformations or growth or mental retardation.

Stochastic effects occur at low doses (doses < 0.5Gy) of radiation, reflect damage to one cell, and may result in carcinogenesis and genetic damage. The severity of the radiation-induced stochastic effects is independent of the radiation dose and there is no associated dose threshold. The radiation dose only affects the probability of the stochastic effects. The important goal of radiation protection is to prevent the occurrence of deterministic effects and minimize the radiation dose, and thus the potentially associated stochastic effects.

The International Commission on Radiological Protection in its 2007 recommendations stated that no deterministic effects of practical significance are likely to occur on the fetus or embryo when exposed to a cumulative dose less than 100mGy [1]. No additional updates from the commission were available at the time of this review. In contrast, there is no dose threshold for stochastic effects of radiation exposure. Stochastic effects reflect damage to one cell, which can lead to carcinogenesis. Exposure of the fetus to radiation up to 1mGy is acceptable given the very low likelihood for carcinogenesis (less than 1/10,000).

Computed tomography studies above the diaphragm and below the knee fall into this category. In addition, during head CT, the fetus is exposed mainly to attenuated scattered rather than direct radiation exposure. The estimated fetal exposure from a head CT is 1.0–10mGy [1, 2]. The most vulnerable stage of the embryo in terms of teratogenesis is between the 2nd and 20th weeks of gestation, particularly the period between the 8th and 15th weeks [3]. Although the use of lead on the pregnant woman's abdomen does not protect from the scattered radiation, most radiology departments recommend its use. In the case of unintended exposure to radiation solely for imaging purposes, the American College of Obstetricians and Gynecologists has stated that abortion is not recommended [4].

Iodinated Contrast Medium and the Effect on the Fetus and Newborn

Diagnostic iodinated contrast media have been shown to cross the human placenta and enter the fetus when given in usual clinical doses. Animal testing has shown no evidence of either mutagenic or teratogenic effects with low-osmolality contrast media. There have been rare reports of hypothyroidism in newborns after the administration of an iodinated contrast medium during pregnancy. However, this occurred only following amniofetography using a fat-soluble iodinated contrast medium. There has been no reported case of neonatal hypothyroidism from the maternal intravascular injection of water-soluble iodinated contrast agents. Given the current available data and routine screening of all newborns for congenital hypothyroidism, no additional precautions are necessary. The American College of Radiology (ACR) does not recommend withholding the use of iodinated contrast agents in pregnant or potentially pregnant patients when it is needed for diagnostic purposes [5].

Iodinated contrast media are excreted into breast milk, however, as high-molecular-weight, non-ionized, and water-soluble drugs have little affinity in binding to milk. Their use in breastfeeding women is considered safe, with an exception placed on women nursing preterm infants, as their immature auto-regulatory thyroid axis puts them at increased risk for transient hypothyroidism. Nursing mothers should be informed and, if concerned, instructed to discard milk for 24 hours. The administration of contrast agents takes into consideration the mother's safety as well. In our institution, the renal function is checked routinely prior to administration of contrast agents.

Magnetic Resonance Imaging

When a pregnant woman undergoes MRI, the fetus is exposed to a strong magnetic field (10,000 times higher than the Earth), an energy deposition that has the potential of causing a minimal increase in body temperature and a high acoustic noise level. The main safety concern is exposure to radiofrequency pulses with subsequent tissue heating. Each excitation and refocusing radiofrequency pulse of an MRI sequence deposits energy into the individual being scanned, which is converted into heat. Heating greater than 2°C can be teratogenic [6].

In practice, fetal temperature cannot be directly measured; instead, the maternal specific absorption rate (SAR) is used to estimate the absorbed radiofrequency power per unit body weight and is measured in Watts per kilogram. Although SAR can be calculated for specific regions, the most commonly reported value is whole-body average SAR. A maternal rise in SAR logically coincides with a risk for embryonic or fetal temperature increases, although models have shown that the fetus receives only approximately 40–70% of the maternal SAR [7, 8]. Magnetic resonance scanners estimate SAR values automatically and warn the operator if regulatory limits are likely to be exceeded.

Acoustic noise in MRI is also a concern as loud noises could potentially damage fetal hearing. Multiple studies have explored potential damage to fetal hearing organs after exposure to 1.5T and 3T MRI during different stages of pregnancy. None of the studies found differences in hearing ability between exposed and nonexposed neonates [9–12].

A retrospective review of a Canadian provincial database including 1.4 million pregnancies published in 2016 found that MRI use in the first trimester was not shown to be harmful to the fetus. Although there has been no documented harm to the fetus so far [13, 14], and the use of MRI is considered safe, caution in the use of this imaging modality during pregnancy has been suggested. The ACR eliminated restrictions related to gestational age in the 2007 update and suggested that the benefits for the mother and fetus must always outweigh the risks and, if necessary, to defer MRI until after the delivery [4].

Gadolinium-Based Contrast Medium and the Effect on the Fetus and Newborn

So far there have been no controlled studies in pregnant women regarding the adverse effects of gadolinium-based contrast on the human fetus. Animal studies use higher doses of gadolinium than usually used in imaging of humans, but they have shown that it may result in aborted fetuses or cause developmental anomalies. The gadolinium-based contrast agents are rated as class C drugs by the Food and Drug Administration (FDA), based on the fact that animal studies have shown adverse effects on the fetus at much higher doses than routinely administered and no controlled studies on women exist.

A retrospective review of a Canadian provincial database of births did not find an increased risk of a congenital anomaly associated with gadolinium exposure during pregnancy. However, it showed that gadolinium MRI at any time during pregnancy was associated with an increased risk of a broad set of rheumatologic, inflammatory, or infiltrative skin conditions and for stillbirth or neonatal death [14]. According to the current ACR recommendation on contrast media (2021) [5], gadolinium-based contrast agents should be administered with caution to pregnant or potentially pregnant patients. Such agents should only be used if their usage is considered critical and the potential benefits justify the potential unknown risk to the fetus. As with the iodine contrast medium, informed written consent should be obtained prior to using a gadolinium-based medium [13].

Gadolinium-based contrast agents are excreted into breast milk. They share similar properties with iodinated contrast media, resulting in minimal binding to milk and plasma proteins and thus minimal delivery to the infant. It is considered safe to continue breastfeeding following gadolinium administration. Again, if the nursing mother is concerned, she may be instructed to discard breast milk for 24 hours, which is the necessary time for the contrast agent to be cleared from the bloodstream. All radiology departments have policies in place as how to appropriately image pregnant and nursing women and minimize the exposure to the fetus of any risk related to modality or contrast medium.

Seizures in Pregnancy-Related Conditions: Neuroimaging

Comorbid conditions in pregnancy, such as the ones discussed next, may affect women otherwise healthy as well as women with epilepsy.

Preeclampsia and Eclampsia

Preeclampsia and eclampsia are the most severe stages of a complex, multisystem disorder that occurs in later stages of pregnancy as well as in the first 6–8 weeks postpartum. Preeclampsia, which occurs in 2–8% of all pregnancies, is a disorder characterized by the onset of hypertension, peripheral edema, and proteinuria in pregnant women after the 20th week of gestation. Patients with preeclampsia may also experience headache, visual changes, confusion, and altered mentation.

Eclampsia refers to complications of seizures or coma, unrelated to other causes superimposed on the preeclamptic status. In reality, women with eclampsia may have variable, if present, hypertension and proteinuria, and thus eclampsia may not represent just the next step of preeclampsia [15, 16]. Delayed eclampsia, following delivery, may not be associated with hypertension or proteinuria [17].

Preeclampsia/eclampsia, also known as toxemia of pregnancy, is associated with posterior reversible encephalopathy syndrome (PRES) [18]. This is a distinct syndrome referring to specific imaging findings in the brain seen in a variety of toxicity settings, not just eclampsia. The pathophysiology is complex and remains unclear in many aspects. However, several observations have been established and are shared among several toxicity settings (eclampsia, severe hypertension, transplantation, infection/sepsis, autoimmune disease, chemotherapy, and cancer). The explanations for brain edema, the hallmark finding in PRES, vary [19]. They are focused on the disruption of the blood–brain barrier and include hypertension with failed auto-regulation and hyper-perfusion [15], with an alternative hypothesis of vascular endothelial damage, hypoperfusion, and vasoconstriction [19, 20]. Regardless, endothelial cell damage and abnormal activation have been proven and are accepted as an inciting factor in the development of eclampsia [21, 22].

T-cell activation and cytokine production (TNF-α, IL-1, INF, IL-6), and systemically increased vascular endothelial growth factor (VEGF) levels are common findings and contribute to the development of brain edema [15, 17, 19, 23]. The diffuse endothelial activation also affects the platelet function, resulting in platelet adhesion, degranulation, hemolysis, protein/fluid leak, and edema. Magnesium, protein, and fluid loss are also encountered as result of glomerular endothelial malfunction [18]. Decreased levels of magnesium have been found in patients with abnormal brain MRI findings [19]. Endothelial cell activation and associated “leakiness,” along with vasoconstriction and hypertension are believed to affect the uteroplacental unit, which becomes dysfunctional.

Neuroimaging can accurately contribute to the diagnosis of PRES. The CT imaging performed in an emergency situation may exclude other etiologies for acute onset of seizures, such as an intracranial hemorrhage, but may also reveal hypo-dense areas in the parieto-occipital regions that are considered manifestations of eclampsia [24]. The imaging modality of choice is MRI, which can be diagnostic for eclampsia and also rule out other potential causes. The pertinent findings on MRI are patchy areas of T2 hyperintensity involving the parieto-occipital regions and distributed along the posterior as well as anterior watershed zones [25]. Other areas of the brain, such as the cerebellum, brainstem, and thalami, may also be involved [26]. The lesions are located at the subcortical white matter with some involvement of the overlying cortex (Figure 14.1). Occasionally they may be associated with micro hemorrhages [27].

The type and etiology of the brain edema in eclampsia has been extensively discussed in the literature. The MRI findings and laboratory data suggest vasogenic-type edema [15, 17, 19, 28, 29] corresponding to the subcortical white matter signal abnormality on MRI. Rarely, focal, cortical-based diffusion-weighted imaging (DWI) abnormalities, surrounded by vasogenic subcortical white matter edema, and associated with either restricted diffusion or pseudo normalization of DWI, have been observed. Both findings are indicative of a severe form of PRES, with the worst outcome linked to the presence of true restricted diffusion, indicative of acute infarct [26–28]. Therefore, DWI contributes in the diagnosis and assessment of severity of PRES in addition to its well-known specificity in the diagnosis of territorial stroke.

The PRES findings are often distributed along the watershed zones or in a random fashion, but do not follow the vascular territory distribution which is the typical presentation of the arterial ischemic stroke. The MRI of the brain obtained soon after seizure activity may demonstrate cortical swelling and restricted diffusion due to seizure activity. The finding is transient

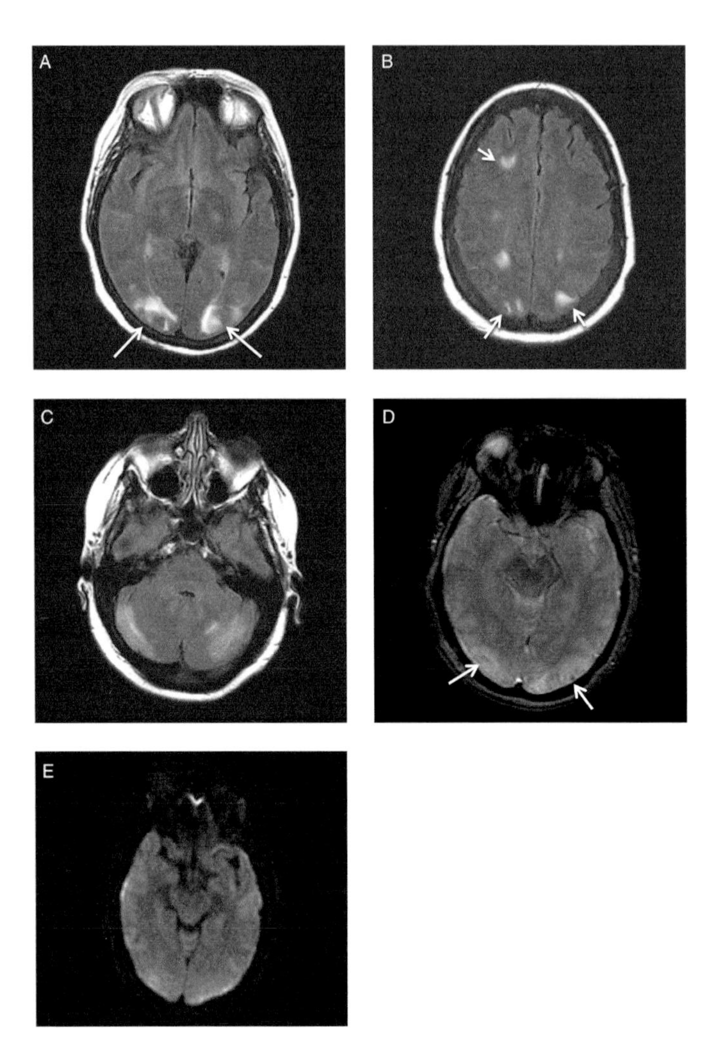

Figure 14.1 Thirty-four-year-old female with eclampsia and seizure. Axial FLAIR sequences demonstrate vasogenic edema in the occipital lobes (Figure A arrows), along the watershed zones in the frontoparietal vertex (Figure B arrows), as well as in the cerebellum (Figure C). Punctate areas of susceptibility artifact suggestive of micro hemorrhage are shown on GRE sequence (Figure D arrows). The DWI showed no evidence of restricted diffusion (Figure E).

without any residual abnormality. The lesions in eclampsia rarely show any enhancement; therefore, unenhanced MRI, which is generally all that can be used during pregnancy, suffices. The suggested MRI protocol should include T1-weighted (T1W), fluid-attenuated inversion recovery (FLAIR), fast spin echo T2-weighted (FSET2), DWI, and gradient echo (GRE) sequences, in order to delineate even the most subtle of the findings (FLAIR, FSET2) and assess for micro hemorrhages (GRE/SWI/SWAN) [30, 31]. The use of DWI is recommended to exclude true ischemic event in more complicated situations (Figure 14.1, E).

Catheter angiography and magnetic resonance angiography (MRA) have shown reversible findings in PRES, such as focal stenosis or diffuse lumen irregularity, pruning, or even a beaded appearance of intracranial vessels. Of course, catheter angiography involves radiation exposure as well as iodine contrast administration, which is not exactly advisable in pregnancy, but can be performed postpartum. The MRA can be performed without gadolinium-based contrast medium and therefore can be part of the protocol. The appearance of PRES on routine unenhanced MRA sequences is almost pathognomonic; therefore, the MRA would be useful in exclusion of other entities rather than contributory to the diagnosis of PRES in a pregnant patient.

Thrombotic thrombocytopenic purpura (TTP), which also occurs in pregnancy, shares similar MRI findings with preeclampsia/eclampsia. Follow-up studies usually show resolution of the abnormalities when patients improve clinically, although TTP may be complicated with infarction or intracerebral hemorrhage. Hemolysis, elevated liver enzymes, low platelets (HELLP) syndrome is another hypertensive disorder of pregnancy sharing much of the pathophysiology with preeclampsia/eclampsia [32–34].

Cerebral Venous Thrombosis

The association of pregnancy and the puerperium with cerebral venous thrombosis is well known, with the majority of the cases occurring during peripartum or postpartum [35, 36]. The estimated risk of cerebral venous thrombosis is 11.6 cases per 100,000 deliveries [28]. Risk factors include hypertension, cesarean delivery, infections, preeclampsia/eclampsia [37], and anemia [36]. Clinical symptoms vary and include headache, seizures, papilledema, focal neurologic deficits, and even coma [38].

The thrombosed venous structures on non-contrast-enhanced CT imaging appear hyperdense. Along the superior sagittal sinus, the clot has the shape of the Greek letter delta, the popularized "delta sign." The contrast-enhanced CT shows enhancement around the relatively hypo-dense clot (empty delta sign) [39]. The MRI is the preferred imaging modality when it comes to assessment of the intracranial venous structures since there is no exposure to radiation when the patient is pregnant and, in most cases, there is no need for administration of gadolinium-based contrast medium in order to confidently reach a diagnosis. Routine MRI of the brain provides clues regarding the patency of major intracranial vessels and dedicated magnetic resonance venogram (MRV) confirms patency or not (Figure 14.2, A, B).

Non-contrast MRV options include time-of-flight and phase contrast techniques. Thrombosed vessels on routine imaging show lack of signal void, a finding quite reliable on sequences such as T2-weighted and T2-FLAIR (Figure 14.3, A, B), and a variable degree of hyperintensity on T1-weighted sequences (Figure 14.2, A). The affected vessels show no detectable flow on MRV (Figure 14.2, B). Pitfalls of MRI do exist. Clots exhibiting very low signal on FSET2W sequences should not be misinterpreted as flow void. Developmentally small dural sinuses may appear as occluded, especially on maximum-intensity projection (MIP) images (Figure 14.4).

Partially thrombosed dural sinus may appear as completely occluded, since MRA techniques overestimate vascular lumen stenosis [40]. Flow artifacts can cause lack of flow voids within the venous sinuses on T2-weighted sequences and T1 hyperintensity on T1-weighted sequences, mimicking thrombus. Careful analysis, however, of routine brain imaging in conjunction with MRV findings allows accurate diagnosis on most occasions. Diagnosis, however, of cavernous sinus thrombosis, often a sign of ongoing infection, requires intravenous contrast administration [30]. A computed tomography venogram (CTV) is not subject to the MRV limitations, but the application includes radiation exposure as well as exposure to an iodinated contrast agent. It is an excellent choice as a follow-up study after the delivery.

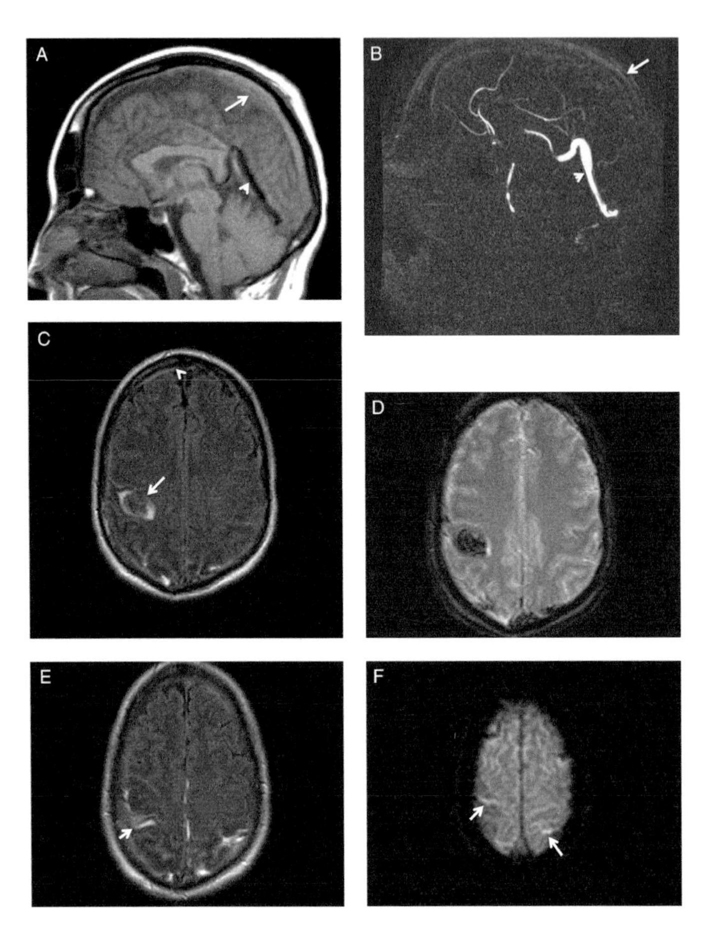

Figure 14.2 Twenty-eight-year-old female with superior sagittal sinus (SSS) thrombosis complicated with hemorrhage in the right posterior frontal lobe. A sagittal T1W image shows lack of flow void along the SSS (Figure A arrows), while the straight sinus remains patent (Figure A short arrow). A corresponding sagittal MIP image of the MRV shows no flow-related enhancement along the SSS (Figure B arrow), but is present along the straight sinus (Figure B short arrow). Parenchymal hemorrhage is noted in the right posterior frontal lobe on FLAIR (Figure C arrow) and GRE (Figure D) sequences. In addition, a thin subdural hematoma is noted (Figure C arrowhead). Further axial FLAIR sequences show cortical edema in the frontoparietal vertex (Figure E arrows). Subtle abnormalities in the same areas on the DWI are suggestive of infarct due to cortical vein thrombosis (Figure F arrows).

Although cerebral venous thrombosis in puerperium has a more benign course than in other patient categories [36], complications may occur and are evident on MRI. Ischemic infarcts, especially in non-arterial territory distribution as well as intraparenchymal hemorrhages, may occur (Figure 14.2, C, D, E, F). Alternatively, these findings may serve as clues to the interpreting radiologist to look for signs of intracranial venous thrombosis or recommend further imaging. The value of DWI in the diagnosis of arterial ischemia is well established. Venous stroke, however, is associated with more variable patterns of DWI and ADC [41]. Three types of lesions have been described [42]: (a) lesions with elevated diffusion suggestive of vasogenic edema that resolved; (b) lesions with low diffusion suggestive of cytotoxic edema found in patients without seizure activity that persisted;

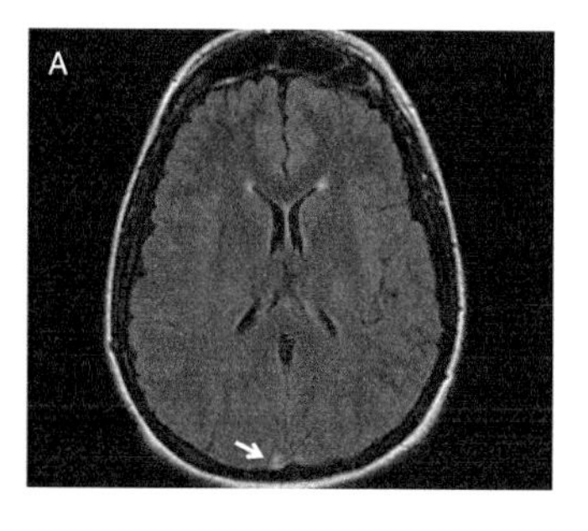

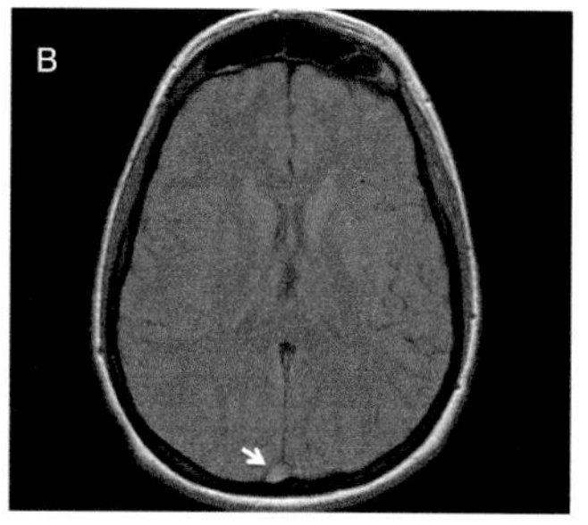

Figure 14.3 Uncomplicated superior sagittal sinus thrombosis. The presence of clot in the SSS is evident on axial FLAIR (Figure A arrow) as well as axial proton density (Figure B arrow). This patient's examination did not include MRV; however the original diagnosis was made based on the routine MRI findings. Sagittal T1W sequences (not shown) also demonstrated lack of flow void.

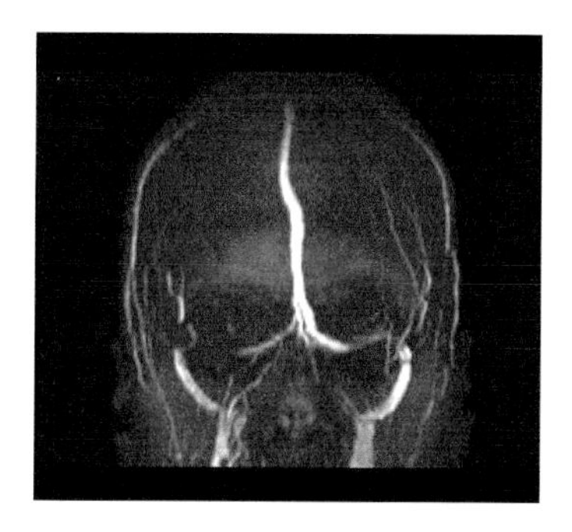

Figure 14.4 MIP images of MRV show narrowing of the transverse sinuses which was not confirmed on the source images. It is a pitfall that can be addressed by carefully evaluating the source images and not to rely on the MIP images only.

and (c) lesions with low diffusion seen in patients with seizure that also resolved [36]. Reversibility of brain abnormalities in a setting of cerebral venous thrombosis has been documented [37, 38]. Following treatment, MRI can be used to assess the brain and monitor the recanalization of dural sinuses. Catheter angiography dynamically assesses the central venous system; however, it is not the first choice of imaging modalities because of increased risks as an interventional procedure and the exposure to radiation in the case of pregnancy.

Postpartum Cerebral Angiopathy

Postpartum cerebral angiopathy is an idiopathic form of the reversible cerebral segmental vasoconstriction syndrome first described in 1988 [43, 44]. It can afflict postpartum women within 1–4 weeks following delivery and is characterized by thunderclap headache, seizure, focal neurologic deficits, and segmental narrowing and dilatation of large and medium-sized cerebral arteries, which is very similar to angiographic findings seen with eclampsia [45]. The MRI of the brain reveals T2 hyperintensities in the white as well as gray matter, often along watershed zones [2] (Figure 14.5, A, B, C). Complication with intracerebral hemorrhages can occur [46, 47]. Tests for cerebral vasculitis are negative; however, MRA, CT angiography, or catheter angiography demonstrate areas of stenosis or dilatation in intracranial arteries, which eventually resolve [38, 41] (Figure 14.5, D, E). Both CT and catheter angiography require intravenous administration of iodine contrast.

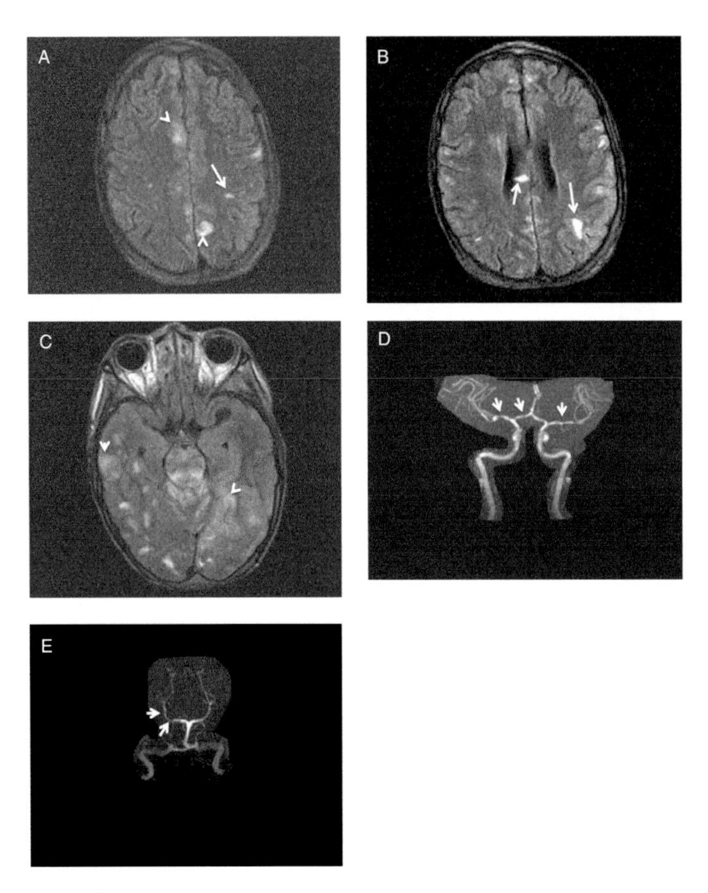

Figure 14.5 Twenty-eight-year-old female presented with severe headache and seizure 2 weeks following delivery. Axial FLAIR multiple abnormalities involving white matter (Figure A, B arrows) as well as gray matter (Figure A, C arrowheads). Midbrain is also involved (Figure C). The MRA shows multiple areas of focal constriction in the anterior (Figure D arrows) as well as posterior circulation (Figure E arrows).

Brain Tumors

Meningioma and choriocarcinoma are tumors that are either influenced or directly related to the pregnancy.

Meningioma

The presence of hormonal receptors found in some meningiomas may promote their growth during pregnancy [48]. Depending on their location, they may present with seizure, along with other symptoms. Meningiomas may calcify, which makes them more easily recognizable on non-contrast-enhanced CT. More often, though, they are isodense to the brain parenchyma. The MRI is far more sensitive in detecting meningiomas, especially in a situation like pregnancy, when an intravenous contrast medium is not advocated. They share the same MRI characteristics with meningiomas found in nonpregnant patients. They are isointense to gray matter on T1 W and moderately hyperintense on T2 W sequences; they also may show restricted diffusion and enhance avidly.

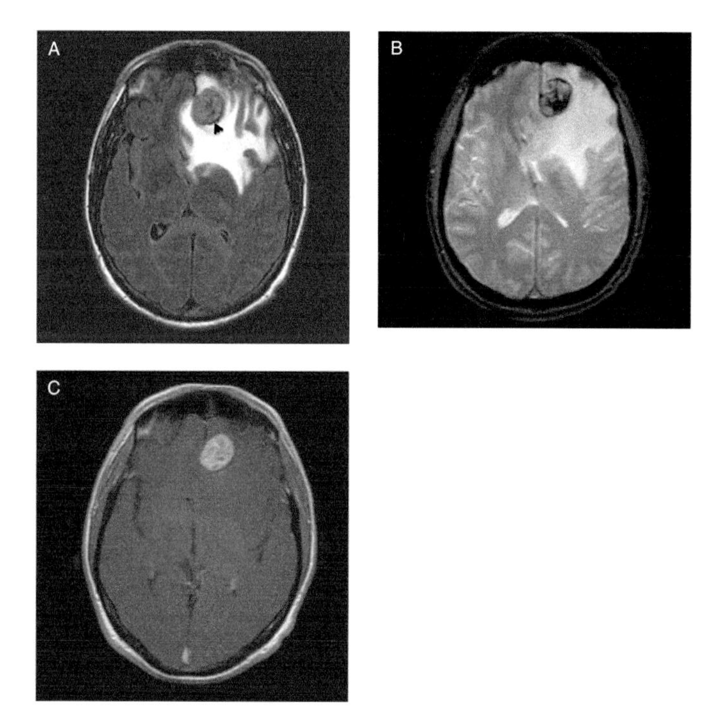

Figure 14.6 Metastatic choriocarcinoma. Axial FLAIR sequence demonstrates a mass in the left frontal lobe surrounded by extensive vasogenic edema (Figure A). There is hemorrhage in the mass as clearly shown on axial GRE sequence (Figure B). Just a subtle rim of hemosiderin can be seen on the FLAIR image (Figure A arrow). The mass enhances avidly on the axial post-contrast T1W sequence (Figure C).

Metastatic Choriocarcinoma

Choriocarcinoma, a malignant trophoblastic tumor specifically associated with pregnancy – normal, molar, or ectopic pregnancy – metastasizes to the brain in 66% of cases [49]. As any other metastasis, choriocarcinoma may manifest with seizure, and, as a highly vascular tumor, it may bleed; this lends the variable signal characteristics of the brain metastasis on MRI. The variability of signal characteristics depends on the age of hemorrhage. The mass enhances and is usually surrounded by extensive vasogenic edema. The MRI should include GRE or other sequences sensitive to susceptibility artifact generated by blood products (Figure 14.6, A, B, C).

Other Primary Brain Tumors

Recent data also suggest that low-grade gliomas may grow faster during pregnancy [50]. Management and treatment of the pregnant woman can represent a challenge, since treatment of the tumor may include radiation and chemotherapy.

Seizures in Non-Pregnancy-Related Conditions: Neuroimaging

Pregnant women may present with seizures for reasons unrelated to pregnancy [51]. In women with an established epilepsy diagnosis, it is likely that a neuroimaging workup has been completed prior to commencement of the pregnancy and appropriate consultation has taken place. In these patients, if the neurological exam is unchanged from baseline and postictal recovery has occurred back to baseline, neuroimaging is usually not warranted. However, even patients with congenital brain anomalies known to represent a substrate for epilepsy may experience first-time seizures later in life. Detailed analysis of these conditions is beyond this chapter's scope; however, it is important for healthcare providers to approach the interpretation of neuroimaging studies from a broader perspective and recognize the imaging findings. Other conditions that evolve over time, such as cavernous hemangiomas, are known to be associated with seizures, which present at any time during the course of life [52, 53].

Pregnant women may also be subject to central nervous system infection. Listeria meningitis, epidural abscesses, or brain infections with space-occupying lesions, such as neurocysticercosis, may present with seizures [54, 55]. Imaging will be challenging, since contrast-enhanced MRI may be necessary to fully disclose the extension of the disease.

Pregnancy sets certain limitations when it comes to imaging. Developmental anomalies in general can be worked up satisfactorily without intravenous contrast administration. Optimization of the protocol with the inclusion of high-resolution 3D images (T1-weighted images and T2-weighted FLAIR images) is all that is needed for accurate diagnosis without exposing the pregnant woman and unborn child to any contrast medium [56]. Diagnosis of vascular malformations and tumors, however, sometimes requires the administration of intravenous contrast medium, either iodinated – for example, catheter angiography – or gadolinium-based contrast for MRI. Postponement of imaging after pregnancy may be entertained, especially if the treatment is postponed as well. The final, often multidisciplinary decision as how to handle these pregnant women will be based on the principle that benefits should outweigh potential risks.

Neuroimaging of Pregnant Women: Protocol Suggestions

This review of the imaging findings of the most frequent medical conditions related to pregnancy that present with epilepsy, in conjunction with the existing safety recommendations, sets the framework for imaging protocols. Every radiology department is required to establish policies on how to handle pregnant or nursing women in terms of safety. Pregnant or nursing women should be informed of potential consequences and be allowed to make the final decision. Written informed consent should be obtained.

Non-contrast-enhanced CT of the brain is accessible and accurately depicts acute intracranial hemorrhage, which may accompany many of the conditions discussed in this chapter. Although often less available, MRI is the preferred imaging modality when it comes to evaluation of neurological conditions. Pregnant women can be imaged on 1.5 T magnets, which are widely available.

The exact MRI sequences to be utilized will depend on the available software, which may differ from one MRI platform to another. However, the absolutely necessary T1 W, FSET2 W, FLAIR, GRE, and DWI sequences are widely available. The addition of GRE or any other (e.g., SWI or SWAN) sequence sensitive to blood by-products provides important information regarding the hemorrhagic nature of a lesion. The DWI is important in detecting acute stroke that may complicate many of the pregnancy-related conditions presenting with seizures or epilepsy. Given the overlapping clinical and imaging findings of the main pregnancy-related conditions with seizure, the addition of MRV may provide important information and thus be part of the routine protocol.

Contrast media, whether iodinated or gadolinium-based, should be avoided during pregnancy. The administration may be considered only if the use is absolutely necessary to reach

Table 14.1 Neuroimaging in pregnancy: Indications according to clinical suspicion

Clinical suspicion	Preferred neuroimaging modality	Alternative neuroimaging modality
Preeclampsia/ eclampsia	Non-contrast MRI including blood-sensitive sequence	Non-contrast CT
Arterial infarct [57]	Where immediately available: Non-contrast MRI, including TOF MRA	CT and CTA if MRI not immediately available
Venous sinus thrombosis	Non-contrast MRI, including venography (TOF and/or phase contrast) and blood-sensitive sequence	CT and contrast-enhanced CT venography
Subarachnoid hemorrhage	CT and, if positive, MRI, including TOF MRI	CT and, if positive, contrast-enhanced CT angiography
Brain metastasis	Contrast-enhanced MRI	Contrast-enhanced CT
Primary brain tumor	MRI with contrast may be necessary in intra-axial lesions but non-contrast MRI is usually enough for symptomatic extra-axial lesions	CT with contrast
Postpartum cerebral angiopathy/reversible vasoconstriction syndrome	Non-contrast MRI, including TOF MRA	CT and contrast enhanced CT angiography
Infection/abscess	Non-contrast MRI, carefully assess need for contrast	CT and post-contrast CT
Developmental anomalies causing seizures	Non-contrast MRI including high resolution 3D T1-weighted images	

a diagnosis that would be beneficial to the pregnant woman as well as the unborn child. The ACR, in its updated *Manual on Contrast Media* for 2022, stated that existing data suggest that it is safe for both mother and infant to continue breastfeeding after contrast agent administration. That includes both iodinated and gadolinium-based contrast (Table 14.1).

References

1. Trop I, Tremblay E, Thérasse E, Thomassin-Naggara I. Quality initiatives: Guidelines for use of medical imaging during pregnancy and lactation. *Radiographics*. 2012;**32**:897–911. https://doi.org/10.1148/rg.323115120.
2. Klein JP, Hsu L. Neuroimaging during pregnancy. *Semin Neurol*. 2011;**31**:361–73. https://doi.org/10.1055/s-0031-1293535.
3. McCollough CH, Schueler BA, Atwell TD, et al. Radiation exposure and pregnancy: When should we be concerned?

Radiographics. 2007;**27**:908–9. https://doi.org/10.1148/rg.274065149.

4. Stuebe A, Auguste T. ACOG Committee Opinion. *Obstet Gynecol*. 2018;**131**:140–50.
5. American College of Radiology Committee on Drugs and Contrast Media. *ACR Manual on Contrast Media*. Reston, VA: American College of Radiology Committee on Drugs and Contrast Media; n.d.
6. Ziskin MC, Morrissey J. Thermal thresholds for teratogenicity, reproduction, and development. *Int J Hyperthermia*. 2011;**27**:374–87. https://doi.org/10.3109/02656736.2011.553769.
7. Hand JW, Li Y, Thomas EL, Rutherford MA, Hajnal J. Prediction of specific absorption rate in mother and fetus associated with MRI examinations during pregnancy. *Magn Reson Med*. 2006;**55**:883–93. https://doi.org/10.1002/mrm.20824.
8. Jabehdar Maralani P, Kapadia A, Liu G, et al. Canadian Association of Radiologists recommendations for the safe use of MRI during pregnancy. *Can Assoc Radiol J*. 2022;**73**:56–67. https://doi.org/10.1177/08465371211015657.
9. Reeves MJ, Brandreth M, Whitby EH, et al. Neonatal cochlear function: Measurement after exposure to acoustic noise during in utero MR imaging. *Radiology*. 2010;**257**:802–9. https://doi.org/10.1148/radiol.10092366.
10. Strizek B, Jani JC, Mucyo E, et al. Safety of MR imaging at 1.5 T in fetuses: A retrospective case-control study of birth weights and the effects of acoustic noise. *Radiology*. 2015;**275**:530–7. https://doi.org/10.1148/radiol.14141382.
11. Jaimes C, Delgado J, Cunnane MB, et al. Does 3-T fetal MRI induce adverse acoustic effects in the neonate? A preliminary study comparing postnatal auditory test performance of fetuses scanned at 1.5 and 3 T. *Pediatr Radiol*. 2019;**49**:37–45. https://doi.org/10.1007/s00247-018-4261-2.
12. Ray JG, Vermeulen MJ, Bharatha A, Montanera WJ, Park AL. Association between MRI exposure during pregnancy and fetal and childhood outcomes. *JAMA*. 2016;**316**:952–61. https://doi.org/10.1001/jama.2016.12126.
13. Kanal E, Barkovich AJ, Bell C, et al. ACR guidance document on MR safe practices: 2013. *J Magn Reson Imaging*. 2013;**37**:501–30. https://doi.org/10.1002/jmri.24011.
14. Ray JG, Vermeulen MJ, Bharatha A, Montanera WJ, Park AL. Association between MRI exposure during pregnancy and fetal and childhood outcomes. *JAMA*. 2016;**316**:952–61. https://doi.org/10.1001/jama.2016.12126.
15. Cipolla MJ, Kraig RP. Seizures in women with preeclampsia: Mechanisms and management. *Fetal Matern Med Rev*. 2011;**22**:91–108. https://doi.org/10.1017/S0965539511000040.
16. Ay H, Buonanno FS, Schaefer PW, et al. Posterior leukoencephalopathy without severe hypertension: Utility of diffusion-weighted MRI. *Neurology*. 1998;**51**:1369–76. https://doi.org/10.1212/wnl.51.5.1369.
17. Bartynski WS, Sanghvi A. Neuroimaging of delayed eclampsia. Report of 3 cases and review of the literature. *J Comput Assist Tomogr*. 2003;**27**:699–713. https://doi.org/10.1097/00004728-200309000-00007.
18. Van Loenen NTVM, Hintzen RQ, de Groot CJM. New onset seizures in pregnancy caused by an unexpected neurologic disorder. *Eur J Obstet Gynecol Reprod Biol*. 2004;**117**:109–11. https://doi.org/10.1016/j.ejogrb.2003.09.046.
19. Bartynski WS. Posterior reversible encephalopathy syndrome, part 1: Fundamental imaging and clinical features. *AJNR Am J Neuroradiol*. 2008;**29**:1036–42. https://doi.org/10.3174/ajnr.A0928.
20. Trommer BL, Homer D, Mikhael MA. Cerebral vasospasm and eclampsia. *Stroke*. 1988;**19**:326–9. https://doi.org/10.1161/01.str.19.3.326.
21. Dekker GA, Sibai BM. Etiology and pathogenesis of preeclampsia: Current concepts. *Am J Obstet Gynecol*. 1998;**179**:1359–75. https://doi.org/10.1016/s0002-9378(98)70160-7.

22. Schwartz RB, Feske SK, Polak JF, et al. Preeclampsia-eclampsia: Clinical and neuroradiographic correlates and insights into the pathogenesis of hypertensive encephalopathy. *Radiology*. 2000;**217**:371–6. https://doi.org/10.1148/radiology.217.2.r00nv44371.

23. Paarlberg KM, De Jong CL, Van Geijn HP, et al. Vasoactive mediators in pregnancy-induced hypertensive disorders: A longitudinal study. *Am J Obstet Gynecol.* 1998;**179**:1559–64. https://doi.org/10.1016/s0002-9378(98)70024-9.

24. Brass SD, Copen WA. Neurological disorders in pregnancy from a neuroimaging perspective. *Semin Neurol.* 2007;**27**:411–24. https://doi.org/10.1055/s-2007-991123.

25. Junewar V, Verma R, Sankhwar PL, et al. Neuroimaging features and predictors of outcome in eclamptic encephalopathy: A prospective observational study. *American Journal of Neuroradiology*. 2014;**35**:1728–34. https://doi.org/10.3174/ajnr.A3923.

26. McKinney AM, Short J, Truwit CL, et al. Posterior reversible encephalopathy syndrome: Incidence of atypical regions of involvement and imaging findings. *AJR Am J Roentgenol.* 2007;**189**:904–12. https://doi.org/10.2214/AJR.07.2024.

27. Hefzy HM, Bartynski WS, Boardman JF, Lacomis D. Hemorrhage in posterior reversible encephalopathy syndrome: Imaging and clinical features. *AJNR Am J Neuroradiol.* 2009;**30**:1371–9. https://doi.org/10.3174/ajnr.A1588.

28. Schaefer PW, Buonanno FS, Gonzalez RG, Schwamm LH. Diffusion-weighted imaging discriminates between cytotoxic and vasogenic edema in a patient with eclampsia. *Stroke*. 1997;**28**:1082–5. https://doi.org/10.1161/01.str.28.5.1082.

29. Schwartz RB, Mulkern R V, Gudbjartsson H, Jolesz F. Diffusion-weighted MR imaging in hypertensive encephalopathy: Clues to pathogenesis. *AJNR Am J Neuroradiol.* 1998;**19**:859–62.

30. Alvis JS, Hicks RJ. Pregnancy-induced acute neurologic emergencies and neurologic conditions encountered in pregnancy. *Semin Ultrasound CT MR*. 2012;**33**:46–54. https://doi.org/10.1053/j.sult.2011.09.002.

31. Acheson J, Malik A. Cerebral venous sinus thrombosis presenting in the puerperium. *Emerg Med J.* 2006;**23**:e44. https://doi.org/10.1136/emj.2006.035550.

32. Bartynski WS. Posterior reversible encephalopathy syndrome, part 2: Controversies surrounding pathophysiology of vasogenic edema. *AJNR Am J Neuroradiol.* 2008;**29**:1043–9. https://doi.org/10.3174/ajnr.A0929.

33. Knopp U, Kehler U, Rickmann H, Arnold H, Gliemroth J. Cerebral haemodynamic pathologies in HELLP syndrome. *Clin Neurol Neurosurg.* 2003;**105**:256–61. https://doi.org/10.1016/s0303-8467(03)00043-x.

34. Stone JH. HELLP syndrome: Hemolysis, elevated liver enzymes, and low platelets. *JAMA*. 1998;**280**:559–62. https://doi.org/10.1001/jama.280.6.559.

35. Srinivasan K. Puerperal cerebral venous and arterial thrombosis. *Semin Neurol.* 1988;**8**:222–5. https://doi.org/10.1055/s-2008-1041381.

36. Cantú C, Barinagarrementeria F. Cerebral venous thrombosis associated with pregnancy and puerperium: Review of 67 cases. *Stroke*. 1993;**24**:1880–4. https://doi.org/10.1161/01.str.24.12.1880.

37. Lanska DJ, Kryscio RJ. Risk factors for peripartum and postpartum stroke and intracranial venous thrombosis. *Stroke.* 2000;**31**:1274–82. https://doi.org/10.1161/01.str.31.6.1274.

38. Angelov A. Intracranial venous thrombosis in relation to pregnancy and delivery. *Pathol Res Pract.* 1989;**185**:843–7. https://doi.org/10.1016/S0344-0338(89)80284-5.

39. Bartynski WS, Boardman JF. Distinct imaging patterns and lesion distribution in posterior reversible encephalopathy syndrome. *AJNR Am J Neuroradiol.* 2007;**28**:1320–7. https://doi.org/10.3174/ajnr.A0549.

40. Provenzale JM, Joseph GJ, Barboriak DP. Dural sinus thrombosis: Findings on CT and MR imaging and

diagnostic pitfalls. *AJR Am J Roentgenol.* 1998;**170**:777–83. https://doi.org/10.2214/ajr.170.3.9490973.

41. Ducreux D, Oppenheim C, Vandamme X, et al. Diffusion-weighted imaging patterns of brain damage associated with cerebral venous thrombosis. *AJNR Am J Neuroradiol.* 2001;**22**:261–8.
42. Mullins ME, Grant PE, Wang B, Gonzalez RG, Schaefer PW. Parenchymal abnormalities associated with cerebral venous sinus thrombosis: Assessment with diffusion-weighted MR imaging. *AJNR Am J Neuroradiol.* 2004;**25**:1666–75.
43. Call GK, Fleming MC, Sealfon S, et al. Reversible cerebral segmental vasoconstriction. *Stroke.* 1988;**19**:1159–70. https://doi.org/10.1161/01.str.19.9.1159.
44. Neudecker S, Stock K, Krasnianski M. Call–Fleming postpartum angiopathy in the puerperium: A reversible cerebral vasoconstriction syndrome. *Obstet Gynecol.* 2006;**107**:446–9. https://doi.org/10.1097/01.AOG.0000187945.61146.e6.
45. Singhal AB. Postpartum angiopathy with reversible posterior leukoencephalopathy. *Arch Neurol.* 2004;**61**:411–16. https://doi.org/10.1001/archneur.61.3.411.
46. Ursell MR, Marras CL, Farb R, et al. Recurrent intracranial hemorrhage due to postpartum cerebral angiopathy: Implications for management. *Stroke.* 1998;**29**:1995–8. https://doi.org/10.1161/01.str.29.9.1995.
47. Zak IT, Dulai HS, Kish KK. Imaging of neurologic disorders associated with pregnancy and the postpartum period. *Radiographics: A Review Publication of the Radiological Society of North America.* 2007;**27**:95–108. https://doi.org/10.1148/rg.271065046.
48. Smith JS, Quiñones-Hinojosa A, Harmon-Smith M, Bollen AW, McDermott MW. Sex steroid and growth factor profile of a meningioma associated with pregnancy. *Canadian Journal of Neurological Sciences Le Journal Canadien Des Sciences Neurologiques.* 2005;**32**:122–7. https://doi.org/10.1017/s0317167100017017.
49. Kobayashi T, Kida Y, Yoshida J, Shibuya N, Kageyama N. Brain metastasis of choriocarcinoma. *Surgical Neurology.* 1982;**17**:395–403. https://doi.org/10.1016/S0090-3019(82)80002-5.
50. Pallud J, Mandonnet E, Deroulers C, et al. Pregnancy increases the growth rates of World Health Organization grade II gliomas. *Ann Neurol.* 2010;**67**:398–404. https://doi.org/10.1002/ana.21888.
51. Larner AJ, Smith SJ, Duncan JS, Howard RS. Late-onset Rasmussen's syndrome with first seizure during pregnancy. *Eur Neurol.* 1995;**35**:172. https://doi.org/10.1159/000117116.
52. Hoeldtke NJ, Floyd D, Werschkul JD, Calhoun BC, Hume RF. Intracranial cavernous angioma initially presenting in pregnancy with new-onset seizures. *Am J Obstet Gynecol.* 1998;**178**:612–13. https://doi.org/10.1016/s0002-9378(98)70449-1.
53. Aladdin Y, Gross DW. Refractory status epilepticus during pregnancy secondary to cavernous angioma. *Epilepsia.* 2008;**49**:1627–9. https://doi.org/10.1111/j.1528-1167.2008.01639.x.
54. Pandian JD, Venkateswaralu K, Thomas S V, Sarma PS. Maternal and fetal outcome in women with epilepsy associated with neurocysticercosis. *Epileptic Disord.* 2007;**9**:285–91. https://doi.org/10.1684/epd.2007.0120.
55. Mylonakis E, Paliou M, Hohmann EL, Calderwood SB, Wing EJ. Listeriosis during pregnancy: A case series and review of 222 cases. *Medicine.* 2002;**81**:260–9. https://doi.org/10.1097/00005792-200207000-00002.
56. Vézina LG. MRI-negative epilepsy: Protocols to optimize lesion detection. *Epilepsia.* 2011;**52** Suppl 4:25–7. https://doi.org/10.1111/j.1528-1167.2011.03147.x.
57. Ladhani NNN, Swartz RH, Foley N, et al. Canadian stroke best practice consensus statement: Acute stroke management during pregnancy. *International Journal of Stroke.* 2018;**13**:743–58. https://doi.org/10.1177/1747493018786617.

Chapter 15

Obstetrical Anesthesia

Fatima Zahir, Jonathan H. Waters, and Janet F. R. Waters

Key Points

- Epilepsy is one of the most common neurological complications encountered in pregnancy and the majority of parturients will have an uneventful pregnancy with an excellent outcome.
- The risk of intubation failure is fivefold higher than in the nonpregnant patient. Mortality is secondary to hypoxia, due to difficult or failed intubation or to pulmonary aspiration of gastric contents.
- There is no contraindication to the use of regional anesthesia, including spinal, epidural, and combined spinal–epidural techniques, in the pregnant epileptic patient who presents in labor.
- Local anesthetic toxicity as a differential diagnosis should be considered when confronted with a newly seizing parturient who has had recent neuraxial anesthesia.
- Close cooperation and communication between the anesthesiologist and obstetric team are required in order to optimize the outcome and minimize perinatal and obstetrical risks.

Obstetric Anesthesia

Airway Management

Breakthrough seizures can occur during delivery in women with epilepsy. They may also occur in the setting of eclampsia. The immediate concern when confronted with an actively seizing patient with impaired awareness is to secure the airway. This may require urgent anesthesiology consult and induction with general anesthetic and intubation. However, most seizures last only 1–3 minutes and induction with general anesthesia may make it difficult to determine if the seizure has ended. General anesthesia can be particularly hazardous in the obstetrical patient given that the risk of intubation failure is fivefold higher than in the nonpregnant patient. It has consistently been shown that maternal mortality is greater with general anesthesia than regional anesthesia. Most deaths are due to hypoxia from difficult or failed intubation, or to pulmonary aspiration of gastric contents [1, 2]. Failed endotracheal intubation and ventilation are a major cause of anesthesia-related maternal mortality occurring during cesarean deliveries, though this may change with the advent and use of video laryngoscopy.

Intubation difficulty can be related to pregnancy-associated edema. One of the hallmarks in the diagnosis of preeclampsia/eclampsia is generalized edema. This edema includes the airway and trachea, making this type of patient notoriously difficult to intubate. Generalized edema of the eclamptic patient is compounded by the normal anatomic changes of the airway that occur during pregnancy. Capillary engorgement leads to increased edema and friability of the mucosal vasculature of the respiratory tract and swelling of the lining of the oropharynx, larynx, and trachea. Therefore, a smaller endotracheal tube is needed to avoid trauma and subsequent swelling of the airway.

While no single method will reliably predict a difficult airway, the Mallampati classification is traditionally used to assess the airway. This classification assesses the visualization of the uvula and soft palate. Better visualization of these structures indicates more room within the oropharynx in which to place a laryngoscope and endotracheal tube. Mallampati classification should be evaluated just prior to anesthetic induction as progesterone-induced water shifts during the course of labor itself can lead to progression of the score even in this brief time period.

Pregnancy-induced weight gain leads to an overall increase in body mass index (BMI). The average patient gains 17% of her body weight during pregnancy. Raised BMI has previously been shown to heighten the risk of difficult intubation [3]. Failure to manage the airway appropriately in a gravid patient threatens not one life, but two, as maternal complications are the leading cause of fetal insult and death [4].

Compounding the difficulty of placing an endotracheal tube, pregnant patients are more likely to desaturate while the airway is being secured due to a combination of parturients' increased oxygen demands in pregnancy and a 20–30% reduction in functional residual capacity (FRC) as a result of upward displacement of the diaphragm by the gravid uterus. The reduction in FRC is attributed to a reduction in expiratory reserve volume by 25% and residual volume by 15%. Therefore, adequate maternal preoxygenation is of the utmost importance prior to securing the airway.

In addition, the pregnant patient has increases in gastric pressure from the mechanic effect of the gravid uterus, decreases in esophageal sphincter tone from hormonal influences, and decreased gastric emptying times. All of these changes make the pregnant patient more prone to aspirate on anesthesia induction. In fact, the first description of aspiration pneumonitis was described in a gravid patient.

The supine position in the parturient can lead to aortocaval compression, decreased venous return to the heart, and an associated decrease in cardiac output, which in turn reduces uterine perfusion pressure. It should be avoided by left uterine displacement. This is achieved by using a wedge made of blankets or towels placed under the right hip to displace the uterus laterally and facilitate venous return to the heart.

Anesthesia and Antiseizure Medications

There is no contraindication to the use of regional anesthesia, including spinal, epidural, and combined spinal–epidural techniques, in the pregnant epileptic patient who presents in labor. Neuraxial anesthesia prevents the hyperventilation that accompanies the pain of labor and its subsequent alkalosis, which could precipitate a seizure by lowering the seizure threshold.

Other factors that may precipitate an episode include hypocarbia and hypoxia, which lower the seizure threshold and result in spontaneous, asynchronous firing of the neurons.

Reduced brain oxygenation itself can trigger a seizure as the neurons are exquisitely sensitive to depletion in their oxygen supply and respond to hypoxia by firing erratically. The seizure threshold may be further lowered by the associated acidity as a result of anaerobic cellular metabolism and lactic acid production. Hypocarbia-associated cerebral vasoconstriction can decrease the blood supply to the brain and aggravate the initial insult.

Hypercarbia, most commonly associated with respiratory failure, can lower the seizure threshold, and its concomitant cerebral vasodilation can increase local anesthetic delivery to the brain. The acidosis caused by hypercarbia can lead to ion trapping and decreased protein binding, which in turn lead to an increase in free local anesthetic in the brain and potentiates central nervous system (CNS) toxicity. Chronic hyperventilation has been noted to increase the incidence of reactive hypoglycemia, reducing the glucose supply to the brain, which does not have its own stores and therefore is highly dependent on normoglycemic conditions. Hypoglycemia has been shown to lower the seizure threshold and trigger "hypoglycemic seizures."

Acute and/or severe electrolyte imbalances can cause seizures, and these seizures may be the sole presenting symptom. Seizures are especially common in patients with sodium disorders, hypocalcemia, and hypomagnesemia. Successful management of seizures begins with the establishment of an accurate diagnosis of the underlying electrolyte disturbance. Correction of the disturbance is necessary to control seizures and prevent permanent brain damage.

While managing the patient with a seizure disorder, the potential influence of these anticonvulsant agents on the response to anesthesia must be kept in mind. Several anticonvulsants, including carbamazepine, phenytoin, and phenobarbital, are known hepatic enzyme inducers. They act on the hepatic microsomal enzymes, specifically on anesthetic drugs. Drugs that compete with phenytoin for a common metabolic pathway, such as diazepam, midazolam, or sulfonamides, will increase phenytoin serum levels. Resistance to neuromuscular blocking agents is observed in patients chronically treated with enzyme-inducing anticonvulsants because of increased hepatic metabolism.

It may be preferable to dose the anticonvulsants parenterally, when possible, in patients who are not allowed oral intake prior to a planned cesarean section. Pain frequently elicits nausea and vomiting, which can also contribute to poor anticonvulsant absorption.

Local Anesthetics

Local anesthetics can be anticonvulsant in low doses, but, when given in high doses, they can be proconvulsant. The proconvulsant properties of all local anesthetics are exhibited with toxic blood levels following inadvertent intravascular injection, or from accumulation following repeated injections. Depending on the route of administration, seizures may present immediately or with a delayed onset. In the laboring obstetrical patient, overdoses generally occur when an epidural catheter is inadvertently placed into a vein. In order to ensure this does not happen, a small dose of local anesthetic is given to test the epidural placement. This "test dose" is typically 1.5% lidocaine with 1:200,000 epinephrine. From this test dose, the patient would exhibit signs of local anesthetic neurotoxicity, or significant changes in heart rate would result from the epinephrine if the catheter was in a vein. Once the test dose is confirmed negative, a larger dose of local anesthetic is given. These larger doses of local anesthetic are necessary to achieve labor analgesia. If the test dose is not given or is misinterpreted, the large dose of local anesthetic necessary to achieve labor analgesia can trigger a seizure. While not proven in humans, data from animals appear to suggest that a lipid emulsion is effective in treating local anesthetic overdoses.

While local anesthetic agents are proconvulsant in high doses, in lower doses, local anesthetics have been shown to have anticonvulsant properties in humans. Their anticonvulsant activity is exhibited at subtoxic plasma levels – for example, 1–2 mg/kg intravenously of lidocaine has been shown to terminate status epilepticus, as well as reduce the duration of electrically induced seizures in electroconvulsive therapy [5]. With this in mind, regional anesthesia is not contraindicated during pregnancy; however, local anesthetic toxicity should be considered as a differential diagnosis when confronted with a newly seizing parturient who has had recent neuraxial anesthesia.

Anesthetic Induction Agents (Benzodiazepines, Ketamine, Etomidate, Propofol)

Benzodiazepines are widely used in the emergency therapy of generalized tonic-clonic seizures because of their potent anticonvulsant properties. Overall, they are effective in controlling status epilepticus in more than 90% of patients with a generalized seizure disorder (see Table 15.1) [6]. Midazolam is as effective in suppressing EEG seizure activity as

Table 15.1 Anesthetic agents and their effect on neuronal excitability.

Agent	Effect
Inhalational agents	Possible proconvulsant
• Nitrous oxide	Terminates status epilepticus
• Isoflurane	Possible proconvulsant role
• Sevoflurane	Terminates status epilepticus
• Desflurane	
Local anesthetics	Proconvulsant at toxic doses
Benzodiazepines	Anticonvulsants
• Etomidate	Proconvulsant; possibly anticonvulsant at higher doses
Propofol	Anticonvulsant
Ketamine	Proconvulsant
Opioids	Possibly proconvulsant after neuraxial administration
• Morphine	Proconvulsant due to normeperidine metabolite
• Meperidine	Possibly proconvulsant after prolonged IV administration
• Fentanyl	Similar to fentanyl
• Sufentanil	Similar to fentanyl
Alfentanil	
• Neuromuscular agents	Atracurium degrades to laudanosine, which can produce seizure activity. None of the other agents are proconvulsant or anticonvulsant.

lorazepam, which is often the first line in the emergency treatment of seizure disorders. If it is not possible to establish intravenous access, intramuscular midazolam and rectal diazepam are acceptable alternative routes of administration. The duration of antiseizure activity with lorazepam is longer than that achieved with intravenous diazepam, reducing the need for frequent redosing. Chronic use of benzodiazepines can lead to a withdrawal syndrome in the neonate, with symptoms including hypotonia, apneic spells, cyanosis, and impaired metabolic responses to cold stress and seizures. The neonatal benzodiazepine withdrawal syndrome has been reported to persist from hours to months after birth [7].

Induction with etomidate in patients with epilepsy is associated with involuntary myoclonic movements that resemble generalized convulsive seizures and positive EEG findings [8]. Because of its proconvulsant properties, etomidate should be avoided while inducing the pregnant epileptic. Higher doses of etomidate suppress the low-dose-induced myoclonus; therefore, dose and rate of administration will determine whether etomidate will exhibit proconvulsant or anticonvulsant properties. It has been used in several instances to control refractory status epilepticus [9].

Ketamine has both proconvulsant and anticonvulsant properties. It seems prudent to avoid use of ketamine in the pregnant epileptic since its ability to activate epileptogenic foci in patients with a known seizure disorder is well established [10]. As ketamine is a racemic mixture, the variability of the EEG pattern produced is attributed to the difference in anesthetic potency of the two isomers. The more potent S isomer causes a greater decrease in EEG amplitude and subsequent burst suppression than the less potent R isomer.

Propofol appears to possess anticonvulsant properties clinically, although it has been reported to cause excitatory activity, including myoclonus, hiccoughs, and muscle tremors during induction of anesthesia. The findings have not been corroborated with positive EEG. Unlike with etomidate, prolonged infusions of propofol have not been associated with persistent myoclonic movements, during or after termination of the infusion [11].

Volatile Anesthetics (Isoflurane, Sevoflurane, Desflurane)

General anesthesia is typically initiated with the induction drugs previously described. Following induction and intubation, maintenance of anesthesia takes place typically with a volatile anesthetic. These volatile anesthetics are halogenated hydrocarbons. Sevoflurane has been associated with seizure-like activities during cesarean delivery [12]. The other volatile agents have not been found to cause seizures in patients with a preexisting seizure disorder; in fact, they have been recommended for treatment of continuous seizures refractory to intravenous therapy. There have been reports of seizure-like activity following concurrent use of nitrous oxide with isoflurane [13].

Neuromuscular Blocking Agents (Rocuronium, Atracurium, Vecuronium)

Neuromuscular blockers, more commonly referred to as muscle relaxants, are pervasive in the anesthetic management of patients. These drugs are used to relax the skeletal muscles to enhance surgical exposure. None of the muscle relaxants used in clinical practice have demonstrated seizure activity. However, atracurium is metabolized to laudanosine, which is known to cause neurotoxicity. Special consideration must be given to patients with hepatic failure in whom the half-life of the metabolite is prolonged [14]. As discussed earlier, anticonvulsant medications will enhance liver metabolism so that muscle relaxants are more rapidly metabolized in the patient taking these drugs. As such, the neuromuscular blocker needs to be redosed more frequently.

Anticholinesterases are routinely used to reverse the effect of neuromuscular blockers. Anticholinesterases have not been reported to cause CNS excitation. Physostigmine is known to cross the blood–brain barrier to reverse the sedative effects of atropine and scopolamine. Rarely, the CNS depressant effects of the centrally acting anticholinergics have been reversed and manifested as excitation and delirium [12]. Sugammadex, which is commonly used to reverse rocuronium and vecuronium, appears to have no effect on the concentrations of antiepileptic drugs.

Opioid Analgesics (Morphine, Hydromorphone, Fentanyl, Alfentanyl, Sufentanyl, Remifentanil)

Pain control for the pregnant epileptic involves the use of opioid analgesics. Meperidine neurotoxicity is well known, manifesting clinically as tremors, myoclonus, and seizures. Its CNS manifestations are thought to be secondary to its biodegradation to its metabolite, normeperidine. The chances of neurotoxicity are increased by repeated administration of meperidine because normeperidine has a significantly longer half-life and will accumulate in the body, leading to toxic levels. The risk is greater with oral administration due to extensive first-pass metabolism of meperidine. The seizures resolve over several days with discontinuation of the agent, as the body excretes the active metabolite. Patients with renal failure are more susceptible to developing neurotoxicity due to decreased metabolism and excretion of normeperidine. There is an increased rate of conversion to normeperidine with use of anticonvulsants [15].

Morphine alone has never been demonstrated to produce seizure activity in humans after intravenous administration. Although animal studies have shown proconvulsant properties, the doses used in clinical practice do not appear to have any effect on the seizure threshold. There have been reports of grand mal seizures after low-to-moderate doses of intravenous fentanyl, sufentanil, and alfentanil [16]. These movements have not been found to be consistent with epileptic activity and are more likely to be non-epileptic myoclonic movements or exaggerated narcotic-induced rigidity.

Although morphine does not exhibit seizure activity when given intravenously, case reports have documented tonic-clonic seizures in patients after administration of epidural and intrathecal morphine [17, 18]. Animal studies have demonstrated seizures after epidural morphine administration, which are naloxone-reversible while intrathecal morphine-induced seizure activity is not. This suggests morphine mediates its seizure activity through both opiate and non-opiate receptors.

Although episodes of generalized tonic-clonic seizure-like activity after intravenous administration of low-to-moderate doses of fentanyl and alfentanil have been reported, current evidence suggests these findings are more consistent with myoclonic movements or exaggerated narcotic-induced rigidity [16]. Prolonged administration of large doses of fentanyl and sufentanil may precipitate seizures and should be used cautiously in the patient with a preexisting seizure disorder [19]. No reports have occurred of seizure activity following intrathecal or epidural administration of fentanyl and its analogs.

The neonate of parturients with chronic opioid abuse may also present with withdrawal symptoms at birth. The predominant manifestations include CNS hyperirritability and autonomic nervous system dysregulation such as sneezing, yawning, sweating, tachycardia, and mydriasis; gastrointestinal dysfunction including diarrhea, nausea and vomiting, and respiratory distress; and abnormal motor movements – for example, tremors, hypertonia, hyper-reflexivity, and repetitive movements. Benzodiazepine withdrawal differs from opioid withdrawal in that it does not cause gastrointestinal dysfunction and abnormal motor movements may be more pronounced [20].

Studies suggest no increase in congenital abnormalities in pregnant patients who underwent surgery during the course of their pregnancy but a greater risk of miscarriage, growth restriction, and low birth weight. These studies concluded that problems resulted from primary disease or the surgical procedure itself rather than exposure to anesthesia [21]. The current consensus is that benzodiazepines are not teratogenic and a single dose appears safe.

Most women with epilepsy will have an uncomplicated pregnancy course with excellent maternal and fetal outcomes. In order to minimize perinatal and obstetrical risks, it is important for the patient to understand that prevention of seizures is the most important goal during her pregnancy. There are complex interactions among the mother, fetus, and epilepsy, as well as the changes associated with pregnancy. Consequently, close cooperation and communication between the anesthesiologist and obstetric team are required in order to optimize the outcome.

References

1. Department of Health and others. *Why mothers die 1997–1999: The Confidential Enquiries into Maternal Deaths in the United Kingdom*. London: RCOG Press; 2001.
2. Hawkins JL, Koonin LM, Palmer SK, Gibbs CP. Anesthesia related deaths during obstetric delivery in the United States, 1979–1990. *Anesthesiology*. 1997;**86**:277–84.
3. Reisner LS, Benumof JL, Cooper SD. The difficult airway: Risk, prophylaxis and management. In Chestnut DH, ed. *Obstetric anesthesia: Principles and practice*. St. Louis, MO: Mosby; 1999, pp. 590–620.
4. Kuczkowski KM, Fouhy SA, Greenberg M, Benumof JL. Trauma in pregnancy: Anaesthetic management of the pregnancy trauma victim with unstable cervical spine. *Anaesthesia*. 2003;**58**:822.
5. Koppanyi T. The sedative, analgesic and anticonvulsant actions of local anesthetics. *Am J Med Sci*. 1962;**244**:646–54.
6. Tassinari CA, Daniele O, Michelucci R, et al. Benzodiazepines: Efficacy in status epilepticus. *Adv Neurol*. 1983;**34**:465–75.
7. McElhatton PR. The effects of benzodiazepine use during pregnancy and lactation. *Reprod Toxicol*. **8**(6):461–75.
8. Kreiger W, Copperman J, Laxer KD. Seizures with etomidate anesthesia. *Anesth Analg*. 1985;**64**:1226–7.
9. Hoffman P, Schockenhoff B. Etomidate as an anticonvulsive agent. *Anaesthesist*. 1984;**33**:142–4.
10. Bennett DR, Madsen JA, Jordan WS, Wiser WC. Ketamine anesthesia in brain-damaged: Electroencephalographic and clinical observations. *Neurology*. 1973;**23**:449–60.
11. White PF. Propofol: Pharmacokinetics and pharmacodynamics. *Sem Anesth*. 1988;7 (Suppl 1):4–20.
12. Duvosin R, Katz R. Reversal of central anticholinergic syndrome in man by physostigmine. *JAMA*. 1968;**206**:163–5.
13. Smith PA, McDonald TR, Jones CS. Convulsions associated with halothane anesthesia. *Anesthesia*. 1966;**21**:229–33.

14. Ward S, Weatherly BC. Pharmacokinetics of atracurium and its metabolites. *Br J Anaesth.* 1986; **58** (Suppl):6S–10S.

15. Pond SM, Kretschzmar KM. Effect of phenytoin on meperidine clearance and normeperidine formation. *Clin Pharmacol Ther.* 1981:**30**:680–6.

16. Bailey PL, Wilbrink J, Zwanikken P, Pace NL, Stanley TH. Anesthetic induction with fentanyl. *Anesth Analg.* 1985;**64**:48–53.

17. Borgeat A, Biollaz J, Depierraz B, Neff R. Grand mal seizure after extradural morphine analgesia. *Br J Anaesth.* 1988;**60**:733–5.

18. Jacobson L. Intrathecal and extradural narcotics. *Adv Pain Res Ther.* 1984;7:199–236.

19. Young ML, Smith DS, Greenberg J, et al. Effects of sufentanil on regional glucose utilization in rats. *Anesthesiology.* 1984;**61**:564–8.

20. Anand KJS, Ingraham J. Tolerance, dependence, and strategies for compassionate withdrawal of analgesics and anxiolytics in the pediatric ICU. *Crit Care Nurs.* 1996;**16**:87–93.

21. Mazze RI, Kallen B Reproductive outcome after anaesthesia and operation during pregnancy: A registry study of 5405 cases. *Am J Obstet Gynecol.* 1989;**161**:1178–85.

Chapter 16

Postpartum Seizure Management and Safety Issues for Women with Epilepsy

Natalia Rincon and Naymee J. Velez-Ruiz

Key Points

- During the postpartum period, physiological changes experienced during pregnancy, which alter drug metabolism, start to normalize and return to prepregnancy states.
- Antiseizure medication plasma levels can become elevated and toxic during the puerperium if pregnancy doses are not appropriately decreased.
- Stress and sleep deprivation in the postpartum period may trigger breakthrough seizures, even in women who have been seizure free for a while.
- The risk of women with epilepsy accidentally harming a newborn is low and depends on the type of seizure, its severity, and its frequency.
- Assistance for the mother with epilepsy is particularly important when she is bathing, carrying, or traveling with the newborn.
- Overall, the antiseizure medication concentrations in blood samples of infants who are breastfed are substantially lower than maternal blood concentrations. In most cases, mothers with epilepsy who are taking antiseizure medications should be strongly encouraged to breastfeed.
- The persons assisting the mother in the newborn's care should be encouraged to help with feeding the child, especially at night, so the mother can sleep.

Introduction

The postpartum period, commonly defined as the 6 weeks after childbirth, is a critical time for a woman and her infant as it sets the stage for long-term health and well-being. During this period, a woman is adapting to multiple physical, psychological, and social changes that can present considerable challenges such as sleep deprivation, fatigue, stress, and exacerbation of mental health disorders [1]. These challenges may be magnified when the woman is also living with epilepsy. She is recovering from childbirth, adjusting to hormonal changes, and caring for a newborn while self-managing her epilepsy.

To ensure the best postpartum outcomes possible, anticipatory guidance and counseling should begin during pregnancy with development of a postpartum care plan that addresses not only the transition to parenthood but also the prevention and management of breakthrough seizures and mood disorders. This chapter will address the postpartum medication plan and safety issues for women with epilepsy (WWE) to assist healthcare professionals in counseling and caring for them during this critical time.

Medication Adjustments in the Postpartum Period

The doses of antiseizure medication (ASM) are often increased during pregnancy to compensate for the effects of associated physiological changes and maintain seizure control. These changes include increased maternal blood volume, renal blood flow, and hepatic metabolism, as well as decreased plasma-binding protein levels and gastrointestinal motility [2]. Maternal ASM plasma levels may fluctuate until the eighth week postpartum. While these fluctuations occur, appropriate adjustments of the ASM must be done immediately to avoid toxicity, unnecessary high drug exposure of the breastfeeding infant, and breakthrough seizures. Adjustments to the ASM doses are primarily accomplished by monitoring drug plasma levels with the purpose of controlling for pregnancy-related alterations in the pharmacokinetics of ASMs. Therapeutic ranges do not guide adjustments in therapy but rather help create an individualized approach for each patient. This involves monitoring for ASM serum levels using a patient's individual optimal plasma level at the lowest effective dose, or reference concentration, which is ideally obtained before pregnancy when the patient is optimally treated [3]. This approach is naturally limited to ASMs amenable to therapeutic drug monitoring; therefore, an empiric approach is required for drugs with no measurable serum levels.

It is also important to recognize that WWE experience significant stressors such as sleep deprivation that may provoke seizures. Postpartum down-titration of ASMs to avoid drug toxicity is balanced by maintaining adequate drug levels to prevent seizures.

New-Generation Antiseizure Medications

Lamotrigine (LTG): Lamotrigine (LTG) is one of the most studied newer-generation ASMs. It is primarily metabolized by glucuronic acid conjugation in the liver with negligible first-pass effect, and excreted renally as a glucuronide conjugate [4]. Individual specific factors influence glucuronidation, including age, smoking, diet, concomitant drugs, ethnicity, genetics, and hormonal changes [4]. Immediately after delivery, the rate of LTG elimination rapidly decreases, reaching prepregnancy levels within 1–3 weeks postpartum. To avoid the risk of toxicity, an anticipated schedule to lower LTG doses after delivery based on the patient's individual serum reference concentration is recommended [5, 6]. For patients who required three or four increases in dosage during pregnancy, the dose should be reduced by 20–25% as early as postpartum day 3 [5, 6]. For all patients, the LTG level should be obtained within the first week after birth. If the LTG level is not increased above the reference concentration, the dose should not be adjusted. If the LTG level increases above the reference concentration after the first week, the dose should be decreased by an additional 20–25%. Lamotrigine levels may be repeated every 2–4 weeks until plasma levels stabilize [5]. Anticipating these changes could decrease toxicities related to elevated plasma levels in the postpartum period.

The extent of LTG elimination may be affected by genetic polymorphism in the uridine diphosphate glucuronosyltransferase (UGT) gene, ethnicity (which has been associated with enzyme activity), and exogenous factors [5, 7]. For example, the increased LTG level in the immediate postpartum period is not seen when LTG is used in combination with enzyme inducers such as phenytoin or carbamazepine [4]. Lamotrigine is transferred into the breast milk with some accumulation in infants likely due to low glucuronidation capacity, though breastfed infants' serum concentrations represent only ~20% of maternal serum concentrations [6, 8]. Overall, breastfeeding is regarded as safe in most cases, with caution advised in patients taking high doses [9].

Levetiracetam (LEV): Levetiracetam (LEV) is readily and completely absorbed after oral administration. It is not bound to plasma proteins, and its excretion is primarily renal with approximately 30% of the dose metabolized by enzymatic hydrolysis [3, 10]. Women experience a significant increase in the excretion of LEV during pregnancy. This is believed to be a result of increased volume of distribution and renal elimination as well as enhanced enzymatic hydrolysis. Studies suggest approximately 47.8% reduction in LEV plasma levels by the seventh month of pregnancy [3, 11], and a more recent study showed that changes in clearance are significant by the first trimester [12]. In the postpartum period, there is an expected elevation of plasma LEV concentrations. One study found LEV plasma levels increased by 30.4% 2 months postpartum compared to prepregnancy levels [11]. Another study suggested that LEV plasma concentrations reach prepregnancy levels within the first week postpartum [13]. Levetiracetam is transferred to breast milk in clinically significant amounts. Therefore, it is advisable to monitor LEV plasma levels in the first weeks postpartum to appropriately adjust the dose in order to decrease toxicity in the mother and to avoid unnecessary exposure to the nursing infant [11, 14]. No adverse reactions have been reported in breastfed children [9]. Serum concentrations in breastfed infants are low and frequently undetectable [8], indicating that LEV is efficiently eliminated by the neonate and the exposure is significantly lower than in utero.

Oxcarbazepine (OXC): Oxcarbazepine (OXC) is a prodrug almost completely metabolized to monohydroxy-carbamazepine (MHD), which has independent anticonvulsant effects. Oxcarbazepine is 40% protein bound, and it is metabolized by glucuronidation, in a similar fashion to LTG. The MHD plasma levels have been shown to decrease by 30–40% during pregnancy. This decrease is secondary to increased metabolic clearance, presumably in the setting of hormonal changes [15]. Post delivery, there is a significant increase in serum drug concentration. The MHD levels may return to prepregnancy levels as early as 1 week after delivery [15]. Clinical response and OXC levels should be monitored throughout pregnancy and the puerperium, and the levels should be adjusted to maintain prepregnancy levels. If the OXC dose is increased during pregnancy, it should be tapered down to the prepregnancy dose during the first 1–2 weeks after delivery [15]. The OXC levels in breast milk are low and not expected to cause adverse effects in the breastfed infant [16].

Gabapentin (GBP): Gabapentin (GBP) is primarily absorbed in the gastrointestinal tract, and it is eliminated by the kidneys. As a result, the main pregnancy-related changes that affect its pharmacokinetics are the ones that cause a change in the glomerular filtration rate (GFR). Small studies have shown minimal changes in maternal GBP plasma concentrations after delivery compared to earlier in the pregnancy. However, the data available are scarce. Studies have been inconclusive regarding the postpartum alteration of GBP pharmacokinetics, and it is difficult to draw conclusions regarding GBP dose adjustments during this period [3].

Topiramate (TPM): The bioavailability of topiramate (TPM) is almost complete after oral administration. Topiramate is primarily eliminated renally. While the data are limited, small samples have indicated similar levels of serum TPM at the time of delivery compared to 2–3 weeks postpartum [3, 17]. Low TPM concentrations have been documented in breastfed infants with no adverse effects noted [9].

Zonisamide (ZNS): Zonisamide (ZNS) accumulates in erythrocytes, and it is approximately 40–60% protein bound. Zonisamide undergoes hepatic biotransformation and it is metabolized by acetylation, glucuronide conjugation, and oxidation [9, 3]. It is mainly eliminated by renal excretion [2]. A small study looking into 144 serum concentrations from 23 pregnancies in 15 individual WWE showed that ZNS concentrations may fall more than 40% during pregnancy, with large interindividual variability [18]. In a recent publication from the Maternal Outcomes and Neurodevelopmental Effects of Antiepileptic Drugs (MONEAD) study, analysis of data from 326 pregnant WWE demonstrated that dose-normalized concentrations during pregnancy were decreased by up to 29.8% for ZNS when compared with postpartum values [19].

Lacosamide (LCS): Data are very limited regarding lacosamide (LCS) use and monitoring during pregnancy and the postpartum period. Lacosamide has low molecular weight and minimal binding to plasma proteins, which is one reason why it is transferred to breast milk. One case series found no adverse reactions from indirect exposure to LCS [20]. It does not seem to induce withdrawal symptoms or psychomotor developmental delays in the breastfed child [20].

Older-Generation Antiseizure Medications

Valproic acid (VPA): Valproic acid (VPA) is extensively used throughout the world despite its known teratogenic effects. To minimize the risks to the fetus, careful surveillance is required during pregnancy. Valproic acid is extensively protein bound, approximately 90% in the nonpregnant state. Pregnancy is known to result in decreased plasma protein binding, and therapeutic VPA monitoring is typically recommended throughout the pregnancy and puerperium. However, the decrease in plasma-free drug concentrations during pregnancy seen with other first-line ASMs is not typically seen with VPA. As a result, dose adjustments during pregnancy and the postpartum period are typically not necessary unless the patient requires dose optimization for clinical reasons such as breakthrough seizures [20].

Phenytoin (PHT): Phenytoin (PHT) is highly protein bound and around 90% metabolized by hepatic CYP isozymes CYP2C9 and CYP2C1913. Studies have shown a decline in the total and free plasma concentrations of PHT that begins in the first trimester and persists through the rest of the pregnancy. Total PHT levels can decrease by 55–61% whereas free PHT, the unbound and pharmacologically active portion, decreases by 16–31%. Both levels need to be monitored to properly adjust the dose. Adjustments based on total levels only can potentially result in neurotoxicity after delivery as protein binding and clearance return to prepregnancy levels [7, 13, 14]. Phenytoin is considered safe during breastfeeding [8].

Carbamazepine (CBZ): Carbamazepine (CBZ) is highly protein bound, approximately 70–80%, and its metabolism is facilitated by hepatic CYP isoenzymes, primarily through oxidation. The data regarding CBZ in pregnancy show very minor variation in plasma levels compared to baseline prepregnancy levels. Free CBZ concentration remains stable, likely due to decreased plasma protein binding [21]. Like when using PHT, it is important to follow unbound free plasma levels, if available, during and after pregnancy to determine the need for subsequent adjustments. Carbamazepine is considered safe for breastfeeding with low estimated levels of exposure through the breast milk [8].

Phenobarbital (Pb): Phenobarbital (Pb) is 50% protein bound and it is eliminated through CYP enzymes. Earlier studies documented significant decreases in the steady-state plasma level during pregnancy. An 85% increase in the prepregnancy dose would be required to compensate for the decline in plasma levels during pregnancy. Prepregnancy levels are reached approximately 4 weeks after delivery, likely due to

Pb's long half-life. Due to the complex pharmacokinetics of Pb during pregnancy and the puerperium, dosage adjustments are not recommended unless required clinically in the setting of breakthrough seizures [21]. In addition, despite the lack of statistically significant data, there is a theoretical risk of detrimental effects in the fetus with exposure to Pb.

Counseling Women with Epilepsy about Postpartum Safety

The safety of mother and child in the setting of seizures is important during pregnancy, and perhaps more so in the postpartum period. However, postpartum safety is usually overlooked in discussions with pregnant WWE [7]. In a study done in the United Kingdom, only nearly 50% of WWE were given information on safety, 86% of whom found it useful [22]. Many healthcare professionals fail to provide safety information to WWE due to lack of time or knowledge to appropriately counsel them. While some information about the learning needs of WWE has been documented [23–26], very little has been written about safety practices in the postpartum phase. In addition, there are no widespread educational tools that healthcare providers can use to facilitate the counseling of WWE on this subject in a time-efficient and efficacious manner. A self-instructional module on childrearing used in a prospective study from the Kerala Registry of Epilepsy and Pregnancy (KREP) did not automatically lead to better childcare practices [27]. A study by the Department of Health Clinical Standards Advisory Group of the United Kingdom on WWE who were educated about childrearing revealed that the proportions that recalled receiving information about childcare and breastfeeding were only 12% and 24% respectively [28]. These studies highlight safety gaps in different groups of people from different countries. While all findings cannot be generalized, these seem to suggest that multiple interventions and/or educational modalities are necessary to effectively counsel WWE about postpartum safety. It is important to consider potential differences in educational background and culture when examining counseling practices.

Postpartum Care Plan for Women with Epilepsy

Optimal management of WWE relies on a multidisciplinary approach to patient care. The woman and her healthcare providers, including her obstetrician and her neurologist, should work together to develop a comprehensive postpartum care plan that includes a well-defined care team. This care team should include the medical providers, who will be primarily responsible for the care of the woman and her infant after birth, as well as family and friends who will provide social and material support in the months following birth [1].

For a woman with epilepsy, the care plan should always identify the neurologist or epileptologist who will assume the treatment of her seizures and other epilepsy-related issues in the postpartum period. It should also include other specialists such as psychiatrists if applicable. Table 16.1 includes a list of the components of a basic postpartum care plan as suggested by the Presidential Task Force on Redefining the Postpartum Visit of the American College of Obstetricians and Gynecologists in 2018, with some adaptations to address the special needs of WWE. A written postpartum care plan should be documented in the medical record, provided to the patient, and communicated to the appropriate members of the postpartum care team.

Table 16.1 Postpartum care plan

Element	Components
Care team (obstetrician, neurologist, etc.)	Name, phone number, and office address of each member
Postpartum visits (obstetrician, neurologist, pediatrician, etc.)	Time, date, location, and phone number to schedule or reschedule if needed
Infant feeding plan	Breastfeeding or formula. If breastfeeding, instructions for use of a breast pump. If formula, brand and instructions for preparation. May also include resources for education on the topic
Reproductive plan and contraception	Timing of next pregnancy if desired, and contraception type and timing if applicable
Pregnancy complications	Conditions that will require treatment and/or follow-up such as gestational diabetes, preeclampsia, or eclampsia
Management of chronic conditions * Epilepsy	Epilepsy syndrome if known, seizure types, seizure frequency, daily medications, and rescue medications with instructions and dosing a. Postpartum adjustment of antiseizure medications if required b. Postpartum antiseizure medication levels if applicable
Mental health	Signs and symptoms of perinatal depressions and/or anxiety. List of resources for education on this topic

Self-Management of Epilepsy in the Postpartum Period

Epilepsy self-management is formally defined as "the sum total of steps a person takes to control seizures and the effects of having a seizure disorder" [29]. Self-management in WWE includes healthy living practices common to many chronic illnesses as well as epilepsy-specific tasks such as seizure tracking and response, ASM management, identification, and treatment of comorbid medical conditions such as mood disorders, lifestyle modifications, and safety precautions. Women with well-controlled epilepsy may face little changes in life after pregnancy. However, safety risks may be higher than prepregnancy, suggesting the need to monitor medications, side effects, and triggers carefully. Women with uncontrolled seizures may experience more safety challenges, medication changes, and comorbidities. All women, regardless of seizure control, will experience needs related to caring for a newborn. Women with epilepsy need to consider additional precautions while feeding, bathing, carrying, and transporting the baby. The following section highlights some of the major self-management components and strategies for WWE.

Antiseizure Medication Management

Managing medications is one of the most important self-management tasks. With new stressors and competing needs, women may need additional help to obtain medications from pharmacies and reminders to take them on schedule, especially since her usual routines have been disrupted. The healthcare professional can help her find new or additional ways to remember medicines, such as electronic reminders or alarms, epilepsy diaries, and pillboxes. The dosing times should be adjusted to her new routines, where association with other tasks such as newborn feedings or her own meals can aid in reminding her to take the ASMs. Family and friends can help filling her prescriptions or picking up medications at the pharmacy, or a mail-order prescription or delivery service can be set up. How help is offered and implemented will depend on the human and material resources available to the WWE, but a plan should be established to help her feel more confident and in control of her life.

Seizure Monitoring and Tracking

It is important that WWE and people within the circle of care document epileptic events and share this information with the healthcare team. Documentation should include a description of the semiology and duration of the event and the postictal state as well as any associated safety concerns. If the use of an intervention such as the administration of a rescue medication or swipe of a vagus nerve stimulation (VNS) magnet is needed, the frequency of use, the effectiveness, and any side effects should also be recorded. This information is crucial when determining the need for medication changes and assessing the safety of mother and child. It is recommended that women use a paper or electronic diary for tracking their seizures during this busy period of their lives. Examples of online epilepsy diaries with mobile applications include the Epilepsy Foundation My Seizure Diary (https://diary.epilepsy.com) and Seizure Tracker (www.seizuretracker.com).

Although current epilepsy care relies on seizure diaries, clinical monitoring may miss seizures. Wearable devices are typically well tolerated and suitable for long-term ambulatory monitoring. The US Food and Drug Administration cleared the Embrace2 wrist-worn smart band for seizure monitoring. This device detects convulsive seizures and instantly alerts caregivers wherever they are. While the use of this device is limited by its cost and accessibility, when possible, its use should be considered.

Women with epilepsy may also develop other pregnancy-related conditions that can present with seizures as a symptom and that should not be overlooked. Although not commonly, medical conditions such as eclampsia, posterior reversible encephalopathy syndrome, and reversible cerebral vasoconstriction syndrome may present de novo in the early postpartum period. Accompanying symptoms, including severe headaches, persistent high blood pressure, and focal neurological complaints, should raise suspicion for one of these conditions and trigger further investigation with head imaging and blood work.

Seizure Action Plan

Every woman with epilepsy should have a seizure response or action plan, ideally recorded in a written document by the healthcare professional taking the lead in her epilepsy care. This document should include information about her typical seizures, ASMs, and rescue interventions, and when to call for additional help. The seizure action plan should be available to the woman with epilepsy, her family, and her healthcare provider, and it should communicate the necessary information for any individual to be able to address breakthrough seizures even when not completely familiar with the woman's epilepsy and comorbid conditions. Plans usually work best when they can be individualized between the woman and her healthcare team and shared among pertinent people involved in her life. People who may be helping the mother and her baby should have access to this information and be taught what to do to prevent a potential emergency. Table 16.2 includes the main components of a seizure action plan for WWE. The Epilepsy Foundation provides basic templates for seizure action plans, which can be modified to accommodate the needs of each patient (www.epilepsy.com/learn/managing-your-epilepsy/seizure-action-plans).

Table 16.2 Seizure action plan

Element	Components
Seizure information	Seizure type, description, duration, and frequency
Seizure response	First aid, rescue medication, emergency contact, when to call 911
Rescue therapy	When and what to do, name and dose of medication, and how to administer
Care after seizure	Type of help needed and length of recovery time
Special instructions	For first responders, for emergency department
Daily seizure medications	Name, dose, and timing
Other relevant epilepsy information	Triggers, allergies, epilepsy surgery (type, date, sequelae), devices (VNS, RNS, DBS, date implanted), dietary therapy (yes/no, type)
Obstetric information	Number of pregnancies, number of deliveries and type, number of weeks, complications (e.g., hyperemesis gravidarum, gestational diabetes, preeclampsia, etc.)
Healthcare contacts	Epilepsy provider, obstetrician, primary care physician, preferred hospital, pharmacy

All WWE need to consider the possibility of having a seizure when they are alone. Establishing a safe environment ahead of time and using appropriate safety precautions can be helpful in this situation. If a woman with epilepsy has an aura or if she is feeling unwell, she should limit the time carrying the baby around by herself. She should stay close to a safe place where she can put the baby if she feels a seizure beginning, and her home should be set up in a way that limits injury from falls or other movements. For women with frequent seizures, it may be advisable to have supports available to help her as much as possible. Besides partners, family members, and friends, other options to consider are babysitters, daycare services, home health aides, and personal care assistants. They can help in the home when the mother is more likely to have seizures or when childcare needs are heaviest. Families with older children may discuss and practice an emergency plan such as calling 911 or a trusted adult for help. Women with persistent seizures may need to establish long-term plans for home and childcare help that extends beyond the 6–8 weeks of the postpartum period.

Lifestyle Modifications for Seizure Trigger Minimization

Many patients report lifestyle or environmental factors that can increase the likelihood of having a seizure. People with epilepsy frequently report as triggers sleep deprivation, stress, and anxiety; some people can self-predict their seizures when sleep deprivation has occurred [30]. Women with epilepsy are at increased risk of seizures during the postpartum period as multiple potential precipitants are occurring at the same time, including hormonal and medication changes, sleep deprivation, and stress. The mother and her caregivers should be educated about these triggers to reduce the risk of seizures and to maintain the safety of the mother and her baby. Women should be counseled on how to modify their lifestyle and environment to minimize the occurrence of these triggers.

In general, an average of 8 hours of sleep within a 24-hour period is recommended for all patients with epilepsy. Sleep is particularly important for WWE in the postpartum period. A typical strategy for a mother who is not getting enough sleep due to breastfeeding or waking up frequently at night may be for her to rest when the baby sleeps [31]. However, short naps can lead to poor-quality sleep and aggravate seizures in WWE sensitive to sleep deprivation. In this case, people within the immediate circle of care such as partners, family, or trusted friends could assist with nighttime feedings and, when possible, babysitters could be hired to allow longer periods of uninterrupted sleep [31]. Avoiding beverages or products that contain caffeine, alcohol, or other foods/fluids that may affect seizures is also important. Managing stress and mood monitoring are other lifestyle modifications that can be beneficial for seizure control in the postpartum period, specially but not exclusively in women with preexisting mood disorders or with risk factors for postpartum depression.

Monitoring Mood during the Postpartum Period

Depression and anxiety are overrepresented in people with epilepsy [32]. Peripartum depression is frequent in WWE and seldom medically treated. A review of depression and anxiety during pregnancy and the postpartum period in WWE revealed a point prevalence of depression from the second trimester to 6 months postpartum of 16–35% in WWE compared to 9–12% in controls. The highest estimates were found early in pregnancy and in the postpartum period [33]. In two of the studies included in this review, the point prevalence of depression 5–8 weeks postpartum was found to be more than three times higher than in healthy control women [34, 35]. The same review found that anxiety symptoms postpartum were reported by 10% of WWE versus 5% of controls [33].

The risk factors for postpartum mood disorders in WWE include previous psychiatric disease, sexual/physical abuse, ASM polytherapy, and high seizure frequency [33]. Identifying these risk factors may help the healthcare provider to closely monitor the WWE at highest risk for developing mood disorders. However, assessing mood should be incorporated into the care of all WWE, particularly at high-risk times such as the postpartum period. Including questions about mood and coping mechanisms during office visits and other interactions may help identify mood symptoms early or detect if preexisting problems are worsening over time. If mood symptoms are present, the mother should be referred to a behavioral health specialist, and, if possible, to both a psychiatrist and a psychologist. Other resources such as educational materials on the subject and support groups may also be helpful. This is discussed in detail in Chapter 2.

Newborn Care by Women with Epilepsy

In a study exploring the fears of WWE, May and colleagues found that WWE have significant concerns regarding safety and parenting needs [36]. Approximately 41% of WWE worried about the child's safety when the mother had a seizure and 36% worried that seizures would frighten their child. Although there is much anxiety about the possible risks to a child from the mother's epilepsy, no data have been published on this topic. The risk of the child being harmed depends on the type of seizure, its severity, and its frequency, and this risk is probably small if time is taken to inform WWE and their family of safety precautions [37].

The women who appear most at risk of injuring the newborn during a seizure appear to be those with uncontrolled juvenile myoclonic epilepsy, because they tend to be especially susceptible to sleep deprivation and their seizures often occur early in the morning upon waking up, which is when they are typically caring for their babies [37]. Some clinicians recommend that mothers with uncontrolled juvenile myoclonic epilepsy have someone else look after the child in the early morning if possible. Advice about safety precautions should be given to all mothers with epilepsy, even those who have been seizure free for a while, because breakthrough seizures are possible in the context of stress and exhaustion during the postpartum period. A collaborative routine for taking care of the baby should be established to minimize the risk of seizures in the mother and injury to the baby. This routine should maximize and not compromise the opportunities for the mother to bond with her child. Table 16.3 provides a list of home safety strategies to aid WWE to care for their newborns in the safest way possible while feeling confident and autonomous.

Breastfeeding and Epilepsy

The benefits of breastfeeding for both the mother and the newborn are well documented. For the child, these include a positive impact on neurodevelopment and decreased risk of infections and sudden infant death syndrome (SIDS). Breastfeeding mothers have a decreased risk of postpartum depression and of breast and ovarian cancer, and have better mother–infant attachment than non-breastfeeding mothers [7, 38]. There has been an increase in breastfeeding trends in the United States with studies over the past decade

Table 16.3 Home safety strategies in the postpartum period

- Keep all baby items in the lower level of the house to minimize the use of stairs.
- Keep the house full of open spaces and avoid rugs and other fall risks.
- Remove or pad objects with hard or sharp edges and avoid glass furniture.
- Change the baby on the floor with the use of portable changing pads.
- Feed the baby while seated on a couch, a padded floor, or the middle of a bed.
- Bathe the baby when someone else is around.
- Use a baby-size bathtub with a minimum amount of water.
- Consider using a stroller inside the house to minimize the time carrying the baby.
- Use strollers when walking outside, and, if possible, walk with another adult.
- Carry personal identification and medical information when outside the house.
- Have a system to call for help – pagers, cell phone applications, or other smart devices.
- Give a house key to a family member or close friend in case of emergency.
- Consider speaking to local first responders about your seizure action plan.

showing approximately 83.9% of infants have been breastfed, and 56.7% have been exclusively breastfed by 6 months of age [8, 39].

Breastfeeding provides a unique opportunity for a woman to bond with her baby. All WWE should be strongly encouraged to breastfeed their babies. Studies have shown that the rate of breastfeeding initiation in WWE is lower than in healthy women without epilepsy (50.9% vs. 87.6%), and WWE are less likely to maintain breastfeeding at 6 weeks (38.2%) [8]. While placental transfer of ASM is out of the control of the mother, breastfeeding is completely optional and therefore deciding to start lactating can generate some anxiety in the new mother with epilepsy [14]. Factors that affect the mother's decision include concerns about harming the child through medication exposure through breast milk, dissuasion by some clinicians, and limited access to counseling from epileptologists [38]. This is true despite data from MONEAD confirming that antiepileptic drug concentrations in blood samples of infants who were breastfed were substantially lower than maternal blood concentrations [8]. Furthermore, there is evidence from previous studies that ASM exposure via breast milk has no adverse neurodevelopmental effect on the children [8]. The only caveat is that women breastfeeding while taking potentially sedating medications, such as barbiturates and benzodiazepines, should monitor their babies for any evidence of adverse effects such as difficulty breathing or feeding, cyanosis, or failure to gain weight. Educating WWE on the benefits and safety of breastfeeding despite taking ASMs can influence their attitudes, decision-making, and behaviors toward breastfeeding. Read more details about information on different medication exposure through lactation in Chapter 17.

For WWE, there are other practical barriers such as tackling the complicated logistics of feeding a newborn and its consequences, including stress, sleep deprivation, and exhaustion. The persons assisting the mother in the newborn's care should be encouraged to help with feeding the child, especially at night, so that the mother can sleep. Breast milk can be obtained using a breast pump so that it can be given at night by a person other than the baby's mother. Another alternative is to supplement breastfeeding with bottle-feeding as the baby grows. Regardless of how the baby is fed, getting adequate sleep is important for the mother's health. These strategies may make it possible for the mother to sleep in a separate room and allow someone else to take the primary night duty.

Developing Postpartum Safety Plans for Women with Epilepsy and Their Babies

Like postpartum care and seizure action plans, safety plans should be individualized and should take into consideration the mother's daily life, activities, seizure type and frequency, and triggers. This information will help the healthcare professional as well as the patient and her family to identify and prevent potential risks as much as possible.

Newborn Feedings, Meal Preparation, and Home Maintenance

If it is necessary for the WWE to do the nighttime feedings herself, there should be an assessment of the character of the woman's seizures and a plan to minimize the risk of injury if she were to have an event in the context of sleep deprivation. Seizures without aura in which the mother loses awareness, wanders, convulses, or has postictal confusion are particularly dangerous.

Assuming no one is available to assist with meal preparation, to lessen the risks of burns or injuries from cooking, the mother may make meals ahead of time when accompanied that can be frozen, easily thawed, and cooked for mealtimes. Stovetop cooking is discouraged in women with frequent seizures or who may be at risk for falls. Using a microwave or crockpot may decrease the risk of burns. The healthcare professionals should encourage the WWE and her family to keep the kitchen stocked with quick and easy food items that can be safely prepared with a minimum amount of time or effort.

Home chores should be reexamined to determine which ones may not be safe for the mother to do for a while. If a woman has had seizure recurrence or has experienced medication side effects during pregnancy or the postpartum period, she may be at greater risk of injury while performing some household chores and driving. Safety plans may include redistribution of these chores within the circle of care and seeking paid assistance when possible.

Conclusions

The postpartum period typically results in most of the attention revolving around the newborn. It is critical for clinicians treating the WWE to recognize the various risk factors, physiological and psychological, that may have an impact in the tolerance of medication as well as frequency or severity of breakthrough events. Furthermore, this is a period of uncertainty for the mother, with choices that have implications in the development of the child, including but not limited to breastfeeding. As a result, patients must be adequately counseled about strategies to mitigate risks and maximize benefits during this time.

Safety in WWE during the postpartum period has profound health and psychosocial implications that will affect a WWE and her baby. It requires a conscious and orchestrated effort by the healthcare providers, the patient, and her family and friends. Planning is the key for success in keeping WWE safe during the postpartum period. Development of a postpartum care plan, seizure action plan, and home safety plan should help in organizing the efforts of all the parts working together to ensure safety.

References

1. Mckinney J, Keyser L, Clinton S, et al. ACOG Committee Opinion No. 736: Optimizing postpartum care. *Obstet Gynecol* 2018;**132**(3):784–5.
2. Kamyar VM, Varner M. Epilepsy in pregnancy. *Clin Obstet Gynecol.* 2013;**56**(2):330–41.
3. Tomson T, Battino D. Pharmacokinetics and therapeutic drug monitoring of newer antiepileptic drugs during pregnancy and the puerperium. *Clin Pharmacokinet.* 2007;**46**(3):209–19.
4. Ohman I, Vitols S, Tomson T. Lamotrigine in pregnancy: Pharmacokinetics during delivery, in the neonate, and during lactation. *Epilepsia* (Copenhagen). 2000;**41**(6):709–13.
5. Sabers A. Algorithm for lamotrigine dose adjustment before, during, and after pregnancy. *Acta Neurol Scand.* 2012;**126**(1):e1–e4.
6. Pennell PB, Peng L, Newport DJ, et al. Lamotrigine in pregnancy: Clearance, therapeutic drug monitoring, and seizure frequency. *Neurology.* 2008;**70** (22Pt2):2130–6.
7. Klein A. The postpartum period in women with epilepsy. *Neurol Clin.* 2012;**30**(3):867–75.
8. Meador KJ, Baker GA, Browning N, et al. Breastfeeding in children of women taking antiepileptic drugs: Cognitive outcomes at age 6 years. *JAMA Pediatr.* 2014;**168**(8):729–36.
9. Reimers A, Brodtkorb E. Second-generation antiepileptic drugs and pregnancy: A guide for clinicians. *Expert Rev Neurother.* 2012;**12**(6):707–17.
10. Tomson T, Palm R, Källén K, et al. Pharmacokinetics of levetiracetam during pregnancy, delivery, in the neonatal period, and lactation. *Epilepsia* (Copenhagen). 2007;**48**(6):1111–16.
11. López-Fraile IP, Cid AO, Juste AO, et al. Levetiracetam plasma level monitoring during pregnancy, delivery, and postpartum: Clinical and outcome implications. *Epilepsy Behav.* 2009;**15**(3):372–5.
12. Voinescu PE, Park S, Chen LQ, et al. Antiepileptic drug clearances during pregnancy and clinical implications for women with epilepsy. *Neurology.* 2018;**91**(13):e1228–e1236.
13. Tomson T, Landmark CJ, Battino D. Antiepileptic drug treatment in pregnancy: Changes in drug disposition and their clinical implications. *Epilepsia* (Copenhagen). 2013;**54**(3):405–14.
14. Pennell PB, Gidal BE, Sabers A, et al. Pharmacology of antiepileptic drugs during pregnancy and lactation. *Epilepsy Behav.* 2007;**11**(3):263–9.
15. Mazzucchelli I, Onat FY, Ozkara C, et al. Changes in the disposition of oxcarbazepine and its metabolites during pregnancy and the puerperium. *Epilepsia* (Copenhagen). 2006;**47**(3):504–9.
16. Drugs and Lactation Database (LactMed®) [Internet]. Bethesda (MD): National Institute of Child Health and Human Development; 2006–. Oxcarbazepine. 2021 Feb 15. PMID: 30000302.
17. Ohman I, Vitols S, Luef G, et al. Topiramate kinetics during delivery, lactation, and in the neonate: Preliminary observations. *Epilepsia.* 2002;**43**(10):1157–60.
18. Reimers A, Helde G, Becser Andersen N, et al. Zonisamide serum concentrations during pregnancy. *Epilepsy Res.* 2018;**144**:25–9.
19. Pennell PB, Karanam A, Meador KJ, et al. Antiseizure medication concentrations during pregnancy. *Jama Neurol.* 2022;**79**(4).
20. Lattanzi S, Cagnetti C, Foschi N, et al. Lacosamide during pregnancy and breastfeeding. *Neurol Neurochir Pol.* 51(3):266–9.
21. Sabers A, Petrenaite V. Pharmacokinetics of antiepileptic drugs in pregnancy. *Expert Rev Clin Pharmacol.* 2008;**1**(1):129–36.

22. Bagshaw J, Crawford P, Chappell B. Problems that mothers with epilepsy experience when caring for their children. *Seizure*. 2008;**17**(1):42–8.
23. Crawford P, Hudson S. Understanding the information needs of women with epilepsy at different life stages: results of the "Ideal World" survey. *Seizure*. 2003;**12**(7):502–7.
24. Vazquez B, Gibson P, Kustra R. Epilepsy and women's health issues: Unmet needs. Survey results from women with epilepsy. *Epilepsy Behav*. 2007;**10**(1):163–9.
25. Friedrich L, Sruk A, Bielen I. Women with epilepsy in childbearing age: Pregnancy-related knowledge, information sources, and antiepileptic drugs. *Epilepsy Behav*. 2018;**80**:122–8.
26. Dierking C, Porschen T, Walter U, et al. Pregnancy-related knowledge of women with epilepsy: An internet-based survey in German-speaking countries. *Epilepsy Behav*. 2018;**79**:17–22.
27. Saramma PP, Sarma PS, Thomas SV. Effect of a self-instructional module on the child rearing knowledge and practice of women with epilepsy. *Seizure*. 2014;**23**(6):424–8.
28. Bell GS, Nashef SK, Kendall S, et al. Information recalled by women taking antiepileptic drugs for epilepsy: A questionnaire study. *Epilepsy Res*. 2002;**52**(2):139–46.
29. Dilorio C. Epilepsy self-management. In Gachman DS, ed. *Handbook of health behavior research II: Provider determinants*. New York: Plenum Press; 1997, pp. 213–30.
30. Haut SR, Hall CB, Masur J, et al. Seizure occurrence: Precipitants and prediction. *Neurology*. 2007;**69**(20):1905–10.
31. Callanan M. Parenting for women with epilepsy. In Morell MJ, Flynn K, eds. *Women with epilepsy: A handbook of health and treatment issues*. New York: Cambridge University Press; 2023, pp. 228–6.
32. Rai D, Kerr M, McManus S, et al. Epilepsy and psychiatric comorbidity: A nationally representative population-based study. *Epilepsia*. 2012;**53**(6):1095–1103.
33. Bjørk MH, Veiby G, Engelsen BA, et al. Depression and anxiety during pregnancy and the postpartum period in women with epilepsy: A review of frequency, risks, and recommendations for treatment. *Seizure*. 2015;**28**:39–45.
34. Turner K, Piazzini A, Franza A, et al. Postpartum depression in women with epilepsy versus women without epilepsy. *Epilepsy Behav*. 2006;**9**(2):293–7.
35. Turner K, Piazzini A, Franza A, et al. Epilepsy and postpartum depression. *Epilepsia*. 2009;**50** Suppl 1:24–7.
36. May TW, Pfäfflin M, Coban I, et al. Fears, knowledge, and need of counseling for women with epilepsy: Results of an outpatient study. *Nervenarzt*. 2009;**80**(2):174–83.
37. Crawford, P. Best practice guidelines for the management of women with epilepsy. *Epilepsia*. 2005;**46** (Suppl. 9):117–24.
38. al-Faraj AO, Pandey S, Herlihy MM, et al. Factors affecting breastfeeding in women with epilepsy. *Epilepsia* (Copenhagen). 2021;**62**(9):2171–9.
39. www.cdc.gov/breastfeeding/data/reportcard.htm.
40. Birnbaum A, Meador KJ, Karanam A, et al. Antiepileptic drug exposure in infants of breastfeeding mothers with epilepsy. *JAMA Neurol*. 2020;**77**(4):441–50.

Chapter

17

Breastfeeding and Use of Antiseizure Medications

Abrar O. al-Faraj and Trudy D. Pang

Key Points

- Breastfeeding is safe and should be encouraged for most infants of mothers taking antiseizure medications, with close infant monitoring.
- Serum concentration of various commonly used antiseizure medications in breastfed infants is below the lower level of quantification.
- Infants breastfed by mothers with epilepsy have better IQ and developmental outcomes compared to non-breastfed infants.
- Women with epilepsy have lower rates of breastfeeding compared to the general population as they face unique challenges, which underscores the need for interventions to support this vulnerable population.

Introduction

In the United States, approximately 1 million women with epilepsy (WWE) are of child-bearing age and 80% of them take at least one antiseizure medication (ASM) [1]. Although most WWE taking ASMs have normal pregnancies and healthy babies, their pregnancies are considered high-risk pregnancies. Management of the expectant mother is focused on close monitoring and delicately balancing seizure control while minimizing ASM exposure to the developing fetus in order to lower the risk of major congenital malformations (MCM) and potential adverse cognitive effects. Therefore, simplification of ASM therapy, use of the lowest therapeutic dose, and tailored selection of ASM with the safest MCM profile are important steps to facilitating a healthy pregnancy in WWE, ideally prior to conception [1].

The decision whether to breastfeed represents a great challenge for WWE and their physicians. While breastfeeding is associated with a wide variety of health benefits for both mother and infant, there is concern regarding the potential of additional adverse effects with ASM exposure via breast milk, especially on long-term neurodevelopmental outcomes. Until recently, there has been a scarcity of data regarding the amount of various ASMs expressed in breast milk and their short- and long-term effects on the infant, especially neurodevelopmental effects, which led to many clinicians, including physicians to discourage breastfeeding in WWE.

However, in the past decade, growing evidence has shown that breastfeeding is safe for many of the commonly used ASMs, and that breastfed infants have additional benefits compared to non-breastfed infants, particularly neurodevelopmental benefits. Despite the newly published data supporting the safety of breastfeeding, breastfeeding recommendations have not kept pace with the evolving literature and recent studies have shown that rates of breastfeeding in WWE remain significantly lower than in the general population [2–4].

A number of factors may contribute to this observed gap. Surveys have shown that neurologists may not be adequately equipped to counsel WWE about breastfeeding due to lack of knowledge and training, particularly regarding safety and long-term neurodevelopmental benefits [5, 6]. Furthermore, counseling is often sought by the patient in the later stages of pregnancy, rather than proactively offered by treating physicians prior to conception or early in the pregnancy process, thereby limiting patients' opportunity to make informed decisions, and this increases the risk of a missed or disrupted opportunity [5]. Additionally, there are patient-specific barriers, which are rarely explored. In a study of 281 Chinese WWE to assess reasons for early cessation of breastfeeding, the authors showed that the most common causes were fear of exposure of the baby to ASMs, uncontrolled seizures, and insufficient milk supply [4]. A recent retrospective study explored potential factors affecting WWE and their breastfeeding practices and showed that early termination of breastfeeding was most commonly due to technical difficulties, followed by concern of negative impact on infant development, and finally dissuasion by other clinicians, including pediatricians and obstetric nurses [3].

Further research is needed to prospectively evaluate factors that may negatively impact breastfeeding practices in WWE, in order to improve breastfeeding overall in WWE. This chapter will provide an overview of the current literature regarding ASM exposure via breast milk, the safety of commonly used ASMs and their reported potential side effects, and recommendations about breastfeeding with regard to specific ASM use in WWE.

Benefits of Breastfeeding in the General Population

Breastfeeding is known to promote optimal health and well-being for both mother and infant. The American Academy of Pediatrics (AAP) recommends exclusive breastfeeding for the first 6 months of life, and the introduction of a complementary diet at 6 months of age and continuation of breastfeeding until 12 months [7]. Benefits for infants include reducing risk of necrotizing enterocolitis, urinary tract infection, otitis media, diarrheal illnesses, and sepsis. Breastfeeding has protective properties against infection due to the presence of secretory antibodies (e.g., IgA) and of antiviral and antibacterial agents in breast milk [8]. Breastfeeding benefits extend beyond the neonatal period, as it lowers the infant hospitalization rate for respiratory illnesses up to 3 years, reduces the risk of diabetes mellitus and obesity in children, and enhances infant cognitive function, including memory performance and problem-solving abilities, in breastfed children compared to children who were not breastfed [9]. Benefits for the mother include improved birth spacing, lowered risk of breast cancer with a 4% risk reduction for every year a woman breastfeeds, and lowered risk for a variety of other conditions, including ovarian cancer, diabetes mellitus, hypertension, hyperlipidemia, and obesity [8].

From an economic perspective, it is suggested that breastfeeding could reduce the economic burden of medical complications, morbidity, and mortality by an estimated $17.2 billion annually and could prevent 823,000 deaths per year in children younger than 5 years of age [9]. Thus, the World Health Organization (WHO) and United Nations advocate increasing the rate of exclusive breastfeeding by developing and implementing policies that support breastfeeding and implementing interventions such as adapting baby-friendly hospitals, breastfeeding counseling, and training by International Board-Certified Lactation Consultants (IBCLCs) and volunteer-based mother-to-mother support organizations [10]. These efforts have resulted in increased overall rates of breastfeeding initiation and continuation. In the United States, the Centers for Disease Control and Prevent (CDC) report card (2018) data showed that the rate of breastfeeding initiation in the general population is at 83.2% and the rate of continuation at 6 months is at 57.6% [11].

Breastfeeding Practices among Women with Epilepsy

Initiation rates of breastfeeding have been shown to be lower in WWE at 50%, compared to 83.2% in the general population, based on the most recent CDC breastfeeding report card [2–4, 11]. Similarly, the duration of breastfeeding in WWE is shorter, with only 36.3% of WWE breastfeeding at 6 months postpartum, compared to 60% of women in the general population [12]. The main factors contributing to lower breastfeeding rates in WWE include lack of knowledge about the amount of ASMs expressed in breast milk, pharmacokinetics of ASMs in infants and their subsequent cumulative effects on the infants, especially neurodevelopmental effects, over the longer term [13]. Other concerns relate to sleep deprivation and the risk of missed medications, which may lead to breakthrough seizures [2].

Recently, a study showed that factors such as delivery mode (spontaneous vaginal delivery versus cesarean section), specific ASMs, and newborn condition at birth are predictive of breastfeeding initiation in WWE [12]. Furthermore, socioeconomic factors, including maternal education, employment, social support, maternal self-esteem, and emotional status, are major determinants of maternal capacity for breastfeeding [10]. Mothers with epilepsy often have lower employment rates and higher rates of postpartum depression and anxiety, which may render them more vulnerable to unsuccessful breastfeeding [14, 15]. Despite the benefits of lactation consultation, WWE are significantly less likely to be offered support from certified lactation consultants, further exacerbating the gap in breastfeeding [3].

Benefits of Breastfeeding for Infants of Women with Epilepsy Taking Antiseizure Medications

Mounting evidence from recent large prospective studies shows that breastfeeding is overall safe when using common ASMs (e.g., lamotrigine, levetiracetam, oxcarbazepine, carbamazepine, phenytoin, and valproate), and breastfeeding should be encouraged for WWE. The Neurodevelopmental Effects of Antiepileptic Drugs (NEAD) study, a prospective observational study that assessed the effect of breastfeeding in children of women taking ASMs (lamotrigine, carbamazepine, phenytoin, and valproate) on cognitive function of breastfed infants at 3 years and 6 years of age [13, 16], showed that the average IQ was higher for infants who were breastfed. Furthermore, the Norwegian Mother and Child Cohort (MoBa) [17] study showed lack of harmful effects in breastfed infants by mothers taking ASMs, and breastfed infants showed slightly better verbal abilities and fine motor and social skills than non-breastfed infants [17].

Determinants of Infant Level of Drug Exposure via Breast Milk

Measuring an infant's level of drug exposure via breast milk is challenging because several factors need to be considered: the drug's physiochemical properties, maternal serum concentrations, milk volume (e.g., drug penetration is usually higher during the colostral period, but it is offset by the low volume of milk), infant's level of absorption, maturation of the drug metabolism system, clearance, and time of serum level sampling to the time of feeding and maternal ASM dosing [18, 19]. One should also consider the drug distribution gradient, which measures drug concentrations in foremilk to hindmilk. Drugs that are active on the central nervous system are more heavily concentrated in hindmilk because of its higher lipid content [18]. Overall, the risk of drug exposure via breast milk becomes lower in infants between the ages of 6 and 18 months because of the reduced ratio of milk to solid food [19].

Drugs' Physiochemical Properties

Drugs' physiochemical properties that facilitate their entry in breast milk are: 1) low molecular weight (<500 Da); 2) low protein binding capacity; and 3) higher pKa (unionized drugs) [18]. Medications considered safe for pregnancy have high protein-binding capacity and molecular weight and are ionized with a short half-life [18].

Indices of Infant Drug Exposure

Oral bioavailability of drugs in breast milk is variable. Some drugs are poorly absorbed, while others are unstable in the gastrointestinal environment due to the proteolytic enzymes and acids that may destroy the medications [19]. Ideally, direct measurement of the infant's drug serum level can determine the amount ingested; however, it is associated with many ethical dilemmas, especially in asymptomatic infants. Many surrogate theoretical markers have been developed to estimate the level of infant drug exposure.

The most widely used measure is the relative infant dosage (RID), which is calculated by dividing the weight-adjusted infant dosage per day (via milk) (mg/kg/day) by the maternal weight-adjusted dosage per day (mg/kg/day). An important consideration when calculating the RID is the infant's age and size. For example, premature infants are at a somewhat increased risk of adverse effects because of lower metabolic capacity. An RID less than 10% is considered safe, while an RID greater than 25% is considered an unacceptable risk [20]. Most used ASMs have an RID less than 10%. Specific RIDs for select ASMs are listed in Table 17.1.

A second method that estimates the amount of drug in breast milk (exposure index) is the ratio of milk to the maternal serum plasma drug concentration. It is measured by the ratio of average concentration of the drug in breast milk to the average concentration of the drug in maternal plasma. An M/P ratio of less than 1 signifies a low level of drug exposure [21]. Specific ASM M/P ratios are listed in Table 17.1 for individual ASMs. This method is subject to variability in maternal drug concentrations because of the altered maternal pharmacokinetics during pregnancy and the postpartum period. One must interpret this ratio with caution because for some drugs, the M/P ratio maybe high but the maternal serum level is low. Thus the amount of the drug that is transferred via breast milk is still low. In addition, the M/P is influenced by the timing of the sample relative to the timing of the

Table 17.1 Clinical parameters for infant drug exposure and breastfeeding safety for selected antiseizure medications

Medication	RID (%)	M/P ratio	T ½ (hours)
Levetiracetam	3.4–7.8	0.76–1.55	6–8
Lamotrigine	9.2	0.057–1.47	29
Oxcarbazepine	1.5–1.7	0.5	9
Zonisamide	28.9–36.8	0.93	63
Topiramate	24.5	0.86–1.1	18–24
Clonazepam	0.33	2.8	18–25
Phenytoin	0.6–7.7	0.4–0.6	6–24
Phenobarbital	24	0.4–0.6	20–133
Primidone	8.4–8.6	0.7	5–18
Ethosuximide	31.4–73.5	0.94	30–60
Gabapentin	1.3–6.6	0.7–1.3	5–7
Carbamazepine	3.8–5.9	0.69	18–54
Diazepam	7.1	0.2–2.7	43
Valproic acid	1.4–1.7	0.42	14

RID: relative infant dose
M/P ratio: ratio of milk to maternal plasma
T ½: drug half-life
RID = weight-adjusted infant dosage (mg/kg/day) x 100 / weight-adjusted maternal dosage (mg/kg/day)

ASM dose and the compartmentalization of the drug in breast milk [21]. Thus this measure alone does not always reflect the actual infant's drug exposure [22].

Infant Drug Metabolism and Clearance

An infant's drug metabolism and clearance may influence the infant's serum drug accumulation. Variability in enzymatic ontogeny age, the infant's comorbidities, and environmental factors influence the infant's drug metabolism systems [20]. The cytochrome P450 (CYP450) enzyme system, which contains various enzyme isomers, represents the main drug-metabolizing system for many ASMs, such as phenytoin, carbamazepine, clobazam, clonazepam, ethosuximide, felbamate, and phenobarbital. There is significant variability in the maturation age of the different isoenzymes [20]. The CYP3A7 is the most abundant CYP isoenzyme at birth, while the CYP3A4 enzyme becomes the most dominant enzyme system in adult life [23]. The second metabolizing system is the glucuronosyltransferases (UGT) system, which is responsible for glucuronidation of some ASMs (e.g., UGT1A4 for lamotrigine, UGT2B1 for valproic acid and oxcarbazepine) [24]. The UGT system is known to have low levels of activity in the neonatal period, and it has significant variability in age of maturation, ranging from 1 year to more than 10 years old [23].

Renal clearance is an additional factor that influences an infant's drug exposure. Renal function in neonates is low (25% of the adult level per body weight), but during the first 2 weeks of life, renal function develops significantly, reaching 50–75% of adult function due to an increase in renal blood flow. All of these factors can significantly impact ASM clearance and half-lives. Specific drug half-lives for individual selected ASMs are listed in Table 17.1.

For most ASMs, the overall exposure to ASMs via breast milk is significantly lower than in utero exposure, at approximately 20–30% [25]. Thus the risk of ASMs exposure via breast milk is overall low and reports of adverse effects related to many of the commonly used ASMs are rare.

Effect of Acute Antiseizure Medication Exposure on Breastfed Infants

Most acute drug adverse reactions due to drug exposure via breast milk occur in the first 2 months of life [25]. This can be explained by infants' low capacity for drug metabolism and clearance, while receiving large doses via breast milk relative to their body weight during that time [25]. Centrally active drugs such as ASMs have higher predilection for adverse effects on the central nervous system (CNS) because of their lipophilic nature and their tendency to cross the blood–brain barrier more readily. The overall reported rate of adverse effects related to ASMs in infants is 11%; commonly reported symptoms include drowsiness, apnea, cyanosis, bradycardia, sedation, vomiting, weight loss, absent suck, and diarrhea [25]. However, one must interpret this in the context of how frequently the drugs are used and how many reports have been made of their use without adverse effects [25].

Specific Antiseizure Medications and Recommendations during Lactation

The American Academy of Neurology practice parameters for 2009 provided limited information about the amount of various ASMs expressed in breast milk [1]. Since then, many case reports, case series, and large observational studies have emerged, providing additional data about the concentrations of commonly used ASMs in breast milk, infants' serum levels, and adverse effects. The most recent was a large observational multicenter study that assessed exposure to commonly used ASMs in breastfed infants of WWE taking various ASMs (lamotrigine, levetiracetam, carbamazepine, oxcarbazepine, phenytoin, valproic acid, zonisamide, and topiramate) [25]. The study showed that 49% of ASM concentrations in infants were less than the lower limit of quantification (LLoQ) except for lamotrigine [26]. The median concentration of the infant to the mother's serum was 0.3–44.2% [26]. Thus these data showed relatively low infant ASM serum concentrations, significantly lower than that of maternal serum concentrations, thereby supporting the safety of these ASMs during breastfeeding. Detailed clinical parameters of infant drug exposure to individual ASMs are listed in Table 17.1.

Safe Antiseizure Medications for Breastfeeding

Levetiracetam

Levetiracetam is one of the ASMs that is most frequently used during pregnancy. It is minimally protein bound and has extensive transplacental transfer and excretion into breast milk [27]. However, breastfed infants' serum concentration is below the LLoQ [25]. Additionally, the median infant-to-maternal serum concentration is low, which suggests rapid renal elimination [26, 28]. Reported adverse effects are extremely rare. There is one case report of hypotonia with poor suck in an infant breastfed by a mother taking levetiracetam; symptoms resolved after stopping breastfeeding [28]. A second case of withdrawal seizure was reported in an infant whose mother was taking a combination of primidone and levetiracetam throughout the pregnancy. The mother was discouraged from breastfeeding after delivery. The infant developed withdrawal seizures 24 hours after discontinuing breastfeeding, which may be attributed to primidone withdrawal rather than levetiracetam [19]. In three additional cases, sedation and poor feeding were reported in infants breastfed by mothers taking combination therapy, levetiracetam and clobazam, and levetiracetam and lacosamide [29, 30].

Breastfeeding is overall encouraged for WWE taking levetiracetam. The infant should be monitored for sedation, drowsiness, adequate weight gain, hypotonia, and poor suck, especially in exclusively breastfed infants and when used in combination with other ASMs, which can cause greater CNS sedation.

Lamotrigine

Lamotrigine's relatively favorable profile, with a low rate of major congenital malformations (MCMs) and side effects, has made it one of the most commonly prescribed ASMs for WWE during their reproductive ages. One must be aware of its highly variable pharmacokinetics during pregnancy, the postpartum period, and excretion in breast milk (maternal serum concentration is a major determinant of the amount expressed and subsequently the infant's serum level) [26]. Overall, lamotrigine is extensively expressed in breast milk with an M/P ratio of 41.2, and the average infant/maternal serum concentration range is 14–40% [26].

In a study that evaluated breastfed infants and maternal serum drug concentrations, lamotrigine was the only drug with an infant serum level above the LLoQ [26]. The high infant/maternal ratio was theorized to be related to the immature metabolic system utilizing glucuronidation, which may mature to adult levels at approximately 2 years of age [19]. All of these factors may theoretically increase the risk of lamotrigine accumulation in the infant's serum and hence may cause adverse effects in the breastfed infant. Several rare adverse effects have been reported in infants exposed to lamotrigine via breast milk. These include an infant who developed normocytic, normochromic anemia with neutropenia that normalized after cessation of breastfeeding [31], and a single case of severe apneic episode requiring cardiac resuscitation that occurred in an infant breastfed by a mother taking an unusually high dose of lamotrigine [32]. Other additional rare reported adverse effects in infants that may be related to lamotrigine exposure via breast milk are skin rash, elevated liver enzymes, crying, and refusal of food [33]. However, the most robust evidence for breastfeeding safety exists for lamotrigine, particularly with regard to neurodevelopmental outcomes [17].

Overall, breastfeeding in women taking lamotrigine has been well tolerated in large patient cohorts without adverse effects. Thus breastfeeding is encouraged for mothers taking lamotrigine, and infants should be monitored closely for rare adverse reactions such as skin rash and bruises, drowsiness, lethargy, and poor weight gain.

Oxcarbazepine

Scarce data about oxcarbazepine and its active metabolite, monohydroxycarbazepine (MHD), have shown extensive transplacental passage and secretion into breast milk [34]. Similar to lamotrigine, oxcarbazepine metabolism occurs via glucuronidation, which is immature in neonates. Thus there is a theoretical risk of drug accumulation in the exposed infant. However, quantitative studies have revealed that levels of oxcarbazepine and its active metabolite are below the LLoQ [26, 35, 36]. The rate of reported immediate and/or delayed adverse effects in infants breastfed by mothers taking oxcarbazepine is extremely low, with only one case report of an infant who developed withdrawal symptoms [37]. Breastfeeding is encouraged, with close monitoring for signs of excessive sedation, irritability, and insufficient weight gain.

Topiramate

Despite the known MCM risk of topiramate during pregnancy, it is considered overall safe in the postpartum period, and breastfeeding is encouraged in women taking topiramate with close monitoring for side effects. It has extensive transplacental passage and expression in breast milk. However, its serum concentration in breastfed infants by mothers taking topiramate is below the LLoQ [26], indicating rapid clearance [38]. There is one case report of frothy, watery diarrhea and weight decline 40 days postpartum in an infant breastfed by a mother taking topiramate 100 mg/day, without an identifiable etiology except for an elevated topiramate level in breast milk [39]. Breastfeeding is encouraged, with close monitoring for signs of excessive sedation, irritability, and insufficient weight gain.

Gabapentin

Gabapentin is excreted in small amounts in breast milk [1]. There are no reports of adverse effects in infants exposed to gabapentin via breast milk. However, general monitoring of breastfed infants for side effects such as drowsiness and sedation is recommended.

Zonisamide

Zonisamide has extensive transplacental transfer as well as significant secretion into breast milk [40]. Zonisamide's long half-life and elevated drug peak concentration (1.5-fold) associated with once-daily dosing may theoretically subject infants to excessive zonisamide exposure and theoretically to drug accumulation, leading to adverse effects [24]. However, the M/P ratio was found to be less than 1, and the infant serum level of zonisamide was below the LLoQ, suggestive of rapid drug clearance [25, 41]. There are three case reports of infants breastfed by mothers taking zonisamide with no adverse effects [40–41]. Breastfeeding for mothers taking zonisamide is encouraged, again with close infant monitoring [41].

Valproic Acid

Despite the higher risk of MCMs with valproic acid during pregnancy, it is excreted in small amounts in breast milk and the measured infant serum concentration is below the LLoQ [26]; thus it is compatible with breastfeeding. It was hypothesized that infants exposed to valproic acid via breast milk are at increased risk of adverse effects, especially liver toxicity, because of their immature glucuronidation systems [25]. There are rare case reports of patchy alopecia and thrombotic thrombocytopenic anemia in breastfed infants, which resolved after cessation of breastfeeding [42–43], and a case of sedation due to combination therapy with primidone [44]. However, the NEAD study showed that despite the negative effects of in utero fetal exposure to valproate, breastfeeding has been shown to be safe, likely due to the lower index of drug exposure via breast milk [16]. Thus, the overall health and neurodevelopmental benefits of breastfeeding outweigh the low risk of minimal valproate exposure via breast milk, and breastfeeding should be encouraged.

Phenytoin

Phenytoin is another ASM considered safe for breastfeeding. It is highly protein bound with a low M/P ratio and the measured infant serum concentration is below the LLoQ [26]. Adverse effects related to phenytoin exposure in breastfed infants are rare; however, when taken with other psychotropic medications, it may result in sedation or withdrawal seizures. A case of excessive sedation and elevated methemoglobinemia was reported in an infant breastfed by a mother taking a combination of phenobarbital and phenytoin [45]. Thus breastfeeding should be offered with close clinical monitoring of the infant for sedation and other side effects, especially in mothers taking phenytoin in combination with other centrally acting depressants.

Carbamazepine

Carbamazepine is a second-generation ASM expressed in larger quantities in breast milk, but the infant serum concentration is below the LLoQ in clinical studies [26]. Infants breastfed by mothers taking carbamazepine were found to have no adverse cognitive effects at 3 and 6 years of age [14, 17]. Adverse reactions are rare in breastfed infants; few cases of excessive sedation, poor suckling, and a case of hepatic dysfunction were reported [45–47]. The latter occurred in patients taking combination therapy. Thus breastfeeding is encouraged for infants of mothers taking carbamazepine, with close monitoring for signs of sedation.

Antiseizure Medications Possibly Hazardous with Breastfeeding

Phenobarbital and Primidone

Phenobarbital excretion in breast milk is variable, but it has a low M/P ratio less than 1 [21]. Unlike phenobarbital, primidone penetrates breast milk extensively and has a long half-life [1]. It also has an elevated free fraction of greater than 90% in some infants, thus causing increased risk of sedation. Cases of lethargy, poor suck, and hypotonia have been described in infants exposed to phenobarbital/primidone via breast milk. Nonetheless, the presence of phenobarbital/primidone in breast milk may mitigate possible neonatal withdrawal symptoms in infants exposed in utero [21]. Commonly reported adverse effects of primidone/phenobarbital exposure via breast milk are hypotonia, lethargy, poor suck, and withdrawal symptoms such as jitteriness, tremor, and sleep disturbances [46]. The decision to breastfeed should be balanced against the risk of excessive sedation and mitigation of the risk of withdrawal symptoms in infants. Thus the APP advocates an individualized approach and recommends breastfeeding with caution and close monitoring of the breastfed infant for lethargy, decreased suckle, and delayed milestones.

Clobazam

Clobazam is a long-acting benzodiazepine with a major active metabolite N-desmethylclobazam, which also has a long half-life. Therefore, there is a theoretical risk of active metabolite accumulation. However, the M/P ratio is less than 1 [47]. Sedation is the main concern with a breastfed infant being exposed to clobazam. Thus breastfeeding may be recommended with caution under the following conditions: the maternal dose and infant exposure are low (partial breastfeeding). Close monitoring of the infant for symptoms of sedation and poor suckling is encouraged [48]. Notably, breastfeeding during the postpartum period may minimize withdrawal effects in the neonate.

Clonazepam

Clonazepam has a low M/P ratio of less than 1, but has the potential to accumulate in the breastfed infant due to its long half-life. Most published reports of infants breastfed by mothers taking clonazepam showed a lack of adverse effects. Only a few cases reported symptoms of sedation, excessive periodic breathing with prolonged apnea and cyanosis, and sedation, especially when clonazepam is taken with other ASMs [48]. Breastfeeding may be recommended with close monitoring of the infant for symptoms of sedation and may minimize the risk of benzodiazepine withdrawal while facilitating the weaning process. An alternative benzodiazepine with a shorter half-life is recommended over clonazepam if possible.

Felbamate

Felbamate is another drug known to be excreted in breast milk because of its low molecular weight and low protein-binding capacity. Felbamate is generally not recommended for women of childbearing potential due to the significant and severe idiosyncratic reactions associated with its use; however, rare instances of felbamate use during pregnancy exist, and it is not clearly associated with severe adverse fetal outcomes, including fetal loss and MCMs [49]. Although no reports of adverse effects or its use in breastfeeding have been published, felbamate is incompatible with breastfeeding because of its known serious adverse effects in adults [50].

Antiseizure Medications with Limited Data

No data have been published about several ASMs regarding the amount of drug excreted in breast milk, infant serum concentrations, or adverse effects. Brivaracetam is a new ASM about which safety data are limited, and there have been no reports of adverse effects in infants. Breastfeeding can be continued with close monitoring of the infant for drowsiness, agitation, and developmental milestones, especially while nursing a preterm infant with exclusive breastfeeding.

Lacosamide has low molecular weight and a low protein-binding capacity [51]. To date, there have been no reports of adverse effects in infants breastfed by the limited number of women taking lacosamide [51]. Thus caution should be exercised during its use by lactating mothers with close monitoring of the breastfed infant.

Perampanel is also associated with limited information during breastfeeding, although there have been no reports of adverse effects in infants such as sedation or feeding difficulties when breastfed by mothers on a combination of perampanel and other ASMs.

Rufinamide is a third-generation ASM; no information is available on the safety of its use during lactation and breastfeeding. Given the complete lack of information on rufinamide, breastfeeding cannot be safely recommended at this time [52].

Additional newer ASMs, including cenobamate, stiripentol, everolimus, and cannabidiol, are associated with no reported data about infant exposure levels or short-term or long-term effects. Thus the decision of whether to breastfeed requires a careful discussion between the patient and the physician.

One of the non-pharmacological treatments of epilepsy is a ketogenic or modified Atkins diet. Data are scarce regarding the safety of ketogenic or modified Atkins diets during pregnancy and breastfeeding. There is one case report of two pregnant WWE on the ketogenic diet without adverse outcomes in their infants. As for breastfeeding, only one woman elected to breastfeed while on the ketogenic diet and no adverse effects in the infant were noted [53]. Therefore, the decision whether to breastfeed should be based on a careful discussion between patients and their physicians. Additional research is needed to fully understand the safety of breastfeeding in WWE treated with a ketogenic or modified Atkins diet.

Breastfeeding and Sleep Recommendations for Women with Epilepsy

New mothers with epilepsy may be at an increased risk of seizures in the first few months postpartum because of sleep deprivation, especially for some types of epilepsy syndromes known to be sleep sensitive. It is important to counsel these patients and their social support systems (partners, family members, or friends) about risk of seizures with sleep deprivation and strategies to minimize it. These strategies may include taking shifts caring for the infant and using a breast pump to store breast milk for nighttime feeding by family or friends to minimize sleep interruption and deprivation [50].

Breastfeeding Counseling and Support for Women with Epilepsy

Breastfeeding counseling by knowledgeable and trained clinicians will likely play an important role in improving breastfeeding practices in WWE, especially when delivered early in the process, preferably in the antepartum period, to prevent missed opportunities for breastfeeding. Women with epilepsy who were counseled by their epileptologists or neurologists were more likely to initiate breastfeeding and to continue it at 6 weeks and 3 months postpartum [3].

New mothers face many challenges in the postpartum period that may hinder breastfeeding practices, especially postpartum psychiatric complications such as anxiety and postpartum depression that are known to shorten the duration of breastfeeding. Women with epilepsy have higher rates of anxiety, depression, and postpartum depression [15], which may render them more vulnerable to failure in initiation or maintenance of breastfeeding. Therefore, identification of these factors will be helpful and allow clinicians to provide additional early psychosocial support.

Consultation with breastfeeding specialists may facilitate breastfeeding initiation and improve breastfeeding duration. Incorporating lactation specialists in postpartum care has been shown to improve rates of breastfeeding initiation and duration in the general population [54]. The WHO practice guidelines incorporate lactation specialists to facilitate counseling and support new mothers as an essential intervention in improving breastfeeding. Women with epilepsy are no exception, as WWE who received lactation consultation were more likely to continue breastfeeding [3] and would most likely benefit from lactation services to support them during this particularly challenging time.

Summary

In conclusion, most commonly used ASMs are compatible with breastfeeding. Thus breastfeeding should be encouraged unless there are clear contraindications. Rates of breastfeeding in WWE remain low, likely due to unique challenges, as well as a variety of patient and clinician factors. Early counseling by knowledgeable physicians plays a key role in helping WWE make informed decisions. With additional support systems, clinicians may help improve the success of breastfeeding for WWE, eventually leading to better long-term health outcomes for WWE and their infants.

References

1. Harden CL, Pennell PB, Koppel BS, et al. Practice parameter update: Management issues for women with epilepsy. Focus on pregnancy (an evidence-based review). Vitamin K, folic acid, blood levels, and breastfeeding. *Neurology*. 2009;**73**(2):142–9.
2. Johnson EL, Burke AE, Wang A, Pennell PB. Unintended pregnancy, prenatal care, newborn outcomes, and breastfeeding in women with epilepsy. *Neurology*. 2018;91(11):1031–9.
3. al-Faraj, AO, Pandey, S, Herlihy, MM, Pang, TD. Factors affecting breastfeeding in women with epilepsy. *Epilepsia*. 2021;**00**:1–9.
4. Hao N, Jiang H, Wu M, et al. Breastfeeding initiation, duration and exclusivity in mothers with epilepsy from south west China. *Epilepsy Res*. 2017;135:168–75.
5. Roberts JI, Metcalfe A, Abdulla F, et al. Neurologists' and neurology residents' knowledge of issues related to pregnancy for women with epilepsy. *Epilepsy Behav*. 2011;**22**:358–63.
6. Vazquez B, Gibson P, Kustra R. Epilepsy and women's health issues: Unmet needs. Survey results from women with epilepsy. *Epilepsy Behav*. 2007;**10**:163–9.
7. Eidelman AI, Schanler RJ. Breastfeeding and the use of human milk. *Pediatrics*. 2012;**129**(3):e827–e841.
8. Meek JY, Feldman-Winter L, Noble L. Optimal duration of breastfeeding. *Pediatrics*. 2020;**146**(5):e2020021063.
9. Victora CG, Bahl R, Barros AJD, et al. Breastfeeding in the 21st century: Epidemiology, mechanisms, and lifelong effect. *Lancet*. 2016;**387**(10017):475–90.
10. Grubesic TH, Durbin KM. A spatial analysis of breastfeeding and breastfeeding support in the United States: The leaders and laggards landscape. *J Hum Lact*. 2019;**35**(4):790–800.
11. Gupta PM, Perrine CG, Chen J, Elam-Evans LD, Flores-Ayala R. Monitoring the World Health Organization global target 2025 for exclusive breastfeeding: Experience from the United States. *Journal of Human Lactation*. 2017;**33**:578–81.
12. Jędrzejczak J, Kopytek-Beuzen M, Gawłowicz J, Stanosz-Sankowska J, Majkowska-Zwolińska B. Knowledge of pregnancy and procreation in women with epilepsy of childbearing age: A 16-year comparative study in Poland. *Epilepsy Res*. 2020;**164**:106372.

13. Meador KJ, Baker GA, Browning N, et al. Effects of breastfeeding in children of women taking antiepileptic drugs. *Neurology*. 2010;**75**(22):1954–60.

14. Figueiredo B, Canário C, Field T. Breastfeeding is negatively affected by prenatal depression and reduces postpartum depression. *Psychol Med*. 2014;**44**(5):927–36.

15. Bjørk M, Veiby G, Engelsen B, Gilhus NE. Depression and anxiety during pregnancy and the postpartum period in women with epilepsy: A review of frequency, risks and recommendations for treatment. *Seizure*. 2015;**28**:33–9.

16. Meador KJ, Baker GA, Browning N, et al. Breastfeeding in children of women taking antiepileptic drugs: Cognitive outcomes at age 6 years. *JAMA Pediatr*. 2014;**168**(8):729–36.

17. Veiby G, Engelsen BA, Gilhus NE. Early child development and exposure to antiepileptic drugs prenatally and through breastfeeding: A prospective cohort study on children of women with epilepsy. *JAMA Neurol*. 2013;**70**(11):1367–74.

18. Pennell PB, Gidal BE, Sabers A, Gordon J, Perucca E. Pharmacology of antiepileptic drugs during pregnancy and lactation. *Epilepsy Behav*. 2007;**11**(3):263–9.

19. Rauchenzauner M, Kiechl-Kohlendorfer U, Rostasy K, Luef G. Old and new antiepileptic drugs during pregnancy and lactation: Report of a case. *Epilepsy Behav*. 2011;**20**(4):719–20.

20. Allegaert K, van den Anker J, Naulaers G, de Hoon J. Determinants of drug metabolism in early neonatal life. *Curr Clin Pharmacol*. 2008;**2**(1):23–9.

21. Anderson PO, Sauberan JB. Modeling drug passage into human milk. *Clinical Pharmacology and Therapeutics*. 2016;**100**:42–52.

22. Ito S, Koren G. A novel index for expressing exposure of the infant to drugs in breast milk. *Br J Clin Pharmacol*. 1994;**38**(2):99–102.

23. Badée J, Qiu N, Collier AC, et al. Characterization of the ontogeny of hepatic UDP-glucuronosyltransferase enzymes based on glucuronidation activity measured in human liver microsomes. *J Clin Pharmacol*. 2019;**59**(S1):S42–55.

24. Pennell PB. Antiepileptic drug pharmacokinetics during pregnancy and lactation. *Neurology*. 2003;**61**(2):35–42.

25. Anderson PO, Manoguerra AS, Valdés V. A review of adverse reactions in infants from medications in breast milk. *Clin Pediatr* (Phila). 2016;**55**(3):236–44.

26. Birnbaum AK, Meador KJ, Karanam A, et al. Antiepileptic drug exposure in infants of breastfeeding mothers with epilepsy. *JAMA Neurol*. 2020;**77**(4):441–50.

27. López-Fraile IP, Cid AO, Juste AO, Modrego PJ. Levetiracetam plasma level monitoring during pregnancy, delivery, and postpartum: Clinical and outcome implications. *Epilepsy Behav*. 2009;**15**(3):372–5.

28. Johannessen SI, Helde G, Brodtkorb E. Levetiracetam concentrations in serum and in breast milk at birth and during lactation. *Epilepsia*. 2005;**46**(5):775–7.

29. Paret N, Gouraud A, Bernard N, et al. Long-term follow-up of infants exposed to levetiracetam during breastfeeding: Comparison to a control group. *Birth Defects Res A Clin Mol Teratol*. 2014; **100**:537–8.

30. Ylikotila P, Ketola RA, Timonen S, et al. Early pregnancy cerebral venous thrombosis and status epilepticus treated with levetiracetam and lacosamide throughout pregnancy. *Reprod Toxicol*. 2015; **57**:204–6.

31. Ohman I, Vitols S, Tomson T. Lamotrigine in pregnancy: Pharmacokinetics during delivery, in the neonate, and during lactation. *Epilepsia*. 2000;**41**(6):709–13.

32. Nordmo E, Aronsen L, Wasland K, Småbrekke L, Vorren S. Severe apnea in an infant exposed to lamotrigine in breast milk. *Ann Pharmacother*. 2009;**43**:1893–7.

33. Yashima K, Obara T, Matsuzaki F, et al. Evaluation of the safety of taking lamotrigine during lactation period. *Breastfeed Med*. 2021;**16**:432–8.

34. Soussan C, Gouraud A, Portolan G, et al. Drug induced adverse reactions via

breastfeeding: A descriptive study in the French pharmacovigilance database. *Eur J Clin Pharmacol.* 2014;**70**(11):1361–6.

35. Btilau P, Paar WD, Von Unruh GE. Pharmacokinetics of oxcarbazepine and l o-hydroxy-carbazepine in the newborn child of an oxcarbazepine-treated mother. *Eur J Clin Pharmacol.* 1988;**34**(3):311–13.
36. Wegner I, Edelbroek P, De Haan GJ, Lindhout D, Sander JW. Drug monitoring of lamotrigine and oxcarbazepine combination during pregnancy. *Epilepsia.* 2010;**51**(12):2500–2.
37. Chen CY, Li X, Ma LY, et al. In utero oxcarbazepine exposure and neonatal abstinence syndrome: Case report and brief review of the literature. *Pharmacotherapy.* 2017;**37**(7):e71–e75.
38. Kacirova I, Grundmann M, Brozmanova H, Koristkova B. Monitoring topiramate concentrations at delivery and during lactation. *Biomed Pharmacother.* 2021;**138**:111446.
39. Westergren T, Hjelmeland K, Kristoffersen B, Johannessen SI, Kalikstad B. Probable topiramate-induced diarrhea in a 2-month-old breast-fed child: A case report. *Epilepsy Behav Case Reports.* 2014;**2**(1):22–3.
40. Kawada K, Itoh S, Kusaka T, Isobe K, Ishii M. Pharmacokinetics of zonisamide in perinatal period. *Brain Dev.* 2002;**24**(2):95–7.
41. Ando H, Matsubara S, Oi A, et al. Two nursing mothers treated with zonisamide: Should breast-feeding be avoided? *J Obstet Gynaecol Res.* 2014;**40**(1):275–8.
42. Ip S, Chung M, Raman G, et al. Breastfeeding and maternal and infant health outcomes in developed countries. *Evid Rep Technol Assess.* 2007;**153**:1–186.
43. Stahl M, Neiderud J, Vinge E. Thrombocytopenic purpura, and anemia in a breast-fed infant whose mother was treated with valproic acid. *J Pediatr* 1997;**130**:1001–3.
44. Govindan K, Mandadi GD. Alopecia in breastfed infant possibly due to mother getting valproate. *Indian J Pediatr.* 2021;**88**(5):519–20.
45. Finch E, Lorber J. Methaemoglobinaemia in the newborn probably due to phenytoin maternal and infant health outcomes in developed countries. *Evid Rep Technol Assess.* 2007;**153**:1–186.
46. Nau H, Rating D. Placental transfer and pharmacokinetics of primidone and its metabolites phenobarbital, PEMA and hydroxy phenobarbital in neonates and infants of epileptic mothers. *Eur J Clin Pharmacol.* 1980;**18**:31–42.
47. Bar-Oz B, Nulman I, Koren G, Ito S. Anticonvulsants and breast feeding: A critical review. *Paediatr Drugs.* 2000;**2**(2):113–26.
48. Fisher JB, Edgren BE, Mammel MC, et al. Neonatal apnea associated with maternal clonazepam therapy: A case report. *Obstet Gynecol.* 1985;**66**(3 Suppl):34S–5S.
49. Meador KJ, Pennell PB, May RC, MONEAD Investigator Group. Fetal loss and malformations in the MONEAD study of pregnant women with epilepsy. *Neurology.* 2020;**94**(14):e1502–e1511.
50. Tomson T, Battino D, Bromley R, et al. Management of epilepsy in pregnancy: A report from the International League Against Epilepsy Task Force on Women and Pregnancy. *Epileptic Disord.* 2019;**21**(6):497–517.
51. Lattanzi S, Cagnetti C, Foschi N, Provinciali L, Silvestrini M. Lacosamide during pregnancy and breastfeeding. *Neurol Neurochir Pol.* 2017;**51**(3):266–9.
52. Drugs and Lactation Database (LactMed) www.ncbi.nlm.nih.gov/books/NBK501922.
53. Van der Louw EJTM, Williams TJ, Henry-Barron BJ, et al. Ketogenic diet therapy for epilepsy during pregnancy: A case series. *Seizure.* 2017;**45**:198–201.
54. Patel S, Patel S. The effectiveness of lactation consultants and lactation counselors on breastfeeding outcomes. *J Hum Lact.* 2015;**32**(3):530–41.

Chapter 18

Management of the Neonate

Clinical Examination and Surveillance

Carlos I. Salazar, Eugene Ng, and Cecil D. Hahn

Key Points

- In deciding whether to begin or continue antiseizure medications (ASMs) in pregnant women with epilepsy (WWE), clinicians must weigh the potential risk of these medications on the health of the fetus in the short and long terms against the complications for both mother and baby due to inadequate seizure control.
- An explanation of these risks and their impact on the newborn will assist mothers in their decision-making process.
- In the immediate postnatal period, management of newborns exposed to ASMs in utero should be focused on facilitation of neonatal adaptation and transition, and monitoring of neurological symptoms.
- The assessment of these newborns should include complete anthropometric measures and a detailed physical examination in search of congenital malformations or signs related to the ASM exposure.
- Longitudinal follow-up of these infants must also include assessment for physical and developmental problems based on current understanding of the potential long-term effects from in utero exposure to ASMs.

Introduction

Epilepsy requiring ongoing medical treatment is the most common neurologic disorder in pregnancy [1]. Data from a number of population-based studies estimate that maternal epilepsy is present in 0.3–1% of all pregnancies [2–7], the vast majority representing women with preexisting epilepsy, and a minority (2–10%) representing women with new-onset epilepsy during pregnancy [8, 9]. The incidence of antiseizure medication (ASM) use is estimated at 0.3–0.4% of all pregnancies, which includes those who are maintained on ASMs for neuropsychiatric disorders such as bipolar and schizoaffective disorders, a practice that has become more common in the past two decades [3–5, 10, 11].

Although most women with epilepsy (WWE) have uncomplicated and uneventful pregnancies and deliver healthy babies, both seizures and in utero exposure to ASMs may have adverse effects on the developing fetus [8, 12, 13]. When caring for a newborn whose mother was maintained on an ASM during pregnancy, a clinician must have a thorough understanding of the potential for these drugs to cause congenital malformations, affect fetal growth and development, affect neonatal adaptation and transition, and, in the long term, affect neurodevelopmental outcomes [14–23]. A variety of adverse effects have been reported with use of ASM monotherapy or polytherapy in pregnant WWE. Table 18.1 summarizes the currently known potential adverse effects of the commonly used ASMs.

Some medications used as monotherapy have been reported to increase the risk for major congenital malformations, especially carbamazepine (CBZ), phenobarbital (PB), phenytoin (PHE), topiramate (TPM), and valproic acid (VPA). However, this increased risk was not observed with lamotrigine (LGT), gabapentin (GBP), levetiracetam (LEV), oxcarbazepine (OXC), and zonisamide (ZNS) [23]. It is likely that individual genetic factors modify these risks for ASM-associated congenital malformations, and these interactions require further study [24].

Although exposing fetuses to potentially teratogenic drugs may generate anxiety and apprehension, the potential developmental effects on the fetus must be weighed against complications related to inadequately controlled epileptic seizures, which may, in turn, compromise fetal well-being. Having seizures of any type during pregnancy increases the risk for preterm delivery, whereas focal seizures are associated with an increased risk for low birth weight [25]. Moreover, seizures during labor may produce fetal hypoxia and acidosis [6]. The objective of this review is to guide clinicians involved in the care of these infants and children, focusing on delivery room stabilization, newborn assessment, and ongoing surveillance during infancy and childhood.

Care of the Newborn in the Delivery Room

It is recommended that pregnant WWE, especially those at risk for peripartum seizures, have their delivery at a birthing unit with facilities for neonatal resuscitation and with a multidisciplinary team available in case of immediate neonatal complications [6]. There is evidence that pregnant WWE have an increased risk for preterm deliveries of around 10% [4, 9, 26]. Although it is difficult to identify the underlying reasons for this, known factors leading to preterm births include preeclampsia, third-trimester vaginal bleeding, a marginal risk of placental complications, and the presence of premature contractions in mothers treated with an ASM. There is also a significant increase in the rate of emergency caesarean sections, premature rupture of membranes, and respiratory distress [12, 27]. Low Apgar scores at 5 minutes of age are also commonly reported in offspring of WWE [3, 25, 27], hence the importance of access to a team with expertise in neonatal resuscitation.

All babies born to WWE taking enzyme-inducing ASMs should be strongly encouraged to receive 1 mg of intramuscular vitamin K prophylactically, as evidence suggests that there may be an increased risk of hemorrhagic disease of the newborn as a result of altered vitamin K metabolism by exposure to hepatic enzyme-inducing ASMs (such as CBZ, VPA, PB, and PHE, among others [28–32].

Neonatal clinicians should be appropriately prepared for the birth of infants of WWE, especially those maintained on ASMs. A prenatal consultation is often helpful so that the pregnancy and medical history can be reviewed and a birth plan devised in the context of potential medical problems that may be encountered in the delivery room and the postnatal period. At the time of delivery, a full neonatal resuscitation team should be available in anticipation of any neonatal complication at birth. For term and preterm deliveries, the neonatal practitioners must be prepared for neonatal depression and respiratory distress.

Table 18.1 Summary of potential adverse effects from in utero exposure to ASM in infants and children

Potential adverse	effects	VPA	CBZ	PHE	PB	TPM	LGT	Prim	LEV	ZNS	Any	No Rx	Poly	Reference
Pregnancy and delivery	Pre-term labor		+								+		+	3, 6, 7, 8, 9
	Pre-eclampsia	+	+								+			3, 7
	Third trimester vaginal bleeding		+				+				+			3
	Placental complications										+			
	Emergency cesarean section										+			3, 6, 7
Newborn	Prematurity		+								+		+	3, 6, 7, 8, 9, 12
	Low 5-minute Apgar score	+		+							+			2, 3, 12, 35, 36
	Respiratory distress										+			12
	Low birth weight	+	+			+	+			+				6, 7, 8, 12, 35, 36
	Hypotonia										+			38
Postnatal	Hemorrhagic disease of newborn (disputed)	+	+	+	+	+		+						26, 27, 28, 29, 30
	Intracranial hemorrhage				+							+		3, 26, 27, 28, 29, 30
	Neonatal seizure										+			3, 12, 62
	Neonatal withdrawal syndrome	+	+	+								+		12, 26, 39, 49
	Neonatal hypoglycemia	+	+											12
	Transient liver toxicity	+					+							14, 15, 50

Table 18.1 (cont.)

Potential adverse	effects	VPA	CBZ	PHE	PB	TPM	LGT	Prim	LEV	ZNS	Any	No Rx	Poly	Reference
Long term	Cognitive impairment	+	+			+ remove								17, 20, 23, 54, 55, 57, 61
	Developmental delay (general)	+	+			+ remove								53, 58, 59, 60
	Behavior disorders	+	+			+ remove			+					21, 60
	Autism Spectrum Disorders	+												61
	Attention Deficit and Hyperactivity Disorder	+												62

VPA, valproic acid; CBZ, carbamazepine; PHE, phenytoin; PB, phenobarbital; TPM, topiramate; LTG, lamotrigine; Prim, primidone; LEV, levetiracetam; ZNS, zonisamide; Any, any anti-seizure medication; No Rx, mothers not on AED during pregnancy; Poly, polytherapy. (+): known effects reported.

Physical Examination of the Newborn

The first step in the physical examination of infants born from WWE is to record anthropometric measures such as weight, length, and head circumference (HC). A recent meta-analysis showed that pregnant WWE have a 1.28-fold increased risk of fetal growth restriction (FGR), and that this risk is even higher when the mother is taking an ASM [12, 26, 33–36]. The FGR may manifest in the newborn as low birth weight below the tenth percentile for gestational age (also defined as small for gestational age [SGA]), but also as symmetric intrauterine growth restriction (IUGR), in which all the anthropometric measures (weight, height, and HC) are below the normal range for gestational age.

The NEAD study was a prospective multicenter study in the United States and United Kingdom that enrolled pregnant women on ASM monotherapy (CBZ, LGT, PHE, or valproate) from 1999 to 2004. The NEAD study reported a higher incidence of SGA and microcephaly (defined as an HC below the third percentile for age) in those exposed prenatally to either CBZ or VPA [37]. Other studies suggest that the use of CBZ, TPM, LTG, or ASM polytherapy may affect fetal development independently, increasing the risk for both IUGR and SGA, even in women taking these medications for neuropsychiatric disorders [26, 38]. Valproic acid is also related to an increase in the risk for craniosynostosis, also contributing to risk for microcephaly [39].

Following the anthropometric measures, the clinician should continue with a full physical examination of the newborn, beginning with inspection, preferably during the awake state to clearly appreciate the newborn's level of alertness. Prenatal exposure to drugs such as PB, VPA, or PHE or to benzodiazepines may produce an increase in apathy or hyperexcitability [40, 41].

The clinician should also assess the newborn's resting posture for hyper- or hypotonia: a normal newborn should have their arms and legs flexed and hips adducted. Muscle tone should be further evaluated by performing vertical and horizontal suspension of the infant, and by assessing the popliteal angle (normal is 90°).

The face should be examined for evidence of facial dysmorphisms such as hypertelorism, a short philtrum, or a cleft lip, and an oral examination for cleft palate must also be included. These malformations have been associated with prenatal exposure to VPA, PB, PHE, TPM, primidone, and ethosuximide [34, 42].

The spine should be examined for signs of neural tube defects, from the more evident ones like myelomeningocele to the more subtle like spina bifida occulta. These anomalies have been strongly associated with VPA exposure [42].

A cardiac examination, including auscultation for cardiac murmurs, is important given the elevated risk of congenital heart disease associated with exposure to VPA, PB, GBP, CBZ, PHE, LTG, and PHE [42, 43].

The skin should be examined for signs of petechiae, especially on the face and upper thorax, which may indicate hemorrhagic disease of the newborn (due to exposure to enzyme-inducing ASMs), as well as other signs of bleeding such as the presence of blood in either the nasogastric tube or the endotracheal tube, or blood in the umbilical stump [32].

In males, inspection of the genitalia and abdominal palpation are important when looking for hypospadias, which is associated with fetal exposure to VPA, GBP, CZP, and prim [43].

Finally, examination of the fingers is important to assess for hypoplasia of fingers and toenails associated with fetal exposure to PHE [44].

In summary, the initial assessment of newborns of WWE must include a complete and detailed physical examination, with particular focus on the common congenital malformations associated with ASM use (Table 18.2). Clinicians must also include anthropometric assessment to identify those that are SGA and those with microcephaly, both of which may have long-term growth and developmental implications. Efforts should be made to diagnose and confirm abnormal physical findings so that appropriate management, including relevant referrals to subspecialists, can be made in a timely fashion.

Table 18.2 Summary of possible physical examination findings in newborns exposed to ASMs

Physical examination	Possible Findings	Related ASM exposure
Weight, length	• Intrauterine growth restriction (IUGR) • Low birth weight	VPA, CBZ, LTG, TPM, ASM polytherapy
Head circumference	• Microcephaly • Craniosynostosis	VPA
Level of alertness	• Apathy • Hyperexcitability • Withdrawal syndrome: drowsiness, irritability, a high-pitched cry, tremors, excitability, hyper or hypotonia, hyperreflexia, apnea, poor feeding, vomiting, diarrhea, seizures	PB, VPA, PHE, benzodiazepines
Muscle tone	• Hypertonia • Hypotonia	VPA, OXC, CBZ, LTG, LEV, TPM, CLB, CZP, GBP
Face	• Facial dysmorphisms: hypertelorism, short philtrum • Cleft lip • Cleft palate	VPA, PB, PHE, TPM
Spine	• Neural tube defects: myelomeningocele, spina bifida occulta	VPA
Cardiac examination	• Cardiac murmurs (congenital heart disease)	VPA, PB, GBP, CBZ, PHE, LTG, PHE
Skin	• Petechiae (especially on the face and upper thorax)	Enzyme-inducing ASM
Genitalia (in males)	• Hypospadias	VPA, GBP, Prim, CZP
Fingers	• Hypoplasia of fingers and toenails	PHE

phenobarbital; CLB, clobazam; CBZ, carbamazepine; OXC, oxcarbazepine; TPM, topiramate; LTG, lamotrigine; LEV, levetiracetam; CZP, clonazepam; GBP, gabapentin; Prim, primidone; ASM, anti-seizure medications

Postnatal Management and Predischarge Assessment

During the initial birth hospitalization, the care of newborns of WWE should primarily be focused on transition and adaptation. Because of the potential challenges in these areas, early hospital discharge (≤24 hours) is generally not recommended. Since the majority of ASMs are considered safe or moderately safe during breastfeeding, early breastfeeding should be encouraged given the physical and emotional benefits for both the mother and infant, particularly the nutritional benefits for those already born SGA [45]. Moreover, adverse effects have not been reported [15]. Some ASMs such as GBP have been associated with decrease in milk production [15].

Clinicians must also be aware of the potential neurologic effects of ASM exposure on the newborns in the immediate postnatal period. Drug withdrawal has been described in relation to maternal use of VPA, CBZ, OXC, PHE, and GBP, alone or in combination with other ASMs during pregnancy [15, 28, 41, 44, 46, 47]. Symptoms have been reported to occur 12–72 hours after birth, and the severity may be dose dependent. Withdrawal symptoms include drowsiness, irritability, a high-pitched cry, tremors, excitability, hyper- or hypotonia, hyperreflexia, apnea, poor feeding, vomiting, diarrhea, and even seizures in severe cases [44, 46, 48], symptoms that are not dissimilar to that of abstinence from narcotics. These symptoms should be monitored when there is known history of the mother taking the previously mentioned ASMs in mono- or polytherapy. There is a case report of a newborn with a withdrawal syndrome and hypomagnesemia secondary to in utero exposure to valproate and CBZ [41]. Two cases of withdrawal syndrome were reported after in utero exposure to OXC, one of them having also hyponatremia [49, 50].

Treatment of withdrawal syndrome is initially non-pharmacological (room lighting, swaddling, positioning, breastfeeding, parental rooming in, skin-to-skin contact, etc.) and in more severe cases, pharmacological treatment includes opioids as first-line (morphine, methadone, or buprenorphine) or non-opioid adjunct therapy (clonidine or PB) [48, 51]. Clinicians must take into account that neonates born to WWE are at risk for prolonged NICU stays due to preterm birth, lower Apgar scores, respiratory problems, or feeding difficulties [12].

There is an increased risk of asymptomatic neonatal hypoglycemia not related to prematurity, growth restriction, or hyperinsulinemia in those exposed to VPA and CBZ in utero [46]. Postulated mechanisms include impaired ketogenesis and decreased liver glycogen synthesis. There have also been reports of transient liver toxicity, manifested by cholestasis and transaminitis, associated with maternal use of CBZ and LGT [15, 52]. Interestingly, hepatic enzyme-inducing ASMs such as PB may reduce the risk of neonatal unconjugated hyperbilirubinemia [27].

Therefore, during the immediate postnatal period, workup should include a complete blood count, serum glucose, liver function tests, coagulation testing, and electrolytes. In addition, neuroimaging such as head ultrasound may be considered given the risk of intracranial hemorrhage in neonates born to WWE, particularly in those with inadequate seizure control during pregnancy, and also in infants at risk for hemorrhagic disease of the newborn [32, 53, 54].

In summary, infants born to WWE on ASMs during pregnancy may face a number of challenges in the immediate postnatal period. Anticipating the potential problems with feeding and reduced breast milk supply, the mother–infant dyad should be provided with ample breastfeeding support even beyond the birth hospitalization. To adequately observe the newborns for neurologic symptoms such as drug withdrawal or seizures, consideration should be given to hospitalization for a minimum of 48 hours after birth.

Long-Term Follow-Up

Although the developing brain is particularly vulnerable to injury in utero during the processes of neuronal migration and organization, brain maturation extends well beyond the neonatal period, encompassing the refinement of synaptic connections and cerebral lateralization, which are crucial for healthy neurocognitive development. Hence the importance of long-term neurodevelopmental follow-up for children born to WWE [55, 56, 16]. In addition, clinical signs and symptoms due to fetal exposure to ASMs may arise during the ensuing months or years of life. Long-term follow-up assessment should consider the following domains.

Growth and Development

Prospective cohort studies have shown that infants born SGA or with IUGR or microcephaly due to in utero exposure to ASMs may have a persistence of low anthropometric measures by the age of 12 months. Fortunately, these measures tend to normalize by age 36 months in most infants, including the head circumference [37]. An older, population-based cohort study in Norway showed a persistence of low anthropometric measures and even a low body mass index until age 20 years in offspring of WWE; however, those patients were exposed to first-generation ASMs only as they were born between 1967 and 1979 with less information about safety profiles at that time [57].

Physical Examination

Physical abnormalities may appear after 6 months of age – for example, dental anomalies like tooth hypoplasia, delayed eruption, malocclusion, and supernumerary teeth. One study reported dental anomalies in 48% of children born to WWE, with a rate of 54% among children exposed to ASMs in utero, and especially in those exposed to VPA [58].

Neurodevelopment

One of the most important considerations for long-term follow-up assessments are the potential effects of ASMs on neurodevelopment. Cognitive outcomes appear to be reduced in children with in utero exposure to ASM polytherapy compared to monotherapy [18]. Follow-up studies from the NEAD study cohort have reported the impact of ASM exposure on neurodevelopment. At age 3 years, verbal performance was lower in children exposed to VPA and CBZ. At age 6 years, children exposed to any ASM showed reduced right-handedness and reduced verbal abilities, suggesting that ASMs could affect the cerebral lateralization process. Prenatal exposure to CBZ, OXC, and clonazepam have been associated with an increased risk of intellectual disability [61].

Exposure to VPA has been associated with worse cognitive functioning, worse verbal and nonverbal outcomes, reduced IQ (7–10 points lower than other ASMs), reduced memory function, and intellectual disability with delayed milestones [16, 20, 23, 59, 60]. Exposure to VPA is also associated with a fivefold increased risk of neurodevelopmental disorders overall at mean age 3.6 years [62], according to a nationwide population-based study in France that included 1,721,990 children, 8,848 of whom were exposed in utero to ASM monotherapy.

Moreover, recent studies have reported an elevated risk for autism spectrum disorders (ASDs) with fetal exposure to VPA [17]. The most important was a population-based study in Denmark with a cohort of 655,615 children showing an ASD risk of 4.15% and a risk of 2.95% for childhood autism (before the new classification by the DSM-V in which both diagnoses were merged into ASD) [63]. Another study from the same Danish national registry showed that in utero exposure to VPA was associated with an increased risk for attention deficit hyperactivity disorder (ADHD) [64]. Furthermore, behavioral problems, particularly attention and social problems, occurred in 32% of those with prenatal exposure to VPA, but also in 14% of those exposed to CBZ, 16% of those exposed LTG, and 14% of those exposed to LEV [21].

On the other hand, recent evidence has shown that periconceptional folate exposure is associated with better verbal outcomes and better cognitive development at 3 and 6 years of age respectively, supporting the practice of folic acid supplementation during pregnancy as a preventive measure to avoid the risk of neurodevelopmental issues in the offspring of WWE [16, 65].

Risk for Seizures

A population-based study in Australia showed that among a cohort of 1,958 pregnancies of WWE, 2.4% of the offspring experienced seizures during their first year of life, 38% of which were febrile seizures. Seizure risk was 3.5% higher in children born to mothers with generalized epilepsy compared to those with focal epilepsy, and even higher (4.83%) in offspring of those who experienced generalized seizures during the course of the pregnancy [66], placing importance on seizure monitoring during the first year of life.

In summary, systematic follow-up for children exposed prenatally to ASMs is necessary for several reasons: to monitor the growth and development of those born with low birth weight or IUGR; to screen for physical findings that may arise beyond the neonatal period; to monitor for early signs of developmental impairment, including the presence of developmental disorders such as ASD or ADHD; and for opportune neuropsychological assessment and further treatment regarding potential learning disabilities at school age.

Conclusion

There are a multitude of clinically relevant effects of maternal epilepsy and, more specifically, maternal treatment with ASMs on their offspring. A large number of congenital malformations are associated with these potential teratogens. Specific care and surveillance of these infants should begin from the time of birth and continue through the neonatal transition and long into childhood, paying particular attention to issues of growth and cognitive and behavioral development.

References

1. Pennell PB. Pregnancy in women who have epilepsy. *Neurologic Clinics.* 2004;**22**:799–820.
2. Olafsson E, Hallgrimsson JT, Hauser WA, Ludvigsson P, Gudmundsson G. Pregnancies of women with epilepsy: A

population-based study in Iceland. *Epilepsia*. 1998;**39**(8):887–92.

3. Veiby G, Daltveit AK, Engelsen BA, Gilhus NE. Pregnancy, delivery, and outcome for the child in maternal epilepsy. *Epilepsia*. 2009;**50**(9):2130–9.
4. Borthen I, Eide MG, Veiby G, Daltveit AK, Gilhus NE. Complications during pregnancy in women with epilepsy: Population-based cohort study. *BJOG*. 2009;**116**(13):1736–42.
5. Brosh K, Matok I, Sheine E, et al. Teratogenic determinants of first-trimester exposure to antiepileptic medications. *J Popul Ther Clin Pharmacol*. 2011;**18**(1):89–98.
6. Royal College of Obstetricians & Gynaecologists. *Epilepsy in pregnancy: Green-top guideline no. 68*. London: Royal College of Obstetricians & Gynaecologists; 2016. www.rcog.org.uk/globalassets/documents/guidelines/green-top-guidelines/gtg68_epilepsy.pdf.
7. Bansal R, Jain G, Kharbanda PS, Goyal MK, Suri V. Maternal and neonatal complications during pregnancy in women with epilepsy. *Int J Epilepsy*. 2016;**3**(2):80–5.
8. Li W, Hao N, Xiao Y, Zhou D. Clinical characteristics and pregnancy outcomes of new onset epilepsy during pregnancy. *Medicine* (Baltimore). 2019;**98**(27):1–5.
9. Johnson EL, Burke AE, Wang A, Pennell PB. Unintended pregnancy, prenatal care, newborn outcomes, and breastfeeding in women with epilepsy. *Neurology*. 2018;**91**(11):e1031–9.
10. Pennell PB. Use of antiepileptic drugs during pregnancy: Evolving concepts. *Neurotherapeutics*. 2016;**13**(4):811–20. http://dx.doi.org/10.1007/s13311-016-0464-0.
11. Giménez A, Pacchiarotti I, Gil J, et al. Adverse outcomes during pregnancy and major congenital malformations in infants of patients with bipolar and schizoaffective disorders treated with antiepileptic drugs: A systematic review. *Psychiatr Pol*. 2019;**53**(2):223–44.
12. Razaz N, Tomson T, Wikström AK, Cnattingius S. Association between pregnancy and perinatal outcomes among women with epilepsy. *JAMA Neurol*. 2017;**74**(8):983–91.
13. Meador KJ, Pennell PB, May RC, et al. Fetal loss and malformations in the MONEAD study of pregnant women with epilepsy. *Neurology*. 2020;**94**(14):E1502–11.
14. Tomson T, Battino D, Bonizzoni E, et al. Dose-dependent risk of malformations with antiepileptic drugs: An analysis of data from the EURAP epilepsy and pregnancy registry. *Lancet Neurol*. 2011;**10**(7):609–17. http://dx.doi.org/10.1016/S1474-4422(11)70107-7.
15. Iqbal, MM, Gundlapalli SP, Ryan WG, Ryals T, Passman TE. Effects of antimanic mood-stabilizing drugs on fetuses, neonates, and nursing infants. *South Med J*. 2001;**94**(3):304–22.
16. Meador KJ, Baker GA, Browning N, et al. Foetal antiepileptic drug exposure and verbal versus non-verbal abilities at three years of age. *Brain*. 2011;**134**(2):396–404.
17. Bromley R, Weston J, Adab N, et al. Treatment for epilepsy in pregnancy: Neurodevelopmental outcomes in the child. *Cochrane Database Syst Rev*. 2014;**2014**(10):CD010236.
18. Meador KJ, Loring DW. Developmental effects of antiepileptic drugs and the need for improved regulations. *Neurology*. 2016;**86**(3):297–306.
19. Veroniki AA, Rios P, Cogo E, et al. Comparative safety of antiepileptic drugs for neurological development in children exposed during pregnancy and breast feeding: A systematic review and network meta-analysis. *BMJ Open*. 2017;7(7):1–11.
20. Cohen MJ, Meador KJ, May R, et al. Fetal antiepileptic drug exposure and learning and memory functioning at 6 years of age: The NEAD prospective observational study. *Epilepsy Behav*. 2019;**92**:154–64. https://doi.org/10.1016/j.yebeh.2018.12.031.

21. Huber-Mollema Y, Oort FJ, Lindhout D, Rodenburg R. Behavioral problems in children of mothers with epilepsy prenatally exposed to valproate, carbamazepine, lamotrigine, or levetiracetam monotherapy. *Epilepsia.* 2019;**60**(6):1069–82.
22. Videman M, Stjerna S, Wikström V, et al. Prenatal exposure to antiepileptic drugs and early processing of emotionally relevant sounds. *Epilepsy Behav.* 2019;**100**:106503. https://doi.org/10.1016/j.yebeh.2019.106503.
23. Huber-Mollema Y, Van Iterson L, Oort FJ, Lindhout D, Rodenburg R. Neurocognition after prenatal levetiracetam, lamotrigine, carbamazepine or valproate exposure. *J Neurol.* 2020;**267**(6):1724–36. https://doi.org/10.1007/s00415-020-09764-w.
24. Voinescu PE, Pennell PB. Management of epilepsy during pregnancy. *Expert Review of Neurotherapeutics.* 2015;**15**:1171–87.
25. Huang C-Y, Dai Y-M, Feng L-M, Gao W-L. Clinical characteristics and outcomes in pregnant women with epilepsy. *Epilepsy Behav.* 2020;**112**:107433. https://doi.org/10.1016/j.yebeh.2020.107433.
26. Hernández-Díaz S, McElrath TF, Pennell PB, et al. Fetal growth and premature delivery in pregnant women on antiepileptic drugs. *Ann Neurol.* 2017;**82**(3):457–65.
27. Pilo C, Wide K, Winbladh B. Pregnancy, delivery, and neonatal complications after treatment with antiepileptic drugs. *Acta Obstet Gynecol Scand.* 2006;**85**(6):643–6.
28. Burja S, Rakovec-Felser Z, Treiber M, Hajdinjak D, Gajšek-Marchetti M. The frequency of neonatal morbidity after exposure to antiepileptic drugs in utero: A retrospective population-based study. *Wiener Klin Wochenschrift.* Suppl. 2006;**118**(2):12–16.
29. Kazmin A, Wong RC, Sermer M, Koren G. Antiepileptic drugs in pregnancy and hemorrhagic disease of the newborn: An update. *Canadian Family Physician.* 2010;**56**:1291–2.
30. Kaaja E, Kaaja R, Matila R, Hiilesmaa V. Enzyme-inducing antiepileptic drugs in pregnancy and the risk of bleeding in the neonate. *Neurology.* 2002;**58**(4):549–53.
31. Harden CL, Meador KJ, Pennell PB, et al. Practice parameter update: Management issues for women with epilepsy. Focus on pregnancy (an evidence-based review). Teratogenesis and perinatal outcomes. Report of the Quality Standards Subcommittee and Therapeutics and Technology Assessment Subcommittee. *Neurology.* 2009;**73**(2):133–41. www.neurology.org/content/73/2/142.abstract.
32. Barroso FVL, Araujo E, Guazelli CAF, et al. Perinatal outcomes from the use of antiepileptic drugs during pregnancy: A case-control study. *J Matern Neonatal Med.* 2015;**28**(12):1445–50.
33. Chen D, Hou L, Duan X, et al. Effect of epilepsy in pregnancy on fetal growth restriction: A systematic review and meta-analysis. *Arch Gynecol Obstet.* 2017;**296**(3):421–7.
34. Galappatthy P, Liyanage CK, Lucas MN, et al. Obstetric outcomes and effects on babies born to women treated for epilepsy during pregnancy in a resource limited setting: A comparative cohort study. *BMC Pregnancy Childbirth.* 2018;**18**(1):1–11.
35. Fonager K, Larsen H, Pedersen L, Sørensen HT. Birth outcomes in women exposed to anticonvulsant drugs. *Acta Neurol Scand.* 2000;**101**(5):289–94.
36. Holmes LB, Harvey EA, Brown KS, Hayes AM, Khoshbin S. Anticonvulsant teratogenesis: I. A study design for newborn infants. *Teratology.* 1994;**49**(3):202–7.
37. Pennell PB, Klein AM, Browning N, et al. Differential effects of antiepileptic drugs on neonatal outcomes. *Epilepsy Behav.* 2012;**24**(4):449–56. http://dx.doi.org/10.1016/j.yebeh.2012.05.010.
38. Bansal R, Jain G, Kharbanda PS, Goyal MK, Suri V. Maternal and neonatal complications during pregnancy in women with epilepsy. *Indian J Rheumatol.*

2016;**3**(2):80–5. http://dx.doi.org/10.1016/j.ijep.2016.09.001.

39. Centers for Disease Control and Prevention, Division of Birth Defects and Developmental Disabilities. *Facts about microcephaly.* Atlanta, GA: Centers for Disease Control and Prevention;2016.
40. Videman M, Tokariev A, Stjerna S, et al. Effects of prenatal antiepileptic drug exposure on newborn brain activity. *Epilepsia.* 2016;**57**(2):252–62.
41. Satar M, Ortaköylü K, Batun İ, et al. Withdrawal syndrome and hypomagnesaemia in a newborn exposed to valproic acid and carbamazepine during pregnancy. *Turk Pediatr Ars.* 2016;**51**(2):114–16.
42. Hernández-Díaz S, Smith CR, Shen A, et al. Comparative safety of antiepileptic drugs during pregnancy. *Neurology.* 2012;**78**(21):1692–9.
43. Veroniki AA, Cogo E, Rios P, et al. Comparative safety of anti-epileptic drugs during pregnancy: A systematic review and network meta-analysis of congenital malformations and prenatal outcomes. *BMC Med.* 2017;**15**(1):1–20.
44. Souza SWD, Robertson IG, Donnai D, Mawer G. Fetal phenytoin exposure, hypoplastic nails, and jitteriness. *Arch Dis Child.* 1990;**65**:320–4.
45. Veiby G, Bjørk M, Engelsen BA, Gilhus NE. Epilepsy and recommendations for breastfeeding. *Seizure.* 2015;**28**:57–65. http://dx.doi.org/10.1016/j.seizure.2015.02.013
46. Ebbesen F, Holsteen V, Rix M, et al. Neonatal hypoglycaemia and withdrawal symptoms after exposure in utero to valproate. *Arch Dis Child Fetal Neonatal Ed.* 2000;**83**(2):124–9.
47. Carrasco M, Rao SC, Bearer CF, Mbbs SS. Pediatric neurology neonatal gabapentin withdrawal syndrome. *Pediatr Neurol.* 2015;**53**(5):445–7. http://dx.doi.org/10.1016/j.pediatrneurol.2015.06.023.
48. Kanemura A, Masamoto H, Kinjo T, Mekaru K. Evaluation of neonatal withdrawal syndrome in neonates delivered by women taking psychotropic or anticonvulsant drugs: A retrospective chart review of the effects of multiple medication. *Eur J Obstet Gynecol.* 2020;**254**:226–30. https://doi.org/10.1016/j.ejogrb.2020.09.008.
49. Chen CY, Li X, Ma LY, et al. In utero oxcarbazepine exposure and neonatal abstinence syndrome: Case report and brief review of the literature. *Pharmacotherapy.* 2017;**37**(7):e71–5.
50. Rolnitsky A, Merlob P, Klinger G. Pediatric neurology in utero oxcarbazepine and a withdrawal syndrome, anomalies, and hyponatremia. *Pediatr Neurol.* 2013;**48**(6):466–8. http://dx.doi.org/10.1016/j.pediatrneurol.2013.02.012
51. Mangat AK, Schmölzer GM, Kraft WK. Pharmacological and non-pharmacological treatments for the neonatal abstinence syndrome (NAS). *Semin Fetal Neonatal Med.* 2019;**24**(2):133–41. https://doi.org/10.1016/j.siny.2019.01.009.
52. Dubnov-Raz G, Shapiro R, Merlob P. Maternal lamotrigine treatment and elevated neonatal gamma-glutamyl transpeptidase. *Pediatr Neurol.* 2006;**35**(3):220–2.
53. Minkoff H, Schaffer RM, Delke I , Grunebaum AN. Diagnosis of intracranial hemorrhage in utero after a maternal seizure. *Obs Gynecol.* 1985;**65**:22S–24S.
54. Sherer DM, Anyaegbunam A, Onyeije C. Antepartum fetal intracranial hemorrhage, predisposing factors and prenatal sonography: A review. *American Journal of Perinatology.* 1998;**15**:431–41.
55. Veiby G, Daltveit AK, Schjølberg S, et al. Exposure to antiepileptic drugs in utero and child development: A prospective population-based study. *Epilepsia.* 2013;**54**(8):1462–72.
56. Vinten J, Adab N, Kini U, et al. Neuropsychological effects of exposure to anticonvulsant medication in utero. *Neurology.* 2005;**64**(6):949–54.
57. Øyen N, Vollset SE, Eide MG, Bjerkedal T, Skjærven R. Maternal epilepsy and

offsprings' adult intelligence: A population-based study from Norway. *Epilepsia.* 2007;**48**(9):1731–8.

58. Güveli BT, Rosti RÖ, Güzeltaş A, et al. Teratogenicity of antiepileptic drugs. *Clin Psychopharmacol Neurosci.* 2017;**15**(1):19–27.
59. Meador KJ, Baker GA, Browning N, et al. Fetal antiepileptic drug exposure and cognitive outcomes at age 6 years (NEAD study): A prospective observational study. *Lancet Neurol.* 2013;**12**(3):244–52.
60. Banach R, Boskovic R, Einarson T, Koren G. Long-term developmental outcome of children of women with epilepsy, unexposed or exposed prenatally to antiepileptic drugs: A meta-analysis of cohort studies. *Drug Saf.* 2010;**33**(1):73–9.
61. Daugaard CA, Pedersen L, Sun Y, Dreier JW, Christensen J. Association of prenatal exposure to valproate and other antiepileptic drugs with intellectual disability and delayed childhood milestones. *JAMA Netw Open.* 2020;**3**(11):e2025570.
62. Coste J, Blotiere PO, Miranda S, et al. Risk of early neurodevelopmental disorders associated with in utero exposure to valproate and other antiepileptic drugs: A nationwide cohort study in France. *Sci Rep.* 2020;**10**(1):1–11. https://doi.org/10.1038/s41598-020-74409-x
63. Christensen J, Grønborg TK, Sørensen MJ, et al. Prenatal valproate exposure and risk of autism spectrum disorders and childhood autism. *JAMA.* 2013;**309**(16):1696–1703.
64. Christensen J, Pedersen L, Sun Y, et al. Association of prenatal exposure to valproate and other antiepileptic drugs with risk for attention-deficit/hyperactivity disorder in offspring. *JAMA Netw Open.* 2019;**2**(1):e186606.
65. Meador KJ, Pennell PB, May RC, Brown CA, Baker G. Effects of periconceptional folate on cognition in children of women with epilepsy. *Neurology.* 2020;**94** (7):729–40.
66. Vajda FJE, O'Brien TJ, Graham JE, et al. Seizures in infancy in the offspring of women with epilepsy. *Acta Neurol Scand.* 2020;**141**(1):33–7.

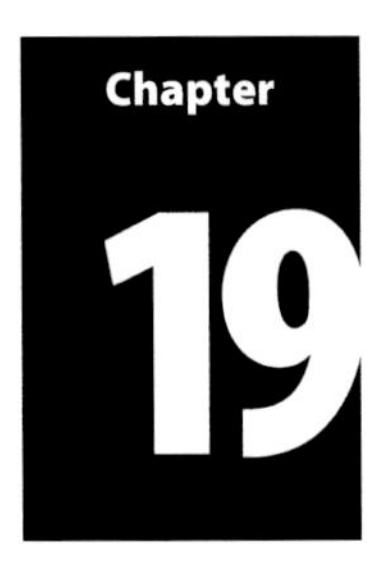

Aging, Menopause, and Bone Health in Women with Epilepsy

Alison M. Pack and Stephanie Shatzman

Key Points

- Limited prospective information is available on the course of epilepsy as women with epilepsy (WWE) progress through the menopausal transition.
- Epilepsy may be associated with early-onset perimenopause and menopause.
- A catamenial seizure pattern may be associated with increased seizures at perimenopause but decreased seizures during and post menopause.
- Perimenopausal WWE likely need monitoring of levels of antiseizure medications (ASMs) to maintain robust therapeutic levels.
- Postmenopausal women, especially those treated with enzyme-inducing ASMs (carbamazepine, phenobarbital, phenytoin), are at increased risk for low bone mineral density (BMD) and fracture.
- Routine screening of 25 hydroxyvitamin D should be considered as routine epilepsy care.
- Vitamin D supplementation may be needed to maintain 25 hydroxyvitamin D levels ≥ 30 ng/mL in women ≥ 50, or in persons at high risk of osteopenia and osteoporosis. Persons taking enzyme-inducing ASMs may need higher doses (≥1,000–4,000IU/day); doses as high as 5,000IU have been found to be safe and well tolerated.

Introduction

Menopause is a time of transition for women. It occurs when the ovarian follicles are depleted, therefore women who bear children tend to have later menopause due to the ovulation-sparing months of pregnancy. This transition occurs gradually over several years and is a normal aging process. It marks the end of the reproductive years and usually occurs during the late 40s or early 50s. The median age at menopause is 51 years and is influenced by various factors including but not limited to genetic and environmental factors such as family history and socioeconomic status, tobacco use, parity, and oral contraception use [1, 2].

Hormonal Changes in Menopause

Ovarian follicles secrete estrogen and progesterone to promote ovulation and endometrial proliferation. Hormonally, as menopause approaches, estrogen levels remain unchanged, may rise steadily, or can surge erratically in response to elevated follicle-stimulating hormone (FSH) levels. The cyclic progesterone elevation, which normally occurs during the luteal phase of the menstrual cycle, gradually becomes less frequent throughout perimenopause, causing increased occurrence of anovulatory cycles [3, 4]. Estrogen and progesterone stabilize at low levels with complete ovarian failure at menopause. When a woman has not had menses for 12 months, she is considered postmenopausal [1].

What makes perimenopause and menopause interesting from an epilepsy standpoint is that estrogen and progesterone and their metabolites are neurosteroid molecules that modulate brain excitability and can influence seizure occurrence. Estrogen and progesterone have opposing effects on neuronal excitability [5, 6], which has been demonstrated in experimental models of epilepsy [5]. Estrogen is thought to primarily exert neuroexcitatory effects by modulating gene expression. Like other steroid hormones, estrogen enters passively into neurons, where it binds to and activates the estrogen receptor, a dimeric nuclear protein that binds to DNA and controls gene expression.

After estrogen binding, the receptor complex forms a transcription factor that binds to hormone receptor elements on genes to modify cellular responses. An example is the estradiol-induced increased density of agonist-binding sites on the N-methyl D-aspartate (NMDA) receptor complex in hippocampal cells [7]. In 2016, Younus and Reddy found that ethinyl estradiol, the primary component of many oral contraceptive pills, significantly hastened epileptogenesis in female mice using the hippocampus kindling model [8]. Estrogen's neuroexcitatory effect, however, is not without complexity; estrogen dose, route of administration, acute versus chronic administration, natural hormonal milieu, and estrogenic species affects estrogen's effect on neuroexcitability, which is predominantly thought to be proconvulsant [9, 10].

Progesterone, in contrast, promotes neuroinhibitory effects primarily through the action of its reduced metabolite, allopregnanolone, a positive allosteric modulator of gamma-amino-butyric acid (GABA) conductance [5, 11]. The neuroinhibitory effect of allopregnanolone is complicated by feedback mechanisms within the receptor. The GABA-A receptor subunit components undergo compensatory alterations in response to changes in the endogenous hormonal neurosteroid milieu and to pharmacological agents that modulate GABA-A receptors, such as benzodiazepines [12, 13]. See Chapter 4 for a more detailed discussion on hormonal influences in women with epilepsy (WWE).

Despite the significant relationship between sex hormones and neuroexcitability, there continues to be a paucity of data or information about the influence of menopause on epilepsy and vice versa. The studies discussed in this chapter are notable for their predominantly retrospective or cross-section designs, often with limited sample sizes and with confounding factors related to variability in subjects.

Early Menopause for Women with Epilepsy

Epilepsy is ultimately an endocrine disruptor, causing hypothalamic-pituitary-gonadal axis dysfunction, which in turn provides opportunities for dysregulation of the maturation of ovarian follicles and loss of mature follicles. This mechanism of follicle wasting is one way in which WWE are thought to be at higher risk for early onset of the menopausal transition. Klein and colleagues provided the first report of early perimenopausal symptoms and premature menopause in WWE, in which 14% of 50 WWE in an epilepsy clinic population had premature ovarian failure (POF) compared with 3.7% of healthy control women (p 0.04) [14].

Consistent with the concept that a portion of WWE has specific reproductive hormone sensitivity, women with POF were more likely to have had catamenial exacerbation of their seizures during earlier reproductive years. The risk for earlier menopause appears to be related to seizure frequency, with increased seizure frequency perhaps indicating a stronger "dose" of endocrine disruption. Harden and colleagues reported a negative correlation between the age at menopause and seizure frequency (p 0.014) [15]. For example, WWE with only rare seizures had a normal age at menopause of 50–51 years, while WWE with frequent seizures experienced earlier menopause at 46–47 years. In this study, no relationship was found between early menopause and specific antiseizure medications (ASMs).

Seizures at Menopause and Perimenopause

What happens at menopause, then, when the cyclic hormonal fluctuations of the reproductive years cease? Unlike puberty and young adulthood, menopause and perimenopause do not appear to be a time of increased epilepsy onset, as the incidence of epilepsy is stable across young and middle-aged adult age groups but increases at age 60 and older, long after menopause has been established in most women [16]. While no prospective information is available on the course of epilepsy as WWE progress through the menopausal transition, retrospective and cross-sectional studies suggest WWE may encounter changes in their seizure disorder with perimenopause and menopause.

A cross-sectional evaluation using mailed questionnaires queried WWE to recall the course of their epilepsy from their reproductive years through perimenopause and menopause [17]. Two-thirds of these perimenopausal WWE reported an increase in seizures during perimenopause. Remarkably, history of a catamenial seizure pattern was significantly associated with an increase in seizures at perimenopause. These findings are consistent with postulated mechanisms for women with hormonally sensitive seizures; the elevated estrogen-to-progesterone ratio may contribute to the increase in seizure frequency at perimenopause. A high percentage of women in the perimenopausal group took synthetic hormone replacement therapy (HRT), and HRT was significantly associated with an increase in seizures ($p < 0.001$) [17].

While a history of a catamenial seizure pattern – defined as cyclic seizure exacerbation in the perimenstrual, periovulatory, or anovulatory phases of the menstrual cycle – was associated with an increase in seizures at perimenopause, it is contrastingly associated with a decrease in frequency during menopause and post menopause, possibly due to the less-epileptogenic estrogen form, estrone, which predominates during menopause and overall lower levels of estrogen post menopause [18, 19].

Hormone Replacement and Epilepsy

The implications for management of symptoms related to perimenopause and menopause necessitate a need for understanding of patients in terms of their history of catamenial seizure patterns, ongoing reproductive state, and whether vasomotor symptoms are interfering with sleep, since this may be an important factor for seizure increase [13]. Management should include increased vigilance for seizure occurrence at perimenopause and a cautious, but lower threshold for relieving vasomotor symptoms that interfere with sleep. Seizure freedom is always a goal of treatment, and for WWE, this may prolong the period of reproductive years to a normal duration.

Harden and colleagues explored whether HRT itself could alter seizure frequency in WWE, due to a possible neurosteroid effect. In a 2002 randomized, double-blind, placebo-controlled trial of Prempro (0.625 mg of conjugated equine estrogens plus 2.5 mg of medroxyprogesterone acetate (CEE/MPA) daily, or double-dose CEE/MPA daily for 3 months), Harden and colleagues found seizure frequency significantly increased with the use of CEE/MPA in a dose-related manner [20]. This is a clinical example of an adverse exogenous neurosteroid effect on seizures in menopausal WWE, although the trial did notably study a small sample size with short duration of treatment (3 months), and results were limited to a single hormone regimen. Regardless, the finding implies that the low and stable hormonal milieu for menopausal WWE is physiologically vulnerable to neuroexcitatory influence.

In 2007, the Women's Health Initiative data on HRT were published, which called for limited use of HRT in only very low-risk-category individuals, as risks of coronary artery disease, stroke, and other morbidity was felt to be higher than the benefit of therapy for most women. Given these findings and the concern for increase in seizures with HRT, alternative therapy is recommended for WWE.

If treatment is needed, a simplified regimen of estradiol only (without the multiple estrogenic compounds in CEE), plus natural progesterone may be a reasonable alternative, especially considering the antiseizure potential of natural progesterone [21]. Topical estrogen for vaginal atrophy could also be considered [22, 23]. Hot flashes may be treated with selective serotonin reuptake inhibitors (SSRIs), serotonin and norepinephrine reuptake inhibitors (SNRIs), and gabapentin. To treat sleep disturbance, sleep hygiene, cognitive behavioral therapy, and gabapentin can be used [24]. Finally, an additional consideration for WWE treated with HRT includes estrogen's interaction with enzyme-inducing ASMs, which may require clinicians to check levels more frequently and make dose adjustments, especially for women on lamotrigine [25].

Bone Health in Perimenopausal Women with Epilepsy

Poor bone health, including low bone mineral density (BMD) and fractures, is increasingly common and contributes to significant comorbidities and healthcare expenditures. Recognized risk factors include menopause, as well as other factors such as glucocorticoid exposure and family history (see Table 19.1). Postmenopausal women are at increased risk

Table 19.1 Factors associated with low bone mineral density

- Ethnicity (Caucasian or Asian)
- Family history of osteoporosis
- Small frame
- Menopause
- Poor nutrition
- Smoking history
- Alcohol use
- Eating disorder history
- Mental retardation
- Cerebral palsy
- Hyperthyroidism
- Hyperparathyroidism
- Liver disease
- Medication use: antiepileptic drugs; glucocorticosteroids; heparin

for comorbidities related to poor bone health because of the effects of ASM exposure superimposed on estrogen-deficient bone loss.

While BMD is an important surrogate for bone health, further investigations are needed to more fully elucidate how hormones and the nervous system, especially in specific biologic states such as menopause, alter this process. Basic physiology and the current breadth of current literature, albeit limited, of hormonal influence on bone is discussed further later in this chapter.

Bone Physiology

Bones are vital to our metabolic homeostasis and functioning, and increasing and maintaining BMD is the result of both bone resorption and formation. The cells responsible for resorption are called osteoclasts, whereas those responsible for formation are called osteoblasts. Any disruption or uncoupling of these processes may result in high or low bone turnover. Peak BMD is obtained between the second and third decade of life, with young women having an average mass of 2,400 g. Women after age 30 typically steadily lose BMD until menopause. In adulthood, the uncoupling results in accelerated bone loss. During the early menopausal years, even more significant bone loss occurs. High turnover bone loss also occurs in the early postmenopausal years. Low turnover bone loss occurs in advanced age.

Bone integrity and homeostasis are highly regulated processes. Bones are repositories for important minerals, including calcium, and play an integral role in the regulation of these minerals. The ionized fraction of calcium is tightly maintained, such that as the concentration of this fraction changes, parathyroid hormone (PTH) levels change in response. For example, if the ionized fraction is low, PTH rises. Parathyroid hormone acts to restore the ionized calcium concentration by increasing distal renal tubule reabsorption and facilitating bone resorption [26].

Vitamin D also plays a critical role in calcium homeostasis and has direct effects on bone, such as promoting differentiation of osteoclasts. Vitamin D metabolism occurs through a series of oxidative pathways involving multiple hepatic and renal cytochrome p450 isoenzymes [27]. In the liver, vitamin D is hydroxylated to 25 hydroxy vitamin D (25OHD), the major circulating form of vitamin D. 25OHD is the most commonly used index of vitamin D status and is further hydroxylated to 24, 25 dihydroxy vitamin D (24, 25(OH)2D) and 1,25(OH)2D in the kidney. 24, 25(OH)2D has little effect on bone whereas 1,25(OH)2D is responsible for most biological effects of vitamin D [26].

Increasing evidence supports nervous system control of bone remodeling [28, 29], mediated both centrally and peripherally by neurotransmitters and neuropeptides. Prolactin, norepinephrine, leptin, serotonin, and inflammatory cytokines have all been documented to influence bone resorption and/or formation [29–38]. Similarly, reproductive hormones directly and indirectly impact bone. Estrogen reduces bone resorption by inhibiting both the formation and the function of osteoclasts [39]. Estrogen receptors have been identified on both osteoclasts and osteoblasts, suggesting direct effects on these bone cells [40].

Mechanisms of Osteoporosis

Researchers have proposed multiple mechanisms to explain why ASMs are associated with low BMD. The principal mechanism relates to induction of the hepatic cytochrome P450 enzyme system. Cytochrome P450 enzyme-inducing ASMs are most consistently associated with abnormalities in bone. Treatment with liver cytochrome P450-inducing ASMs increases activity of hepatic mixed-function oxidases, resulting in accelerated vitamin D metabolism and subsequent less biologically active or inert vitamin D. Reduced active vitamin D leads to decreased intestinal calcium absorption, decreased serum ionized calcium concentration, and increased serum PTH concentration. If hyperparathyroidism persists, bone turnover increases and BMD ultimately decreases.

Basic studies evaluating the effect of enzyme-inducing ASMs on the expression of cytochrome P450 isoenzymes involved in vitamin D metabolism support these clinical observations. Phenobarbital, phenytoin, and carbamazepine are xenobiotics that activate a nuclear receptor known as either the steroid and xenobiotic receptor (SXR) or pregnane X receptor (PXR) [41]. One study found that xenobiotics upregulate 25 hydroxyvitamin D3 -24-hydroxylase (CYP24) in the kidney through activation of PXR. This enzyme catalyzes the conversion of 25(OH)D to its inactive metabolite, 24 (25 OH)2D, rather than to its active metabolite, 1,25(OH)2D [42].

Other investigators found that xenobiotic activation of PXR did not upregulate CYP24 but did increase expression of a different isoenzyme, CYP3A4, in the liver and small intestine [43]. This enzyme converts vitamin D to inactive metabolites. Although valproate is typically considered a cytochrome P450 enzyme-inhibiting ASM, in vitro studies find that valproate induces the cytochrome P450 isoenzyme CYP3A4 at clinically relevant concentrations, as well as CYP24, leading to disturbances in vitamin D and calcium homeostasis [44, 45].

Although some studies support this hypothesis, not all observations are consistent. Carbamazepine, a known inducer of cytochrome P450 enzymes, is not always associated with decreased BMD [46–48]. Although in vitro studies suggest that valproate may also be an inducer of the cytochrome P450 isoenzymes CYP3A4 and CYP24, low active vitamin D metabolites are not consistently described in association with valproate use (see Figure 19.1) [47, 49]. In addition, significant osteopenia and other convincing evidence of increased bone turnover has been found in a series of persons treated with ASMs, even though 25(OH)D and PTH levels were normal [50]. Other mechanisms have been proposed and investigated, including impaired calcium absorption, impaired response to PTH, vitamin K reduction, hyperparathyroidism, calcitonin deficiency, elevated homocysteine, reduced reproductive hormones, genetic predisposition, and a direct effect of epilepsy and seizures on bone [51].

Fracture

Postmenopausal WWE receiving ASMs are likely at greater risk for adverse effects on bone than the general population, as the effects of ASMs are superimposed upon estrogen-deficient bone loss. Children and adults with epilepsy treated with ASMs are described as having a twofold to sixfold increased risk of fracture [51, 52]. Multiple factors, including increased risk of falling, as well as reduced BMD, likely contribute to this increased fracture risk. A meta-analysis by Vestergaard and colleagues demonstrated that while BMD was reduced among persons with epilepsy taking ASMs, the reduction in BMD alone was not enough to explain the elevated fracture risk [89].

A significantly reduced BMD at the femoral neck has been described in postmenopausal women on ASMs as compared to drug-naive controls [53]. One study on Caucasian women

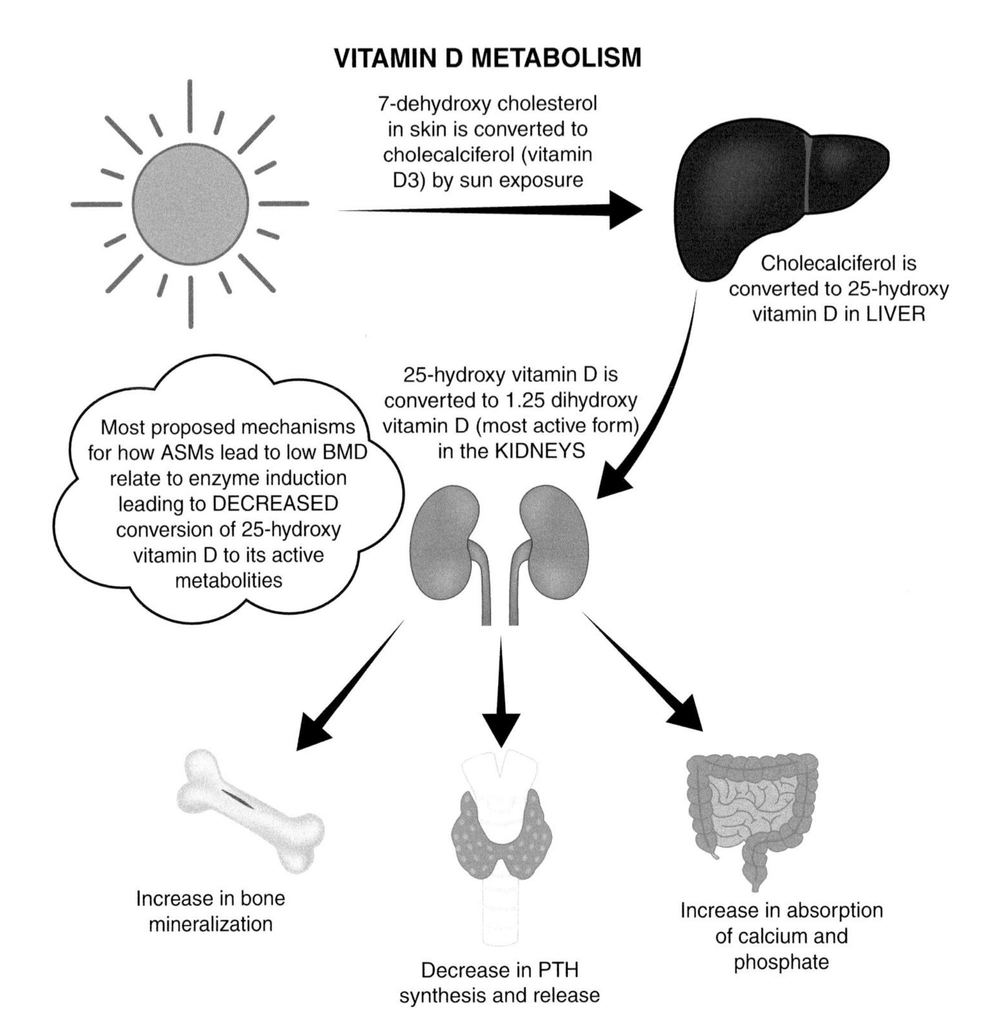

Figure 19.1 Vitamin D metabolism

older than 65 years receiving ASMs found an especially high risk of hip fracture [54]. The Study of Osteoporotic Fractures [55] was a population-based study that measured serial BMD determinations at both the hip and calcaneus, together with many clinical risk factors for low BMD, in more than 6,000 postmenopausal women. After adjustment of multiple confounders, including health status, walking for exercise, smoking status, and estrogen status, the average rate of decline in total hip BMD steadily increased from −0.70%/year in non-ASM users to −0.87%/year in partial ASM users, to −1.16%/year in continuous ASM users (p value for trend 1/4 0.015) [55].

Exposure to ASMs potentially independently increases fracture risk. Using the General Practice Research Database (GPRD) from the United Kingdom and a nested case-control study design, long-term ASM use was associated with an increased fracture risk, particularly in women [52]. Similarly, a case-control study using data from the Funen County, Denmark, hip fracture register found that ASM use increased fracture risk [56].

Independent predictors of fracture included the use of cytochrome P450 enzyme-inducing ASMs as well as higher daily doses of current and recent ASMs. Results from a pharmacoepidemiologic, population-based case-control study, also in Denmark, suggests that ASMs differentially affect fracture risk [57]. Carbamazepine, clonazepam, phenobarbital, and valproate were all associated with an increased fracture risk after adjusting for significant confounders such as a diagnosis of epilepsy. A dose relationship was found for these specific ASMs.

Persons with epilepsy are also more likely to fall because of seizures, as well as the direct effects of ASMs. Increased risk of falling contributes to fracture risk. In a population-based study of older women, those prescribed ASMs had an increased risk for frequent falls (multivariate odds ratio 2.56, 95% confidence interval [CI] 1.49–4.41) [58]. This increased risk of falls may be explained in part by balance impairment secondary to ASM exposure. In a study of 29 ambulatory community-dwelling twin and sibling pairs, balance performance was found to be impaired in the ASM users compared to the siblings not taking ASMs [59].

Seizures themselves may result in fractures. In a large case-control study of 3,478 patients with epilepsy [60], seizure severity was associated with fracture. The type of seizure may influence the fracture risk. Generalized tonic-clonic seizures are associated with a higher fracture risk than focal seizures [61]. Population-based studies, however, find that trauma related to seizures is not associated with fractures [62]. Although seizures likely do contribute to the risk of fracture, studies evaluating the direct effects do not reveal consistent findings.

Screening

While there are published guidelines for bone health screening of at-risk individuals and women older than 50 years of age from the American Association of Clinical Endocrinology and American College of Endocrinology, there are no standardized guidelines for vitamin D screening in WWE. Teagarden and colleagues studied 596 patients with epilepsy and found 45% of subjects had low vitamin D levels of less than 20 ng/mL (54% of subjects from the enzyme-inducing group and 37% from the non-enzyme-inducing group) [63]. Given rates of vitamin D deficiency are significantly higher in patients with epilepsy as compared to the general US population, the authors suggest routine screening of vitamin D for all patients with epilepsy [63].

The most sensitive predictor of fracture, however, is BMD. Therefore, it is reasonable to also consider obtaining BMD measurements using DEXA scans in persons at risk every 2 years [10, 64], though standardized guidelines establishing appropriate times to begin such screening have yet to be established. Both Erel and colleagues and Elliot and colleagues, who reviewed current literature on menopause, bone health, and epilepsy, suggest DEXA scans for persons with childhood exposure to ASMs and 5 years of exposure to adult ASMs (especially enzyme-inducing ASMs), and for women over the age of 50, regardless of the length of use [20, 65].

The World Health Organization additionally developed a fracture risk assessment tool, FRAX®, to calculate a 10-year fracture probability [90]. This tool combines BMD with clinical risk factors known to increase the risk of low BMD to determine this risk. A family history of osteoporosis and fracture and an individual history of glucocorticoid steroid use, rheumatoid arthritis, and tobacco or chronic alcohol use are among the factors this tool addresses. In practice, these risk factors should be addressed in addition to the potential impact of epilepsy and ASMs. Routine screening of 25 hydroxyvitamin D and calcium, particularly in persons treated with enzyme-inducing ASMs, should be considered once or twice per year [10].

Treatment

Based on the American Association of Clinical Endocrinology and American College of Endocrinology clinical practice guidelines, 25 hydroxyvitamin D levels ≥ 30 should be maintained with vitamin D supplements, at least 600IU. For persons on ASMs, or those with osteopenia or osteoporosis, 1,000–2,000IU of Vitamin D is more frequently needed to maintain adequate levels. Even higher maintenance doses may be needed for older individuals or persons with obesity or malabsorption. In 2006, Mikati and colleagues found from two randomized control trials in 72 adults and 78 children that high-dose vitamin D supplementation (4,000IU), but not low-dose (400IU) supplementation in adults, led to an increase in BMD in patients with epilepsy on ASM therapy [66].

In 2018, DeGiorgio and colleagues further determined high-dose vitamin D supplementation (5,000IU) was safe and well tolerated by individuals with drug-resistant epilepsy who were followed for a 12-week treatment period. All subjects with vitamin D insufficiency had vitamin D levels that normalized within the 12-week treatment time without exceeding toxic levels [67]. For women ≥ 50 years of age, adequate calcium intake is also recommended, which may require supplementation to achieve a total intake of 1,200 mg/day [10, 64]. Counseling women to limit alcohol and tobacco use is recommended, as is encouraging activity with weight-bearing and strength-building exercises.

For persons with osteopenia/osteoporosis, pharmacologic therapy may be indicated. Grade A evidences support the use of bisphosphonates and denosumab, a monoclonal antibody, in persons at high risk of fracture, including those with osteopenia and a history of fragility fracture, and those with osteoporosis. Parathyroid hormone, teriparatide, may also be considered in persons who are unable to tolerate oral therapy. Raloxifene, a selective estrogen receptor modulator (SERM), is another alternative therapy with grade A evidence and spine-specific efficacy. Like other estrogens, it has been shown to have neuroprotective effects but may also have anticonvulsant properties, as demonstrated by Pottoo and colleagues, who found in a mouse model significantly reduced mean seizure severity ranks mimicking epilepsy in postmenopausal women treated with raloxifene [68]. Finally, for persons on high-risk ASMs such as phenytoin, phenobarbital, and carbamazepine, switching to an alternative ASM should be considered [10].

Specific Antiepileptic Drugs

Carbamazepine: Carbamazepine treatment increases fracture risk and may reduce BMD [57, 67]. In a Danish pharmacoepidemiologic study, the adjusted risk of fracture among carbamazepine users was elevated (OR 1.18, 1.10–1.26) [57]. Two pediatric studies reveal differing results regarding the impact of carbamazepine treatment on BMD. In a cross-sectional study, 13 otherwise healthy children with epilepsy treated with carbamazepine did not have significantly reduced BMD at either the radius or lumbar spine when compared to controls [46], whereas BMD at the lumbar spine in another cross-sectional study was significantly lower in subjects on carbamazepine when compared to controls [70].

Adult studies also reveal conflicting results. Bone mineral density was significantly reduced at the right calcaneus in 10 adults [71] who were followed longitudinally for 6 months. In contrast, 21 outpatients treated with carbamazepine did have reduced BMD [72]. Carbamazepine is associated with increased risk of fracture, but there are conflicting reports in both pediatric and adult studies regarding the effect of carbamazepine on BMD.

Gabapentin: Gabapentin use resulted in increased fracture in a Canadian population-based study [69]. Several studies have evaluated BMD among adults taking multiple ASMs, including gabapentin [73–75], finding that gabapentin may cause bone loss.

Lamotrigine: No studies support an effect of lamotrigine on fracture risk, whereas there are studies evaluating BMD among lamotrigine users. The data regarding lamotrigine's effects on BMD are mixed. Lamotrigine treatment in children and for more than 2 years was associated with shorter stature and lower BMD [76]. Physical inactivity, however, was the major predictor of lowered BMD. Another study among children found no difference in BMD between controls and those with epilepsy treated with lamotrigine [58]. Similarly, premenopausal women treated with lamotrigine did not have significant reductions in BMD at baseline [47] or after 1 year of follow-up [27].

Levetiracetam: Results from an animal study found that levetiracetam therapy may affect bone quality [77]. Rats treated with low-dose levetiracetam also had reduced bone strength and bone formation, but no changes in bone mass. While Koo and Nam found that among drug-naive subjects (mean age 31.0 ±13.1 years), there were no reductions in BMD after approximately 1 year of levetiracetam treatment, Haggar and colleagues found that, for 24 subjects on levetiracetam monotherapy and polytherapy with valproic acid, there was reduction in BMD in both groups at 6 months [78].

Oxcarbazepine: Oxcarbazepine has been found to increase fracture risk and may decrease BMD. In a Danish fracture study [57], oxcarbazepine was associated with a significantly elevated risk of fracture (OR 1.14, 1.03–1.26). Bone mineral density was significantly lower among 14 healthy children with idiopathic epilepsy treated with oxcarbazepine for at least a year when compared to healthy controls [79, 80, 81]. In another study of 34 newly diagnosed subjects treated with oxcarbazepine for 18 months, BMD was decreased by 8% at the lumbar spine and femoral neck [80]. A Turkish study of 28 subjects did not, however, find any differences in oxcarbazepine-treated subjects in BMD when compared to controls [81]. These studies suggest that oxcarbazepine may be associated with a limited increase in fracture. Ultimately, findings are not consistent regarding effects of oxcarbazepine on BMD.

Phenobarbital: Phenobarbital is associated with increased fracture risk and reduced BMD. A Danish pharmacoepidemiological, population-based, case-control study found an adjusted increased fracture risk (OR 1.79, 1.64–1.95) [57] among those taking phenobarbital. A Canadian population-based, retrospective, matched cohort study of adults older than age 50 also reported increased fracture risk in association with phenobarbital use. Reduced BMD was seen among 130 evaluated consecutive subjects in a tertiary care epilepsy center treated with phenobarbital [82]. These studies support the theory that phenobarbital use results in poor bone health.

Phenytoin: Phenytoin use results in increased fracture risk and reduced BMD. In a Canadian population-based study of older persons [69], phenytoin was associated with the highest risk of fracture among the studied ASMs (1.91 [95% CI, 1.58–2.30]). Cross-sectional and longitudinal studies have found reduced BMD at multiple sites. A cohort of more than 6,000 postmenopausal women who were continuous users of phenytoin had an adjusted 1.8-fold greater mean rate of loss at the calcaneus compared to non-ASM users and an adjusted 1.7-fold greater mean loss at the total hip compared with non-ASM users [57].

Phenytoin is consistently associated with adverse effects on bone, including increased fracture risk and low BMD.

Topiramate: In a population-based study of ASMs in the elderly that included a total of more than 2,000 subjects with a median age of 71 years, topiramate was not associated with increased fracture risk (OR = 0.47) [83]. In a study investigating the effects of topiramate on BMD, 36 women on long-term (at least 1 year) topiramate monotherapy were compared with women taking carbamazepine, valproate, and age- and sex-matched controls [84]. This study found no significant reductions in BMD among topiramate-treated women.

Valproate: Findings regarding the effects of valproate on fracture risk and BMD are contradictory. One study found a limited increased risk of fracture in association with valproate therapy [57], whereas another study did not find an increased risk [69]. Cross-sectional studies in adults and children treated with valproate find decreased BMD in some studies but not in others. One prospective study of 14 premenopausal women treated with valproate monotherapy demonstrated no bone loss after 1 year of treatment [27]. These studies reveal mixed findings regarding the association between valproate and an effect on bone.

Zonisamide: There are no studies evaluating the association between zonisamide and fracture risk. In terms of bone metabolism, one study of 59 patients with new-onset, drug-naive epilepsy who were started on zonisamide monotherapy revealed no significant changes in BMD or markers of bone metabolism after 13 months of treatment [85]. In rats, however, administration of zonisamide significantly decreased BMD at the tibial metaphysis and the diaphysis [86].

Overall Aging and Epilepsy

For WWE, menopause certainly represents a unique biological state with its own health implications and uncertainties. As is the case for menopause, the topics surrounding aging with a focus on WWE and on subjects such as cognition, sexuality, quality of life, independence, and many others, remain inadequately studied. As previously described, elderly WWE are at particularly high risk for fracture, which is enhanced by increased fall risk from ASM side effects, and, often, polypharmacy in this population. The etiology of cognitive impairment in the elderly with epilepsy is similarly poorly understood, as neurodegenerative disease can lead to new-onset epilepsy and patients with chronic epilepsy are vulnerable to accelerated aging from chronic brain disease, long-term ASM use – which also affects nutrition and metabolism – and lifestyle limitations to social and physical activity [24, 87]. Limitations to driving and comorbid mental health disease uniquely affect quality of life in this age group as well [24, 87]. Topics in aging in WWE certainly offer much to explore.

References

1. Nelson HD. Menopause. *Lancet.* 2008;**371**(9614):760–70. https://doi.org/10.1016/S0140-6736(08)60346-3.

2. McNeil MA, Merriam SB. Menopause. *Annals of Internal Medicine.* 2021;**174**(7):97–112. https://doi.org/10.7326/AITC202107200.

3. Prior JC. The endocrinology of perimenopause need for a paradigm shift. *Frontiers in Bioscience.* 2011;**S3**(2):474–86. https://doi.org/10.2741/s166.

4. Burger HG. Hormonal changes in the menopause transition. *Recent Progress in Hormone Research.* 2002;**57**(1):257–75. https://doi.org/10.1210/rp.57.1.257.

5. Reddy DS, Gould J, Gangisetty O. A mouse kindling model of perimenstrual catamenial

epilepsy. *Journal of Pharmacology and Experimental Therapeutics*. 2012;**341**(3): 784–93. https://doi.org/10.1124/jpet.112.192377.

6. Majewska MD, et al. Steroid hormone metabolites are barbiturate-like modulators of the GABA receptor. *Science*. 1986;**232**(4753):1004–7. https://doi.org/10.1126/science.2422758.
7. Pack AM, Reddy DS, et al. Neuroendocrinological aspects of epilepsy: Important issues and trends in future research. *Epilepsy & Behavior*. 2011;**22**(1):94–102. https://doi.org/10.1016/j.yebeh.2011.02.009.
8. Younus I, Reddy DS. Seizure facilitating activity of the oral contraceptive ethinyl estradiol. *Epilepsy Research*. 2016;**121**:29–32. https://doi.org/10.1016/j.eplepsyres.2016.01.007.
9. Velíšková J. Estrogens and epilepsy: Why are we so excited? *Neuroscientist*. 2007;**13**(1):77–88. https://doi.org/10.1177/1073858406295827.
10. Sazgar M. Treatment of women with epilepsy. *Continuum*. 2019;**25**(2):408–30.
11. Frye CA. Effects and mechanisms of progestogens and androgens in ictal activity: Progestogens, androgens, and epilepsy. *Epilepsia*. 2010;**51**:135–40. https://doi.org/10.1111/j.1528-1167.2010.02628.x.
12. Smith SS, et al. Neurosteroid regulation of GABAA receptors: Focus on the A4 and δ subunits. *Pharmacology & Therapeutics*. 2008;**116**(1):58–76. https://doi.org/10.1016/j.pharmthera.2007.03.008.
13. Gulinello M, et al. Short-term exposure to a neuroactive steroid increases A4 GABAA receptor subunit levels in association with increased anxiety in the female rat. *Brain Research*. 2001;**910**(1–2):55–66. https://doi.org/10.1016/S0006-8993(01)02565-3.
14. Klein P, et al. Premature ovarian failure in women with epilepsy. *Epilepsia*. 2001;**42**(12):1584–89. https://doi.org/10.1046/j.1528-1157.2001.13701 r.x.
15. Harden CL, et al. Seizure frequency is associated with age at menopause in women with epilepsy. *Neurology*. 2003;**61**(4):451–5. https://doi.org/10.1212/01.WNL.0000081228.48016.44.
16. Kotsopoulos IAW, et al. Systematic review and meta-analysis of incidence studies of epilepsy and unprovoked seizures. *Epilepsia*. 2002;**43**(11):1402–9. https://doi.org/10.1046/j.1528-1157.2002.t01-1-26901.x.
17. Harden CL, Pulver MC, et al. The effect of menopause and perimenopause on the course of epilepsy. *Epilepsia*. 1999;**40**(10):1402–7. https://doi.org/10.1111/j.1528-1157.1999.tb02012.x.
18. Koppel BS, Harden CL. Gender issues in the neurobiology of epilepsy: A clinical perspective. *Neurobiology of Disease*. 2014;**72**:193–7. https://doi.org/10.1016/j.nbd.2014.08.033.
19. Roste LS, et al. Does menopause affect the epilepsy? *Seizure*. 2008;**17**(2):172–5. https://doi.org/10.1016/j.seizure.2007.11.019.
20. Harden CL, et al. Hormone replacement therapy in women with epilepsy: A randomized, double-blind, placebo-controlled study. *Epilepsia*. 2008;**47**(9):1447–51. https://doi.org/10.1111/j.1528-1167.2006.00507.x.
21. Erel T, Guralp O. Epilepsy and menopause. *Archives of Gynecology and Obstetrics*. 2011;**284**(3):749–55. https://doi.org/10.1007/s00404-011-1936-4.
22. Sveinsson O, Tomson T. Epilepsy and menopause: Potential implications for pharmacotherapy. *Drugs & Aging*. 2014;**31**(9):671–5. https://doi.org/10.1007/s40266-014-0201-5.
23. Cardozo L. Meta-analysis of estrogen therapy in the management of urogenital atrophy in postmenopausal women: Second report of the Hormones and Urogenital Therapy Committee*1. *Obstetrics & Gynecology*. 1998;**92**(4):722–7. https://doi.org/10.1016/S0029-7844(98)00175-6.
24. O'Neal MA, editor. *Neurology and psychiatry of women: A guide to gender-based issues in evaluation, diagnosis, and treatment*. 1st ed. Cham: Springer International; 2019. https://doi.org/10.1007/978-3-030-04245-5.

25. Adis Medical Writers. Be aware of the potential effects of menopause on epilepsy and its treatment. *Drugs & Therapy Perspectives*. 2015;**31**(5):161–3. https://doi.org/10.1007/s40267-015-0192-2.

26. Verrotti A, Coppola G, Parisi P, et al. Bone and calcium metabolism and antiepileptic drugs. *Clinical Neurology and Neurosurgery*. 2010;**112**(1):1–10. https://doi.org/10.1016/j.clineuro.2009.10.011.

27. Pack AM, et al. Bone health in young women with epilepsy after one year of antiepileptic drug monotherapy. *Neurology*. 2008;**70**(18):1586–93. https://doi.org/10.1212/01.wnl.0000310981.44676.de.

28. Karsenty G. The central regulation of bone mass: Genetic evidence and molecular bases. In *Bone regulators and osteoporosis therapy*. Vol. **262**. Stern PH, ed. Cham: Springer International; 2020, pp. 309–23. https://doi.org/10.1007/164_2020_378.

29. Qin W, et al. Evolving concepts in neurogenic osteoporosis. *Current Osteoporosis Reports*. 2010;**8**(4):212–18. https://doi.org/10.1007/s11914-010-0029-9.

30. Nicks KM, et al. Reproductive hormones and bone. *Current Osteoporosis Reports*. 2010;**8**(2):60–7. https://doi.org/10.1007/s11914-010-0014-3.

31. Wongdee K, et al. Prolactin alters the MRNA expression of osteoblast-derived osteoclastogenic factors in osteoblast-like UMR106 cells. *Molecular and Cellular Biochemistry*. 2011;**349**(1–2):195–204. https://doi.org/10.1007/s11010-010-0674-4.

32. Elefteriou F. Regulation of bone remodeling by the central and peripheral nervous system. *Archives of Biochemistry and Biophysics*. 2008;**473**(2):231–6. https://doi.org/10.1016/j.abb.2008.03.016.

33. Karsenty G. The central regulation of bone mass: Genetic evidence and molecular bases. In *Bone regulators and osteoporosis therapy*. Vol. **262**. Stern PH, ed. Cham: Springer International; 2020, pp. 309–23. https://doi.org/10.1007/164_2020_378.

34. Ducy P, Amling M, Takeda S, et al. Leptin inhibits bone formation through a hypothalamic relay: A central control of bone mass. *Cell* 100(2):197–207.

35. Elefteriou F, et al. Serum leptin level is a regulator of bone mass. *Proceedings of the National Academy of Sciences*. 2004;**101**(9):3258–63. https://doi.org/10.1073/pnas.0308744101.

36. Yadav VK, Ryu, JH, et al. Lrp5 controls bone formation by inhibiting serotonin synthesis in the duodenum. *Cell*. 2008;**135**(5):825–37. https://doi.org/10.1016/j.cell.2008.09.059.

37. Yadav VK, Oury F, et al. A serotonin-dependent mechanism explains the leptin regulation of bone mass, appetite, and energy expenditure. *Cell*. 2009;**138**(5):976–89. https://doi.org/10.1016/j.cell.2009.06.051.

38. Zhao B, Ivashkiv LB. Negative regulation of osteoclastogenesis and bone resorption by cytokines and transcriptional repressors. *Arthritis Research & Therapy*. 2011;**13**(4):234. https://doi.org/10.1186/ar3379.

39. Reid IR. Menopause. In *Primer on the metabolic bone diseases and disorders of mineral metabolism*. Rosen CJ, ed. Hoboken, NJ: Wiley; 2013, pp. 165–70. https://doi.org/10.1002/9781118453926.ch21.

40. Ross FP. Osteoclast biology and bone resorption. In *Primer on the metabolic bone diseases and disorders of mineral metabolism*. Rosen CJ, ed. Hoboken, NJ: Wiley, 2013, pp. 25–33. https://doi.org/10.1002/9781118453926.ch3.

41. Pack AM. Treatment of epilepsy to optimize bone health. *Current Treatment Options in Neurology*. 2011;**13**(4):346–54. https://doi.org/10.1007/s11940-011-0133-x.

42. Pascussi JM, et al. Possible involvement of pregnane X receptor–enhanced CYP24 expression in drug-induced osteomalacia. *Journal of Clinical Investigation*. 2005;**115**(1):177–86. https://doi.org/10.1172/JCI21867.

43. Zhou C. Steroid and xenobiotic receptor and vitamin D receptor crosstalk mediates CYP24 expression and drug-induced osteomalacia. *Journal of Clinical Investigation*. 2006;**116**(6):1703–12. https://doi.org/10.1172/JCI27793.

44. Cerveny L, et al. Valproic acid induces CYP3A4 and MDR1 gene expression by

activation of constitutive androstane receptor and pregnane X receptor pathways. *Drug Metabolism and Disposition*. 2007;**35**(7):1032–41. https://doi.org/10.1124/dmd.106.014456.

45. Vrzal R, et al. Valproic acid augments vitamin D receptor-mediated induction of CYP24 by vitamin D3: A possible cause of valproic acid–induced osteomalacia? *Toxicology Letters*. 2011;**200**(3):146–53. https://doi.org/10.1016/j.toxlet.2010.11.008.
46. Sheth RD, et al. Effect of carbamazepine and valproate on bone mineral density. *Journal of Pediatrics*. 1995;**127**(2):7.
47. Pack AM, Morrell MJ, et al. Bone mass and turnover in women with epilepsy on antiepileptic drug monotherapy: Bone metabolism and turnover. *Annals of Neurology*. 2005;**57**(2):252–7. https://doi.org/10.1002/ana.20378.
48. Kafali G, et al. Effect of antiepileptic drugs on bone mineral density in children between ages 6 and 2 years. *Clinical Pediatrics*. 1999;**38**(2):93–8. https://doi.org/10.1177/000992289903800205.
49. Verrotti A, Agostinelli S, et al. A 12-month longitudinal study of calcium metabolism and bone turnover during valproate monotherapy: Increased bone turnover with valproate therapy. *European Journal of Neurology*. 2010;**17**(2):232–7. https://doi.org/10.1111/j.1468-1331.2009.02773.x.
50. Verrotti A, Greco R, Latini G, et al. Increased bone turnover in prepubertal, pubertal, and postpubertal patients receiving carbamazepine. *Epilepsia*. 2002;**43**(12):1488–92. https://doi.org/10.1046/j.1528-1157.2002.13002.x.
51. Pack AM, Walczak TS. Bone health in women with epilepsy. *International Review of Neurobiology*. 2008;**83**:305–28. https://doi.org/10.1016/S0074-7742(08)00018-4.
52. Souverein PC, et al. Incidence of fractures among epilepsy patients: A population-based retrospective cohort study in the General Practice Research Database. *Epilepsia*. 2005;**46**(2):304–10. https://doi.org/10.1111/j.0013-9580.2005.23804.x.
53. Stephen LJ, et al. Bone density and antiepileptic drugs: A case-controlled study. *Seizure*. 1999;**8**(6):339–42. https://doi.org/10.1053/seiz.1999.0301.
54. Cummings SR, et al. Risk factors for hip fracture in white women. *New England Journal of Medicine*. 1995;**332**(12):767–73. https://doi.org/10.1056/NEJM199503233321202.
55. Ensrud KE, et al. Antiepileptic drug use increases rates of bone loss in older women: A prospective study. *Neurology*. 2004;**62**(11):2051–7. https://doi.org/10.1212/01.WNL.0000125185.74276.D2.
56. Tsiropoulos I, et al. Exposure to antiepileptic drugs and the risk of hip fracture: A case-control study. *Epilepsia*. 2008;**49**(12):2092–9. https://doi.org/10.1111/j.1528-1167.2008.01640.x.
57. Vestergaard P, et al. Fracture risk associated with use of antiepileptic drugs. *Epilepsia*. 2004;**45**(11):1330–7. https://doi.org/10.1111/j.0013-9580.2004.18804.x.
58. Ensrud KE, et al. Central nervous system: Active medications and risk for falls in older women. *Journal of the American Geriatrics Society*. 2002;**50**(10):1629–37. https://doi.org/10.1046/j.1532-5415.2002.50453.x.
59. Petty SJ, et al. Balance impairment in chronic antiepileptic drug users: A twin and sibling study. *Epilepsia*. 2010;**51**(2):280–8. https://doi.org/10.1111/j.1528-1167.2009.02254.x.
60. Souverein PC, et al. Use of antiepileptic drugs and risk of fractures: Case-control study among patients with epilepsy. *Neurology*. 2006;**66**(9):1318–24. https://doi.org/10.1212/01.wnl.0000210503.89488.88.
61. Persson HBI, et al. Risk of extremity fractures in adult outpatients with epilepsy. *Epilepsia*. 2002;**43**(7):768–72. https://doi.org/10.1046/j.1528-1157.2002.15801.x.
62. Annegers JF, et al. Risk of age-related fractures in patients with unprovoked seizures. *Epilepsia*. 1989;**30**(3):348–55. https://doi.org/10.1111/j.1528-1157.1989.tb05308.x.
63. Teagarden DL, et al. Low vitamin D levels are common in patients with epilepsy. *Epilepsy Research*. 2014;**108**(8):1352–6.

https://doi.org/10.1016/j.eplepsyres.2014.06.008.

64. Camacho PM, et al. American Association of Clinical Endocrinologists and American College of Endocrinology clinical practice guidelines for the diagnosis and treatment of postmenopausal osteoporosis: 2016. *Endocrine Practice*. 2016;**22**:1–42. https://doi.org/10.4158/EP161435.GL.

65. Elliott JO, et al. Homocysteine and bone loss in epilepsy. *Seizure*. 2007;**16**(1):22–34. https://doi.org/10.1016/j.seizure.2006.10.001.

66. Mikati MA, Dib L, Yamout B, et al. Two randomized vitamin D trials in ambulatory patients on anticonvulsants: Impact on bone. *Neurology* 2006;**67**(11):2005–14. https://doi.org/10.1212/01.wnl.0000247107.54562.0e.

67. DeGiorgio CM, et al. Safety and tolerability of vitamin D3 5000 IU/day in epilepsy. *Epilepsy & Behavior*. 2019;**94**:195–7. https://doi.org/10.1016/j.yebeh.2019.03.001.

68. Pottoo FH, et al. Raloxifene protects against seizures and neurodegeneration in a mouse model mimicking epilepsy in postmenopausal women. *European Journal of Pharmaceutical Sciences*. 2014;**65**:167–73. https://doi.org/10.1016/j.ejps.2014.09.002.

69. Jetté N, et al. Association of antiepileptic drugs with nontraumatic fractures: A population-based analysis. *Archives of Neurology*. 2011;**68**(1). https://doi.org/10.1001/archneurol.2010.341.

70. Kumandas S, et al. Effect of carbamazepine and valproic acid on bone mineral density, IGF-I and IGFBP-3. *Journal of Pediatric Endocrinology & Metabolism*. 2006;**19**(4):529–34

71. Kim SH, et al. A 6-month longitudinal study of bone mineral density with antiepileptic drug monotherapy. *Epilepsy & Behavior*. 2007;**10**(2):291–5. https://doi.org/10.1016/j.yebeh.2006.11.007.

72. Hoikka V, et al. Carbamazepine and bone mineral metabolism. *Acta Neurologica Scandinavica*. 2009;**70**(2):77–80. https://doi.org/10.1111/j.1600-0404.1984.tb00806.x.

73. Andress DL. Antiepileptic drug-induced bone loss in young male patients who have seizures. *Archives of Neurology*. 2002;**59**(5):781. https://doi.org/10.1001/archneur.59.5.781.

74. el-Hajj Fuleihan G, et al. Predictors of bone density in ambulatory patients on antiepileptic drugs. *Bone*. 2008;**43**(1):149–55. https://doi.org/10.1016/j.bone.2008.03.002.

75. Vestergaard P, et al. Anxiolytics, sedatives, antidepressants, neuroleptics and the risk of fracture. *Osteoporosis International*. 2006;**17**(6):807–16. https://doi.org/10.1007/s00198-005-0065-y.

76. Guo CY, et al. Long-term valproate and lamotrigine treatment may be a marker for reduced growth and bone mass in children with epilepsy. *Epilepsia*. 2002;**42**(9):1141–7. https://doi.org/10.1046/j.1528-1157.2001.416800.x.

77. Nissen-Meyer LSH, et al. Levetiracetam, phenytoin, and valproate act differently on rat bone mass, structure, and metabolism. *Epilepsia*. 2007;**48**(10):1850–60. https://doi.org/10.1111/j.1528-1167.2007.01176.x.

78. el-Haggar, SM, et al. Levetiracetam and lamotrigine effects as mono- and polytherapy on bone mineral density in epileptic patients. *Arquivos de Neuro-Psiquiatria*. 2018;**76**(7):452–8. https://doi.org/10.1590/0004-282x20180068.

79. Babayigit A, et al. Adverse effects of antiepileptic drugs on bone mineral density. *Pediatric Neurology*. 2006;**35**(3):177–81. https://doi.org/10.1016/j.pediatrneurol.2006.03.004.

80. Cansu A, et al. Evaluation of bone turnover in epileptic children using oxcarbazepine. *Pediatric Neurology*. 2008;**39**(4):266–71. https://doi.org/10.1016/j.pediatrneurol.2008.07.001.

81. Çetinkaya Y, et al. The effect of oxcarbazepine on bone metabolism. *Acta Neurologica Scandinavica*. 2009;**120**(3):170–5. https://doi.org/10.1111/j.1600-0404.2008.01148.x.

82. Lado F, et al. Value of routine screening for bone demineralization in an urban population of patients with epilepsy. *Epilepsy*

Research. 2008;**78**(2–3):155–60. https://doi.org/10.1016/j.eplepsyres.2007.11.003.

83. Cheng HH, et al. Anti-epileptic drugs associated with fractures in the elderly: A preliminary population-based study. *Current Medical Research and Opinion*. 2019;**35**(5):903–7. https://doi.org/10.1080/03007995.2018.1541447.

84. Heo K, et al. The effect of topiramate monotherapy on bone mineral density and markers of bone and mineral metabolism in premenopausal women with epilepsy: Effect of topiramate on bone. *Epilepsia*. 2011;**52**(10):pp. 1884–9. https://doi.org/10.1111/j.1528-1167.2011.03131.x.

85. Koo DL, Nam H. Effects of zonisamide monotherapy on bone health in drug-naive epileptic patients. *Epilepsia*. 2020:**61**(10):2142–9. https://doi.org/10.1111/epi.16678.

86. Takahashi A, et al. Effects of chronic administration of aonisamide, an antiepileptic drug, on bone mineral density and their prevention with alfacalcidol in growing rats. *Journal of Pharmacological Sciences*. 2003;**91**(4):313–18. https://doi.org/10.1254/jphs.91.313.

87. Kotloski RJ, et al. Epilepsy and aging. In *Handbook of clinical neurology*. Vol. **167**. Elsevier; 2019, pp. 455–75. https://doi.org/10.1016/B978-0-12-804766-8.00025-X.

88. Breuer LEM, et al. Cognitive deterioration in adult epilepsy: Clinical characteristics of "accelerated cognitive ageing." *Acta Neurologica Scandinavica*. 2017; **136**(1):47–53. https://doi.org/10.1111/ane.12700.

89. Vestergaard, P. Epilepsy, osteoporosis and fracture risk: A meta-analysis. *Acta Neurologica Scandinavica*. 112(5):277–86. https://doi.org/10.1111/j.1600-0404.2005.00474.x.

90. Unnanuntana, A, Gladnick BP, Donnelly E, Lane JM. The assessment of fracture risk. *Journal of Bone and Joint Surgery. American Volume*. 2010;**92**(3):743–53. https://doi.org/10.2106/JBJS.I.00919.

Index

Page numbers in "*Italics*" refer to figures; page numbers in "**bold**" refer to tables.

Printed in the United States
by Baker & Taylor Publisher Services